T0260734

CHARLES A. JANEWAY
Pediatrician to the World's Children

CHARLES A. JANEWAY

Pediatrician to the World's Children

Robert J. Haggerty
Frederick H. Lovejoy, Jr.

BOSTON
CHILDREN'S HOSPITAL
HARVARD MEDICAL SCHOOL
Distributed by Harvard University Press
2007

ISBN 13: 978-0-674-02380-2
ISBN 10: 0-674-02380-3

Contents

Illustrations appear in two groups, between Chapters 9 and
10 and 12 and 13.

FOREWORD

HAYDN WROTE of himself, "Since God has given me a cheerful heart, He will forgive me for having served him cheerfully."[1] Dr. Charles Alderson Janeway, who served the children of the world cheerfully and well for more than three decades, was endowed with a cheerful temperament and a strong sense of commitment. Reared in the security of a mother's love and a legacy of many generations of successful and community-oriented ministers and physicians, he lived a life of service. As an outstanding medical scientist, he created one of the first departments of pediatrics with specialty divisions at what is now known as Children's Hospital, Boston and at Harvard Medical School, a department based on laboratory science as well as clinical expertise, and he educated a generation of leaders in pediatrics there and all over the globe. At that then primarily WASP institution he labored to add persons of different religious belief and varying views. He also rejuvenated the worldwide organization of pediatrics—the International Pediatric Association, which he served in so many capacities—and dreamed of having it serve as a focus for an international corps of pediatricians for peace.[2] At the same time he served his local community as a champion for fluoridating the public water supply, led a peace march on Boston Common during the Vietnam War, and was a faithful, concerned and involved husband and father. And he did it all cheerfully.

Dr. Janeway truly was, as one of his colleagues dubbed him, "Pediatrician to the World's Children." But he was so much more than that. He was a scientist, a clinician, a teacher, an administrator, a humanist.

Most of all, he was a wonderful human being. Knowing firsthand that he was a role model for all who worked with him, we thought we could write a biography of Dr. Janeway because both of us had long associations with him. This biography began when one of the authors (RJH) was a visiting professor at Children's Hospital, Boston in 1985. When shown a patient who had an immunological problem, one of Janeway's specialties, I mentioned how Dr. Janeway would have approached it. The blank looks on the residents' faces revealed that they were not sure who Dr. Janeway was, and this was only four years after Janeway's death! Later, I took the group of residents to the lobby, where Dr. Janeway's picture hung, and began to tell them about the man who had been chief of pediatrics at the hospital for twenty-eight years. Realizing that memories fade quickly, especially in a hospital where residents usually spend only three or four years, I resolved to collect information on Janeway's remarkable life in order to preserve for the future his contributions and to inspire those who, unlike the authors, did not have the benefit of his personal contact. Thus, this book is not only an attempt to preserve his legacy; it is our tribute to our teacher and friend.

I (RJH) had my pediatric residency under Janeway and spent nine years as a member of Janeway's faculty. My wife, Muriel, and I lived for a time in the town of Weston, where Dr. Janeway lived, and we maintained contact with Janeway and his wife, Betty after I left the Harvard faculty. When I returned to Boston (1975 to 1980), Muriel and I once again saw the Janeways frequently. After Dr. Janeway's death in 1981, we maintained contact with Betty in Weston and later in Kendall at Dartmouth, a congregate living establishment she resided in during the last years of her life. The biographic effort continued at a more serious pace after RJH asked FHL to join in the work. I (FHL) accepted the task gladly; I had known Dr. Janeway from the time I was a boy until Janeway's death. My family had a summer home in Annisquam, Massachusetts, next to the Janeways', where I knew Charles Janeway as a father figure and a friend. Later I had my pediatric residency under Janeway, spent a fellowship year at Children's Hospital, and served as Janeway's chief resident for four years. I have remained on the staff of the hospital ever since.

In pursuit of our goal, we collected as many of Dr. Janeway's papers and as much of his correspondence as was available. Most of the material (including his correspondence and diaries) was at his home, and we were given free access to it by Betty, who, along with the children, was most gracious and helpful in telling us their experiences in the Janeway family. We also found Janeway-related papers and correspondence at the Countway Library at Harvard and at Dr. Janeway's alma mater, The Johns Hopkins Medical Institution. The Countway collections proved to be a valuable source of official records from Harvard Medical School, such as search committee reports and appointments and promotion documents within the pediatrics department. Altogether we assembled several four-drawer files full of pertinent information, which will be deposited in the archives of the Children's Hospital when this work is completed.

In addition, we interviewed and corresponded with other family and colleagues about Dr. Janeway's life and work. We conducted many of these interviews and exchanged many of these letters years ago, in the 1980s and early 1990s, and it is fortunate that we did, for many of the people cited here have since passed away. Everyone we interviewed or corresponded with was most cooperative and wanted, as much as we did, to illuminate Dr. Janeway's life. In carrying out our task, we have followed the advice of Dr. Richard Goldbloom, chair of pediatrics at Dalhousie University in Halifax, Nova Scotia and a former pediatric resident at Children's Hospital Boston, who wrote, when asked for his recollections, "I hope you won't paint Charlie as 101 per cent saintly perfection, as such tributes occasionally do."[3] Goldbloom certainly was aware of our admiration for Dr. Janeway, and perhaps we should have been more diligent in looking for Janeway's failings, but we rarely stumbled on such "feet-of-clay" facts in the course of our research, because we mostly found that Dr. Janeway's life was exemplary. Our research made us realize, even more than we had before, that Charles A. Janeway was what he outwardly appeared to be: a good and decent man who treated others with unfailing respect, and so was respected in turn. Janeway led several lives simultaneously. He was a master clinician, a leading researcher, the leader of a large clinical department, a mentor, a committed "one worlder," a family man, and a community participant. Each of these lives required description and explanation. This we have tried to do.

The subtitle of this biography, "Pediatrician to the World's Children," describes Dr. Janeway well, but another might also have been appropriate. Janeway trusted young people. He was confident that they would have or would acquire the wisdom and courage to make the world a better place. When I (RJH) was leaving Boston in 1980 to take the presidency of The William T. Grant Foundation in New York City, Muriel and I spent an evening with Charles and Betty at their home in Weston, at a time when Janeway was in the terminal stages of his ultimately fatal disease. During the evening he was quite inattentive, although hospitable as usual. I asked him for advice as to the focus for the foundation, for which I had essentially been given a blank slate. Dr. Janeway said little when asked questions directly, but as we were leaving, he put his arm around my shoulder and said. "Bet on young people, Bob." That credo of his would have made a good title, too.

Our story will be largely chronological, albeit with much overlap as we discuss Dr. Janeway's commitments to his early career as a researcher, his work as a pediatrician and teacher of pediatrics in Boston, and his involvement with the children of the world. We have decided to write it that way because we believe that a man is ultimately a product of his genes and the culture and traditions in which he was reared. As in all men, the combination of inheritance, early life, and broader context molded Charles A. Janeway. From these influences came the superb scientist, the careful and caring clinician, the committed internationalist, and the man of peace. We think that it was essentially these factors that made him a giant in his time. We hope that recording this remarkable life will inspire others, as it has inspired us, to reach for the stars, to seek to fulfill our potential, to do good, and to do it well

Acknowledgments

The construction of this biography of Charles Janeway has been based mainly on two sources. The first category comprises the voluminous correspondence, diaries and other unpublished materials that were generated or collected and maintained by Dr. Janeway throughout his life, and which have been made available to us by his family as well as by several institutions that hold them. The second group is made up of interviews with Dr. Janeways associates, students, friends and other contacts he interacted with throughout his professional life, or the authors' correspondence with them. One of the joys of working on this biography has been the opportunity to talk or correspond with many people who knew Dr. Janeway during his distinguished career. It seems that once he touched somebody, the contact or associatiion was never forgotten. We began to communicate with such sources more than fifteen years ago, inteiwing and sharing letters with CAJ's family, friends and colleages wherever and whenever we could. And, as was noted before, it is fortunate that we did, for it is likely that their unique memories and recollections of the chief would have otherwise been lost forever.

First and foremost, we are immensely indebted to Elizabeth Bradley Janeway, more familiarly Betty, Dr. Janeway's wife, who generously gave of her memory as well as well as access to CAJ's personal files, pictures, letters and his extensive and meticulously detailed diaries of his foreign trips. We also thank Charlie and Betty's children, Anne, Charles, Jr., Elizabeth and Barbara, as well as CAJ's younger sister, Francesca Keeler, for filling out our dimensions of their father's (or brother's) life and adding immensely to the telling of it. Others who have done the same by providing reminiscences, anecdotes and details of their contacts and experiences with Dr. Janeway include many of his associates and students at the Children's Hospital in Boston as well as physicians and others he met abroad in his international work. Their memories illustrate the humanity and warmth of the man as well as his outstanding qualities as practitioner and teacher of pediatrics. Because our list of such individuals contains the names of over fifty individuals, extending from the letters A to Z (beginning with Joel Alpert and ending with Mohsen Ziai, and touching most of the letters of the alphabet in between) we have omitted their names here, directing readers to the endnotes in this volume where their names may be found along with citations to interviews, correspondence and other pertinent research materials they contributed.

However, we must single out and acknowledge the special assistance of a few individuals. Foremost among these is Dr. Fred Rosen, who maintained a great interest in our project. It was a profound disappointment to the authors that his death in 2005, coming as it did before the publication of this book, did not allow him to see the final product of our work, in which he was so intimately involved. We must also acknowledge with grateful thanks the help of Dr. Richard Janeway, a distant cousin and former Dean and Vice President of Health Affairs at Bowman Gray Medical School, who shared with us the genealogy he amassed of his long and glorious family since the arrival of the Janeways in America 300 years ago. We are also grateful to Mr. Erwin Levild, Archivist of the Rockefeller Archives Center in Pocantico Hills, New York, for generous access to all of the Center's meticulously archived files, where we found information on the grants from the foundation to fund many of CAJ's trips as well as support CAJ's father, Theodore, at the Johns Hopkins Medical School early in the twentieth century. Other institutions that contributed significant records were the Children's Hospital, Boston, and the Countway Library of Medicine at Harvard. The latter, through its holdings of the Harvard Medical Archives, enabled us to document much of Dr. Janeway's administrative background while an officer of the Children's Hospital and a member of the Harvard medical faculty. We are also grateful to Dr. William Preston for his guidance and advice throughout the composition of this work and to Richard J. Wolfe, late of the Countway Library at Harvard, who edited the final manuscript and saw it through press and into book form.

Assistance to finance this project was provided by Dr. Gary Fleisher, Dr. Janeway's present successor as Pediatrician in Chief of Children's Hospital, Dr. James Mandell, President of Children's Hospital, and, Dr. Fred Rosen, President of The Center of Blood Research at the time of his death.

Robert J. Haggerty
Frederick H. Lovejoy, Jr.

1 Roots, Family, Beginnings

THE JANEWAYS were, and are, a distinguished family. The family, however, is not rich in monetary wealth, nor is it noted for political power or social status; rather, it is a family rich in social accomplishments. In a letter of condolence to Charles A. Janeway's widow, Betty, following her husband's death in 1981, Dr. Thomas Stapleton, of England, remarked that Dr. Janeway had been born with a silver spoon in his mouth. Betty was nonplussed by Dr. Stapleton's remark. When replying to him she wrote, "I don't think Charlie was born with a silver spoon in his mouth, at least not in the way that Dr. [James L.] Gamble [of the wealthy Proctor and Gamble family] was, but I think he lived his life that way and I am grateful." Stapleton, stung by Betty's misunderstanding of his words, replied that in England the phrase did not refer to money but to brains and opportunity—and opportunity taken. Indeed, he added, a friend, William Wallace, had backed him up on this point, for Wallace said of Janeway, "he had used it for the benefit of humanity."[1] In that sense, Dr. Stapleton was right. The Janeway family history encourages one to believe that destiny resides in one's genes.

Although the Janeway family's traceable odyssey in America dates from seventeenth-century England, tradition has it that the Janeways were originally named Genovese and were from northern Italy, with one version telling that, later, as Huguenots, they emigrated to England from France, possibly following the Edict of Nantes in 1685. An-

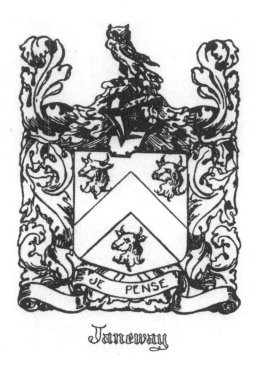

The Janeway family coat-of-arms.

other, more likely account dates their migration to the period following the Saint Bartholomew's Day Massacre in 1572. In either event, the fact that later Presbyterian clerical leaders in the Janeway family were known for their close theological ties to Calvinism and Huguenot codes of strict moral behavior, and the high moral standards inherited by Charles Janeway and his forebears, clearly indicate that this was an old family tradition. In addition, the high intelligence of the family is borne out by the family coat of arms, which features three ox heads and, more significantly, an owl at the top. At the bottom is the motto, *Je Pense* (I think).[2] The strength of the ox, the wisdom of the owl, and the thinking person have characterized so much of the Janeway family history that one can believe that psychological insights can reside in family coats of arms.

An unpublished family history in the keeping of Dr. Timothy

Janeway, a distant relative and contemporary of Charles Janeway, states that "The Janeway family has consisted of but two lines in America through 1850. The first [and the one leading to the subject of this biography] arrived in the person of William Janeway, an officer in the British navy in 1693. In 1696 he married a New York woman, and bought property and settled there."[3] The history also relates that there were many Janeways in and around London in the 1500s, and, while the genealogical records state that the family originally came from Genoa, Italy, they do not speak of a Huguenot connection.

Later Janeways are descended from Reverend William Janeway, who, the records of the church in Kelshall, Herts., near London, indicate, was born in 1600 and died in 1654.[4] Of his eleven children, the direct line to the current Janeways traces to his first-born child, William, born in 1631, who married a woman named Elizabeth (family name unknown). This son was also a minister in the Church of England, assuming the father's position upon the senior's death. His seventh and last child, named William, born in 1659, was the naval officer who emigrated to the American colonies in 1693. That William died in 1708, having fathered the first of many subsequent generations of Jacob Janeways in America.

William's only son, Jacob, was born in 1707. He married Sarah Hoagland in 1738. The fifth-generation Janeway, Captain George, whose birth occurred in 1742, married Effie Marie Ten Eyck. Frances Whitney, a distinguished New York artist and first cousin of Charles A. Janeway, has in her possession a map showing that Captain George Janeway owned land north of what is now City Hall in New York City. She also has a copy of a writ of 1719 that orders an earlier Janeway to remove a windmill on his property that had been adjudged a public nuisance.[5] Captain George Janeway produced the first Janeway cleric in this country, Rev. Jacob Jones Janeway, born in New York City in 1774. He married Martha Gray Lieper, born in 1783. Frances Whitney informed the authors that Liepers's grandmother, Martha Ibbetson, who was born in England, was taught medicine by her father, becoming the first of the Janeway clan to have been in medicine, albeit as a nurse, not a physician. She cared for a number of Revolutionary War soldiers.[6]

Reverend Jacob Jones Janeway was a noted Presbyterian clergyman;

he was graduated from Columbia College and studied for the ministry with Dr. John H. Livingston. He became assistant to Dr. Ashbel Green of the Second Presbyterian Church of Philadelphia, and, when Green was made president of Princeton College, Jacob assumed the sole pastor position, occupying it for nearly thirty years. He subsequently served as a professor at Western Theological Seminary in Pittsburgh before returning to Philadelphia as pastor of the Dutch Reformed Church and later in a parish in New Brunswick, New Jersey. After only one year in New Brunswick, he became pastor of the Market Street Reformed Church in New York City. In 1839 he resigned from that church to become a trustee of Princeton College and president of the Board of Directors of Princeton Theological Seminary. At his death he was president of the Board of Missions of the Presbyterian Church. He wrote extensively on the Bible. Both he and his wife lived long lives for that period, Jacob dying in 1858 at age eighty-four, and Martha in 1850, at age sixty-seven. They had eight children. Their first-born, Thomas Lieper Janeway, also became a noted clergyman; their second, George Jacob Janeway, was the first Janeway physician. Among their other children and their subsequent offspring were numerous other clergymen.

George Jacob Janeway, born October 14, 1806, married Matilda Smith. He was a prominent New York physician and, together with Francis Delafield and J.W. Southwick, was appointed co-curator of Bellevue Hospital. Janeway, Delafield, and Southwick are credited with establishing the first effective medical record-keeping system in this country. George Jacob fathered two sons who became physicians, Edward Gamaliel and Jacob Jones IV. One of the latter Jacob's sons, Henry Harrington Janeway, was a distinguished physician, a New York radiologist for whom the American Radium Society named its annual Janeway gold medal and lecturer. He is described as "a great American pioneer in the therapeutic use of radium"[7] H.H. Janeway's son, Jacob Jones Janeway V, sired two physician sons, Dr. Charles McKeown Janeway, a graduate of the University of Rochester School of Medicine and Dentistry and later a gastroenterologist in Seattle, Washington, and Dr. Timothy Janeway, an orthopedic surgeon in Pittsburgh who was an undergraduate at the University of Rochester. Charles

McKeown Janeway's son, David, is also a physician, a 1998 graduate of the University of Rochester medical school. In the current generations, descended from other cousins, are Dr. Richard Janeway, former Vice President of Health Affairs at Bowman Gray University Medical School, and one of his physician sons, Dr. David Van Zant Janeway.

George Jacob's other son, Edward Gamaliel, was Charles Janeway's distinguished grandfather. He was born August 31, 1841 in New Brunswick, Middlesex County, New Jersey, and died February 10, 1911 in Summit, New Jersey.[8] For reasons unknown he was always known as Gamaliel rather than Edward. He married Frances Strong Rogers (born June 1, 1841). His name, an old Biblical one, came from a maternal grandfather. Gamaliel graduated from Rutgers College in 1860 with a Bachelor of Arts degree and added an A.M. in 1863. He served during the Civil War as a medical cadet in a U.S. Army hospital in Newark (1862–1863), and was graduated from the College of Physicians and Surgeons in New York in 1864. Medical education then was at most two years in length, and he apparently was given credit for his army service.

Starting in 1866, Gamaliel spent six years performing autopsies on all patients who died at Bellevue Hospital. It was from this experience that he became extremely skilled at understanding the pathological correlates of clinical diseases. From this experience he rapidly built a large consulting practice in New York and was said to be the first physician to limit himself to consultations. He also taught at Bellevue Hospital Medical School, the predecessor of New York University School of Medicine, where he held the titles of Professor of Pathology and Practical Anatomy from 1872 to 1879, and Professor of Mental and Nervous Systems from 1881 to 1886. Following the death of the eminent Dr. Austin Flint, he became chair of the department and professor of medicine in 1886, serving until 1892, and later became dean at Bellevue's medical school in 1898, serving in that capacity until 1905.[9] He held appointments to several other New York Hospitals as well, and had his office at 36 West 40th St., New York City. Gamaliel was also Commissioner of Health of New York City (1875–1882) and president of the New York Academy of Medicine (1897–1898). He was president of the Association of American Physicians in 1900 and president of the

National Association for the Study and Prevention of Tuberculosis in 1910.

In 1901, as a delegate to, and vice-president of the British Congress on Tuberculosis, he made his only trip to Europe. He did not go to Europe early in his career, which was then considered necessary for success in academic medicine, but was self taught thanks to his meticulous autopsies and correlating autopsy findings with clinical observations. Frances Whitney, the daughter of Gamaliel's daughter Frances, noted that her grandfather, in addition to all his other accomplishments, heroically coped with an epidemic of smallpox on Ward's Island and encouraged Edward Trudeau to establish a sanitarium at Saranac Lake, New York, as a place to care for patients with tuberculosis.[10] Gamaliel is perhaps best remembered for his description of what are now known as "Janeway spots," diagnostic of bacterial endocarditis.

Gamaliel's role as a consultant was legendary. He was said to give half-hour consultations all day long for the last twenty years of his life and charged fees so low that all social classes could come to him. A biography states, "To know the lessons of disease as the greatest clinician, and none but the greatest have known them in the past, led to his uncanny skill, with which in later life he would sometimes solve a difficult diagnostic problem by a few simple observations, which made men say that he could see inside a patient".[11] Although Gamaliel professed not to enjoy writing, and disliked speaking in public, when he did, it was an extensive and complete exposition of the subject. He wrote sixty-six papers but never allowed his name to be attached to papers by his associates.

One measure of Gamaliel's prominence was his attendance at the secret operation on President Grover Cleveland on a boat in the East River in 1895. An article describing the event referred to him as "the foremost diagnostician in New York."[12] He was later called to see President McKinley, who had been shot in 1901 while in Buffalo, New York, a report of which follows in the florid language of the day:

> It was known that Dr. Janeway, the famous specialist, was on his way from New York. Who could tell but that the skill and knowledge of

the great physician might turn back the force of death and give the President to his people again? Oh the agony of the hour . . . Suddenly the stillness was broken by a distant sound of a galloping horse's feet . . . the voiceless multitude parted as an open carriage . . . swept up to the house of sorrow. A man leaped from the carriage and ran to the house at the top of his speed. It was Dr. Janeway. Alas! No. The President was beyond the help of human hands.[13]

Like his grandson after him, Gamaliel was parsimonious with words. The few he spoke, however, indicated his clinical acumen. A letter in Charles Janeway's files illustrates this. "A story was told how Janeway arrived at Buffalo late at night and saw McKinley after he was shot. Janeway examined him [i.e., the President], said not a word and went to bed. Next day at breakfast a friend asked him how the President was. Janeway said he would die. 'Why?' 'Pulse too fast.' That was about all he would say"[14]

J.B. Clark, who published his personal recollections of Dr. Janeway six years after Gamaliel's death from kidney failure in 1911, noted that he was self-contained and self-controlled; that he was modest and humble in spirit, although absolutely confident in his judgment when he had reached a decision within the realms of science; and that he was a man of great wisdom who, as a Calvinist, held strict religious standards of conduct. But there were some things which kindled his religious wrath to a state of militant activity, among them, newspaper reporters who tried to get inside information on a prominent patient.[15]

Gamaliel was noted for being generous to young physicians, as the following reminiscence of his student and later biographer J. B. Clark illustrates. "Soon after I graduated I was in the Adirondacks near Dr. Janeway's camp when an elderly lady of a well known family was suddenly taken ill. I was hurriedly called to see her and, on arriving at her cottage, was told that Dr. Janeway had been sent for and would be there soon; but they were anxious to have me go to the patient at once." When Janeway arrived, he continued. "it would be hard to describe the difference between this man I now saw examining the sick woman, and the Dr. Janeway I had known before," while a guest at his cottage. "There was a light in his eyes and an alertness in his voice . . . as he deftly built up his diagnosis, pointing out this physical sign and that, until the complete pathological picture seemed to stand out as on a page of a book." Then he told the family, "Now the doctor and I wish to have a little consultation together" . . . He proceeded to go over what Clark should say to the family. Clark was concerned about his ability, being so young, to do so but Janeway said, "If things don't go well just come up and see me anytime and we will have a little talk."[16]

Charles A. Janeway was reminded of his grandfather's clinical acumen by his colleague, Dr. Thomas Cone, who recalled a comment made by Dr. Abraham Jacobi in which Dr. E.G. Janeway had the following experience. The coffin containing the body of a woman who had died of cerebrospinal meningitis was opened and a strand of her hair cut off. This strand was taken home and frequently handled by a child living in the same house. The child developed meningitis, but nobody else in the house was affected. Gamaliel understood the importance of an environmental history to help establish a diagnosis.[17]

Gamaliel had one son, Theodore Caldwell Janeway, who was born November 2, 1872 in New York City. Theodore attended Yale University, where he shared first honors in the college's Sheffield Society; he was graduated in 1892 with a Bachelor of Philosophy degree. William Welch, later to be Theodore's dean at Johns Hopkins, wrote to Gamaliel, congratulating him on the success of his son at Yale.[18] Theodore then attended Columbia University's College of Physicians and Surgeons, graduating in 1895. He practiced with his father in New York and was appointed a professor of medicine at Columbia. In an era when most physicians learned either by apprenticing themselves with another physician or going to a two-year medical school, having a four-year college background before medical school was unusual and was a factor in Theodore's scientific and research approach to medicine. Dr. George Engel, professor in the medical school at Rochester, New York, shared with Charles Janeway information concerning his uncle, the famous Emanuel Libman (describer of Libman-Sachs non-infective endocardial vegetations). Libman had been a favorite pupil of Gamaliel's and was jealous of Theodore because the latter stepped into his father's prestigious practice at a time when it was difficult to establish a practice in New York.[19]

In 1895 Theodore married Eleanor Caroline Alderson of Philadelphia. Theodore and Eleanor ultimately produced five children. Their fourth child, Charles A. Janeway, made his appearance in the world on May 26, 1909. Their youngest child, Francesca, told the authors that her parents met at St. Hubert's at the Ausable Club, then as now an Adirondack retreat for well-to-do Easterners, and where Eleanor's father had bought land and later Theodore did also.[20] Theodore was described by Dr. W. S. Thayer, Theodore's successor as Professor of Medicine at Hopkins, as "A delicate looking, thin fellow with a dark, sallow complexion . . . and a conscience which was his one failing. Failing? No. One must not call it a failing, for it was a beautiful characteristic . . . Like Laennec, he was a lover of music and more times than once I have stopped on the threshold of his study and listened to the strains of his violin."[21] Elsewhere Theodore was described as a slight, well knit, alert figure, graceful in his movements. His eyes sparkled with animation as he talked. As a public speaker he began slowly and with hesitation but soon warmed up and presented his subject in a clear and logical manner.[22]

Theodore was the first in New York City to teach medicine from the standpoint that disease is a deviation from the physiological normal. While at Columbia he produced the major study for which he is known, "The Clinical Study of Blood Pressure," which described essential hypertension,[23] and devised the sphygmomanometer to measure human blood pressure at the bedside. His moral values were ever high, as was later to be seen in his son, Charles, for Theodore resigned in 1905 from Bellevue City Hospital when it would not implement reforms that he championed. In addition to his large medical practice in New York, he was recognized as an academic. In 1908 he was appointed to the editorial board of the *Archives of Internal Medicine* and in 1909 he was appointed Bard Professor of Medicine at Columbia. In 1911 he was made a member of the Scientific Directors of the Rockefeller Institute for Medical Research.[24] He wrote about the need to integrate medical schools and hospitals into the structure of universities, and is credited with being the individual most responsible for bringing Presbyterian Hospital and the College of Physicians and Surgeons into Columbia University.[25]

Theodore was deeply committed to excellence. From 1908 to 1914 he was consumed with the difficulties of being the ideal clinician-investigator-teacher that he wished to be, owing mainly to the demands of clinical practice. He was an intense man, worried by anything less than perfection. Dr. W.S. Thayer, in a statement read at a memorial service after Theodore's death, noted that, "if only he could have obeyed mother's injunction, 'let not the crooked things that cannot be made straight, encumber you.' But he could not. He gave himself heart, soul and body to his country and his duty."[26] In 1913, Theodore was hospitalized in Stockbridge, Massachusetts, and was treated by Dr. Austin Riggs for a "nervous breakdown," according to his daughter-in-law, Elizabeth Janeway.[27] Apparently his institutionalization did not last long, as soon thereafter he was appointed to chair the department of medicine at Hopkins.

Dr. Dana Atchley, at the time of his receipt of the Gold-headed Cane award from the University of California School of Medicine, San Francisco in 1959, devoted his acceptance speech to the contributions of Theodore and other distinguished physicians he had known. Atchley was a fourth-year medical student when Theodore Janeway went to Hopkins as chief. He was impressed that Janeway taught from the pathophysiological point of view, not only from the post-mortem autopsy view (which, interestingly, was his father's great skill). Atchley quotes Janeway as writing, "When we comprehend a disease . . . we see it not as an entity, not static, but something as a process . . . the science of disease [is] the only sure basis for successful practice." Atchley acknowledged that Theodore's view was considered "by most of my associates as little short of heresy and a silly theory at that."[28] Janeway clearly did not have an easy time selling his then revolutionary view. If he could witness medical education and practice today he would see that, while prophets are without honor in their own countries and in their own times, in his son's time and beyond, his approach had become dominant.

Theodore made an eloquent appeal for the full-time system that he felt was necessary to avoid the problems he then saw in the system, where most professors had to earn their salary from practice. In fact William Osler, the first chair of medicine at Hopkins, who had earned most of his income from patient care, had left Hopkins to go to Oxford because he felt that there he could teach and write without the necessity of seeing patients. Theodore was able to test the full-time system when he accepted appointment as the first full-time professor of medicine at Johns Hopkins School of Medicine in 1914, at a salary of $12,500 per year. This was to come from a grant of the General Education Board of the Rockefeller Foundation in the amount of $1.5 million to pay full-time faculty at that institution and others that would adopt the full-time plan. Abraham Flexner noted in a letter to Welch that Halstead (surgeon), Howland (pediatrics), and now Janeway were all full-time professors.[29] The revolution Flexner had proposed in his famous report was slow but continuing. Columbia did not give up Theodore without a fight, appealing to his loyalty by stressing his moral duty to stay, but he was so committed to the full-time system that he felt morally bound to test it.[30] This testing produced the gravest trial to his tranquility as he struggled to balance his commitment to excellence in clinical medicine, research, and teaching with the needs of supporting his growing family .

Theodore entered into the job at Hopkins with his usual attention to detail. In a letter to Dr. Lewellys Barker, who had been acting chair of the department of medicine at Hopkins but had decided to go into practice, he went into a number of details about the teaching program. The financial problems were already apparent to him, such as, "Mr. Phipps has cut his subscription to the tuberculosis dispensary in half. That takes away the other half of Moss's salary." He noted that he planned to come to Baltimore the following week and "expected to live in the hospital, in order to get into closer touch with the resident staff and work out their duties for next year."[31]

After three years as a full-time professor at Hopkins, Theodore had become disillusioned with this system. A paper he published in 1917 spelled out his disappointments with the full-time system.[32] He made clear that he was talking about medical faculties in universities, not those in the still numerous proprietary schools. He wrote, "The ideal medical school should have men [he never mentions women; there were none as faculty then] of equally true university type in the practical clinical chairs, medicine, surgery . . . these men should be masters of their subjects . . . always suggesting [to their students] the unsolved problems for the future and arousing enthusiasm for honest work toward their solution." He raised the question of "whether outside professional engagements for clinical teachers constitute an obstacle to its realization" He wrote about the qualities that such professors should have: [they should be] master clinicians, investigators, and in this regard he noted, "Great advance cannot be made now without the methods of exact science." While he advocated the necessity for research for clinical professors, he also noted that they "must be a practitioner of his branch . . . no matter how able an investigator [i.e., basic scientist] he be, he is not a clinician. The subject matter of his [i.e., the clinician's] investigation must be the sick human being." He then went on to his major thesis, that outside professional engagements, which he previously felt interfered with the role as professors, were necessary to maintain this clinical competence. He was concerned that by restricting consulting work, especially in the full-time system, where all money received from practice went to the school rather than to the professor, it diminished the "sense of deep individual responsibility so essential in making and fostering a good physician, and which is assured by the acceptance of money for his services."

He acknowledged that the old system of large private practice was not conducive to the triple-threat professor he envisioned. His solutions were, 1. To select clinical teachers because of their possession of the same qualities which govern other university positions—"the best man being called wherever he may be found"; 2. Provision of adequate laboratory facilities; 3. Salaries sufficiently ample to make outside practice for a living unnecessary; 4. Entire freedom for every member of the staff to develop into a practitioner, consultant, teacher, or investigator, as may best suit his bent; 5. All clinical faculty, including the professor, have term limits and be judged for reappointment by their contributions to the institution's mission. These provisions would allow some private practice but within the restrictions that if one wanted to continue as a faculty member, it must not interfere with his university obligations. However, the faculty member must be permitted to "sharpen his wits on a case that has puzzled some physician" and,

> If he is to do this, it is unnatural and repugnant to the patient's sense of justice that he should not receive the usual fee for such service . . . I would conclude, therefore, that outside professional engagements may be desirable for most members of medical faculties . . . Uniformity of environment is not the distinctive feature of the university, but unity of purpose. This alone should the university require of the teacher, that he live knowledge and devote himself whole heartedly

to its spread and increase. All else is detail of his life, which he himself should be trusted to regulate wisely.

Altogether the paper represents a carefully reasoned change from his previous espousal of the full-time system and must have caused him pangs of conscience, given his devotion to moral values. But it was also characteristic of his honesty that he would present publicly this eloquent rationale for his change of mind, not heart, to stay at Hopkins, knowing that this was his Achilles heel. But he had been committed to the "experiment" and only wanted to modify it to make it work better. In 1915, after all, he had written Flexner that the full-time experiment was going well.[33] He looked forward to the completion of laboratories that would allow him three whole afternoons per week to do his own work, but even then decried the lack of money to expand them more. He also deplored the separation of the "colored" wards from those designed for the white patients. Lack of money, both for personal and family needs and for the department plagued Theodore during his entire time at Hopkins.

In a letter to Dean Welch, Theodore advocated trying to get the Education Board to soften its stand against outside practice.[34] In a subsequent letter to Dr. Alexander Lambert, a physician at Hopkins, he wrote, "I rebel more and more at earning money for the institution," but he went on to say that some standards should apply to clinical chiefs.[35] Welch knew that Theodore was burning the candle at both ends; he wrote to him, "Again you must not break down in trying to carry too big a load. You are too valuable both here and there [as a consultant to the U.S. Army] to break down under the strain."[36] (With the onset of U.S. participation in what was then called the Great War, Theodore served as a major in the army and toured army hospitals to improve the care being provided; he also recruited leading physicians to serve in the army.) Always one to work to exhaustion, Theodore was said to work until dead tired and then sleep for only three hours.

By the time Theodore was corresponding with Welch, he realized that he could not support his growing family on the full-time salary being provided by Hopkins. He wrote a letter of resignation to take effect July 1, 1918. He noted, "The experiment has now cost me all I can, with any justice to my wife and family, sacrifice to it . . . Someone with less obligations and more resources" should succeed him, he said.[37] His resignations from Hopkins, which was not accepted,[38] and from the army, which was, were moot: he died of pneumonia on December 27, 1917. He was only forty-five years old. He had burned himself out in his devotion to duty. The president of Johns Hopkins University, Frank Goodnow, then asked Abraham Flexner of the General Education Board to grant to Mrs. Janeway Theodore's salary for the rest of the academic year. The Board agreed. On January 29, 1919 the Surgeon General of the U.S. Army awarded the Distinguished Service Medal to Theodore Janeway for especially meritorious service to his country.

Theodore Janeway's legacy was long-lived at Johns Hopkins, even though he was at the institution for only a few years. In 1979, Victor McKusick, then chair of medicine at Hopkins, wrote to Charles A. Janeway, asking if he was coming to Baltimore, since the institution was dedicating five "Firms" in honor of the first five chairs of medicine: Osler, Barker, Janeway, Thayer, and Longcope.[39] The tradition also lives on at Children's Hospital in Boston, where a Janeway Firm was established on the inpatient service for adolescent medicine.

After Theodore's untimely death the Janeway family returned to New York City, where they lived at 131 East 60th Street. Charles, although only eight years old when his father died, always remembered the Hopkins dilemma his father faced. He often spoke of his father's espousal of the full-time system that had led to his Hopkins appointment, and how Theodore had changed his mind after three years there. As we shall see, Theodore's son also was conflicted about private practice. He did some, but was reluctant to charge appropriately, as was true of his grandfather. In spite of honors the world bestowed upon him, Charles Janeway never received an income from Harvard sufficient to live in luxury; again, so similar to his father, Charles rarely spoke to the family of his relation to his father. Indeed, he probably did not remember much about him, but his response to Theodore's death was evident when he developed acute appendicitis the day after Theodore died. Charles's daughter, Anne, remembered that even in later years he was sad on December 27, the anniversary of his father's death.[40]

It is interesting to speculate about the influence of this early adversity on Charles Janeway's quiet drive to succeed. Other biographers have suggested that early adversity, if overcome, is one of the driving forces in many successful careers. Certainly Charles's biological endowment of a strong body, an outstanding intellect, and a stable, upbeat, optimistic personality were keys to his success, but we think it likely that early deprivation of paternal love and support due to his father's early death, also contributed to his strengths.

Charles's mother, Eleanor Caroline Alderson, was the daughter of one of the founders, and later the comptroller of the Lehigh Valley Railroad. Eleanor's father came from Derbyshire, England. Eleanor went to school in Geneva, Switzerland for a time but never went to college; she considered herself uneducated as a result but was in fact cultured, interested in music, and liberal politically. Eleanor was a strong-minded person. She needed to be, to raise the five children after Theodore's death. Mr. Franklin Kirkbride (called Uncle in many of Charles's letters to him) was, with his wife, a dear friend of Charles's mother Eleanor and invested her money for her, and friends helped to support her. The Janeway family did not seem to be destitute, however, since Charles went to Milton Academy and traveled abroad several times.[41] Charles was the oldest Janeway child at home at the time of his father's death. His older sisters, Eleanor and Agnes, were married by then, and his older brother, Edward, was attending college. Charles felt, in his wife's words, "that he had to take his father's place,"[42] and in particular to look after his mother and younger sister, Francesca. Some of Charles's empathy and sense of duty towards others undoubtedly came from the traumatic time of his father's death.

The eldest child in the Janeway family, Eleanor (Nora), married a well-known Philadelphia pediatrician, Dr. John McKay Mitchell. After service in World War II, Mitchell became dean of the University of Pennsylvania Medical School and later the executive director of the American Board of Pediatrics. Nora became the Board's and her husband's executive assistant. Her skills in that position became legendary. When Nora died, Dr. Waldo Nelson, editor of the *Journal of Pediatrics,* paid tribute to her organizational skills for the Board and her person-to-person skills to reduce the anxiety of candidates while they awaited their oral examinations.[43] Nora died at the young age of sixty, following a cerebral hemorrhage owing to hypertension secondary to chronic pyelonephritis.

The second child was Edward Gamaliel Janeway, who, after attending Yale, started work as a broker in New York at his wife's father's investment firm, White-Weld. Edward developed tuberculosis in 1925 and had a recurrence during World War II while he was a Lieutenant Commander in the U.S. Navy and commanding officer of the Thames River Amphibious Base, a take-off point for the invasion of Europe. As a result of his tuberculosis, Edward decided to settle in Vermont after the war, where he became a dairy farmer. He was active in the Republican party in Vermont and was elected to terms in the lower and upper houses of the Vermont legislature. He was active in many other aspects of political life in Vermont: school committee, town moderator, and chairman of the Eisenhower Republican Campaign Committee for Vermont; and was also a trustee of the Experiment in International Living. It is interesting to note how different were the trajectories of political positions taken by the two brothers: Edward, the conservative Republican, Charles, the liberal democrat, with a small "d." (Charles's wife, Betty, in commenting on these differences, told the authors that her husband really was too busy for serious politics; he was a registered "independent.") Despite his party affiliations, however, Edward was as much a conservation enthusiast and internationalist as was Charles. He and his wife were also active in the Vermont Arts Council.[44] In contrast, Charles's only official political position was his service on the Board of Health for the town of Weston. He shared his brother's great interest in the Experiment in International Living, an interest carried on by his eldest daughter, Anne.

The third child of Theodore and Eleanor Janeway was Agnes. She married a surgeon, Dr. Robert Wise, who, after serving in the military in World War II, was chief of surgery at the Veterans Hospital in Portland, Oregon and later served as chief of surgery in the Nemazee Hospital in Shiraz, Iran, to which, as we will see later, Charles devoted so much effort. Agnes and her husband became internationalists during their military time in London, where they made close friends and to which they returned often after World War II. Agnes died in 1974 of carcinoma of the pancreas. Charles's younger sister, Francesca, was married to a Presbyterian minister, Martyn Keeler, who attended Yale

a few years before Charles did. They lived in Buffalo, New York for
many years and retired to Vermont. Francesca moved to a retirement
home in Shelburne, Vermont after her husband died. As was true of
Charles, Theodore and Eleanor's other children were high achievers.
They set a daunting example for the next generation.

Eleanor Janeway lived until 1956. Charles doted on her and wrote
long letters to her regularly, copies of which were in his files at home
when he died. There was some friction between Eleanor and her
daughter-in-law, Betty, who was equally strong-minded. In 1956 Eleanor became ill and, after an operation for cancer of the bile ducts, was
nursed by Betty at Charles and Betty's Weston home before being able
to return to her home in Philadelphia for a short time before her death.
When Dr. Edwards Park, a long-time friend of the family, learned of
her illness he wrote, "I was much depressed to learn of your mother's
illness. I am so sorry it is what it is and where it is . . . she has had a
wonderfully happy life, marred only by the untimely death of your father. She has been a wonderful personality, diffusing *joie de vivre* spirit
like a radiating cloud of light where ever she went."[45]

Charles A. Janeway was devoted to his mother and siblings. A large
folder in his home contained copies of numerous letters he wrote to all
his siblings as well as to his mother; the letters date from the late 1930s.
He wrote to physicians for all the relatives to arrange consultations
when they were ill, reported his knowledge of their medical conditions, thanked each physician for helping one or more of his relatives,
and frequently hosted family when they were in Boston for medical
care. He was scrupulous in not asking for special consideration from
these physicians, on one occasion telling a physician that his brother
was a "non medical family" and should be billed as a regular patient. It
did not hurt, however, that almost all the physicians to whom he referred family members were those he knew on a first-name basis. In
the case of his mother, the surgeon who operated upon her late in life
was the son of one who had operated on her thirty years before for carcinoma of the breast, and another was at one time his father's partner
in practice in New York.

The Janeway family history relates a number of serious illnesses. On
Betty's side there was a strong history of migraine headaches; her father's trigeminal neuralgia could well have been migraine, and Betty

and all three of Charles and Betty's daughters suffered from this disease. On Charles's side were a number with cancer. His mother had two breast cancers, twenty years apart, and a carcinoma of the bile duct as a terminal affair. As noted, one sister died of cancer of the pancreas, and Charles and his son, Charles Jr., died of different types of lymphomas.

Dr. Fred Rosen captured the context of the Janeways' life in his remarks at the memorial service that followed Charles Janeway's death, when he said that Dr. Janeway was born in "that gilded age when good and decent people still owned America, when the burghers of Murray Hill and Turtle Bay could still afford domestic help and leisurely travel." Rosen was certain that "the Janeway family, basking in their Protestant prosperity and scintillating achievement, had little notion that the latest addition to their clan was to be an architect of that American influence over the globe some decades later."[46] It is indeed difficult for us, at this remove, to imagine what the world was like when Charles A. Janeway was born in New York City in 1909. It was the very end of the Victorian age, or the Edwardian age, as people in England came to call it. In retrospect, it seems an almost idyllic time. America was at peace. The major international news in those years were of events in far-off places, such as the deposing of a Turkish sultan and news of a new Shah in what was then called Persia. Little disturbed the American psyche unless it was Freud's lectures in the United States on the revolutionary theory of psychoanalysis and the controversial sexual theories that it expounded. In medicine, German dominance was epitomized by Ehrlich's development of Salvarsan for the treatment of syphilis, the first successful chemotherapeutic anti-infective agent, preceding by twenty-eight years the development of sulfanilamide that would launch Charles A. Janeway's scientific career.

Charles was born at home. Oddly enough, he had no birth certificate. When at age sixty-four he began to assemble material for his application for Medicare and Social Security, he sought assistance from the family financial advisor, Mr. David Kirkbride, who was unable to come up with a birth certificate but was able to find a copy of the 1910 Census that listed Charles A. Janeway as eleven months old and residing at 131 East 60th Street in Manhattan, New York City. Mr. Kirkbride's application was accompanied by a statement from the Census Bureau that this record is usually accepted in lieu of a birth certificate.

Little is known of Charles's early years. As the fourth child, soon to be followed by a sister, his was a warm and loving family. He moved with the family to Baltimore in 1914, when he was only five and started his formal education in the Calvert School in that city. Sixty-five years later he remembered vividly the "walk with Father on a warm September morning in 1914 from our house on the corner of St. Paul and Madison streets, past the Washington monument and up the hill on Charles St. to where the Calvert School awaited the start of my educational career. That was a special day, so I was dressed in my best white sailor suit with short pants and a whistle on a cord around my neck tucked into my breast pocket." [47] He was photographed with a tangle of clothesline, truly a "Gordian Knot," and was asked to untangle it (which he said he didn't quite manage). That picture was famous in the Janeway family; it was used on the Calvert School's brochure for missionaries and was labeled "Concentration." The picture captures what most of us saw throughout Dr. Janeway's career: thoughtful, concentrating on the task at hand but with a friendly, open gaze nonetheless.

A special place in Charles Janeway's early life and in the years afterward was the time spent at the Janeway family's summer home at St. Hubert's in the Adirondack mountains. Eleanor's father, while hunting in the Adirondacks, saw the land and fell in love with it. Mr. Alderson banded together with several others to form the Adirondack Mountain Reserve and save the Ausable Lakes from being lumbered. Eleanor first visited the property in 1887. Charles's grandfather, Edward Gamaliel, also summered there and his son Theodore purchased what was named Felsenheim. It was from the Reserve, in fact, that Gamaliel set out for Buffalo to attend President McKinley when he was shot. Alderson's daughter and Gamaliel's son, who summered in nearby properties, met on the Reserve.

According to a letter found in Charles's files,[48] Theodore Janeway, who had summered there since the late 1890s, initially bought the family property at St. Hubert's in 1914; he purchased about four acres from a minister named Dubois. They named the place "Felsenheim." Eleanor inherited the property after Theodore died and gave an acre to her daughter Francesca, who subsequently turned it over to her own daughter, Martha. Eleanor willed the remainder to Charles to keep in trust for the family. In a hand-written letter to "Doctor Charles A. Janeway to be opened after my death, Eleanor C. Janeway," she wrote, "It is easier for everyone that real estate be left to *one* person, so I am asking you to administer 'Felsenheim' for the family . . . Francesca has her piece of property here but I want her to have a say too and share. I hope some of you can use this home Father and I made for you all. If for some reason it must be sold let every one take something which will be a memento of 'Felsenheim'."[49] In 1957 Charles transferred the property to Edward's wife because Edward's Vermont home was closer and he was better able financially to keep the entire property.[50] Charles kept one acre, which he sold to his nephew, William Wise (son of his sister, Agnes), who built a home known as "Whistlewood." Charles bought back Whistlewood in 1966.

Charles reported to Mr. George Schaefer[51] that he started to go to St. Hubert's as a boy of five. He came to know the history of the Reserve at first hand because his father, Theodore, initiated the formation of the Ausable Club. Edward, his older brother, converted the Janeway property into a family trust. The Ausable Club is located on some 40,000 acres of land. The property still exists and includes a camp on a lake as well as a house. St. Hubert's was a favorite place for Charles throughout his life, as he had spent many happy days there as a boy and young man. It was there that his father's Hopkins colleague, Dr. Edwards Park, taught him to tie flies for fly-fishing and became something of a surrogate father to the boy. It is there also that Charles's ashes are scattered (see chapter 5), as are his mother's. The Janeways' neighbors, members of the Ausable Club, were an Eastern elite. Henry Stimson, Secretary of State under President Hoover and Secretary of War under President Franklin Roosevelt, was a friend of the family.

Charles's mother had her own cabin at St. Hubert's, and he had his. Every morning, when the family were summering there, Charles would go see his mother, at which time she would give him the schedule for the day. This pattern continued for a time after Charles and Betty were married, but Betty soon grew to dislike it; before too long they stopped spending as much time there and instead spent most of the summers at Betty's family place at Annisquam.[52] The strength of Eleanor's character is apparent in one of her letters to her second son, wherein she left instructions "to be cremated and my ashes taken to St. Huberts and left anywhere by the River Trail which I and Theodore loved so dearly." She then quoted a prayer from John Henry Newman that she wanted read but, "no funeral service."[53] Eleanor was the last survivor of the original Reserve members.[54]

After Theodore Janeway's death the family moved back to the New York brownstone home where Charles had been born. Charles went to Buckley School in New York in 1919 and 1920, and to Brunswick School at Greenwich, Connecticut, in 1921 before entering Milton Academy at Milton, Massachusetts as a day student in 1922. He remained at Milton Academy for his high-school years, being graduated in 1926.[55] His roommate at Milton was a young man named John Whitcomb. By the Milton years the three older children were out of the home; accordingly, Eleanor Janeway moved to Milton and lived at Milton Hill House with Francesca to be near her son. Eleanor, whom Whitcomb remembered as "handsome and dominant,"[56] remained very close to Charles then, as she did throughout her life.

Charles recalled that at Milton he co-captained the football team with Barry Wood (who later achieved All-American status at Harvard), and with whom he would maintain a life-long friendship. He described the time at Milton as "five happy years," and attracted the interest of the faculty. He never forgot that Arthur Perry, who ultimately became headmaster, "in my last year at Milton took time out of a busy schedule to read aloud to me daily during a period when I was convalescing from lobar pneumonia." He noted further that it was during this period that "I acquired a sense of becoming a New Englander, which has lasted till now."[57] During the Milton years he was a counselor at Camp Gannett, where, in Whitcomb's terms he," turned to the left." The camp was run by Freda Regolsky and had predominantly Jewish students from Boston. Whitcomb felt that this association had an important influence on Charles's liberal views. Whitcomb said the CAJ was head of the science club at Milton Academy and graduated with distinction and with high scholarship.[58]

We believe that Dr. Janeway's international interest had several origins, Camp Gannett likely being one of them. Others probably included the Christian tradition of missionaries, which he probably heard about as he grew up, and the trips abroad as a youth. He was a

German and history major at Yale and made several trips to Europe, especially to Germany, during college. But even before this there may have been two other influences, as his sister Francesca remembered.

> A man named George Whipple . . . ran a lecture agency in Boston and one of his lecturers was a man who was one of the first in this century to get into Tibet . . . Whipple was a friend of mother's and we saw him socially [and] frequently when we were all in Milton. The other connection was B. Preston Clark, head of Plymouth Cordage, whose hobby was a certain kind of moth or butterfly species and he had collectors from all over the world working for him. Charlie was fascinated. Whether it was the beauty of the moths or where they came from I know not. The Clarks came to St. Hubert's in the summer, and Charlie, aged 10 to 12, spent a lot of time with Mr. Clark.[59]

Thus it appears that many seeds of internationalism were planted in young Janeway's fertile mind. Francesca and Charles were the only two left at home when the family moved back to New York; they remained very close. Francesca said that her brother was always a "very good boy," but on one occasion he and a friend got a live alligator and teased her by dropping it down her back! This is one of the few remembrances she has of his ever acting prankish or improper.[60]

Even at an early age Charles Janeway was an environmentalist. Among his papers is an English thesis for the fall term, probably written during his Milton Academy years. At the top is the title, "Trout," by Charles A. Janeway. Also at the top is the mark, "A." In its introduction he wrote,

> I hope that I may convince my readers of the necessity for helping to promote fair play among anglers. Thank fortune that the sportsmanlike way to take trout, fly fishing, often proves more successful than the crude ways of many men, who know nothing of the fishes' wariness. Several good laws have already been passed to protect the inhabitants of our streams and lakes. One of these laws, prohibiting the sale of trout for eating, has done a great deal of good, and I hope that you will help in the great campaign to have more such laws passed.[61]

Janeway describes the habits of both the brook trout (with a draw-

ing of the fish) and the rainbow trout. His love of the trout is based on
his experience, for he describes, "In a pool of the Ausable River, there
lives a rainbow trout who weighs nearly four pounds, and people have
spent hours beside the river trying to catch him. Nobody has found any
fly or bait yet, which he will deign to touch." He clearly prefers the native brook trout, however, describing in loving terms a male fish swimming "around and around his mate in order that she may see his
gorgeous robe of olive, red and gold." In the section entitled "Conservation," he admits that fisheries are necessary but the real conservation
must be to "better their living conditions [i.e., for the trout] and not
plant fish anywhere." He then went on to describe fish culture, show
drawings of hatching troughs, and describe in detail the methods of
hatcheries. He was a hooked fisherman, but a conservationist. Surely
today he would be a catch-and-release fisherman.

After graduation from Milton Academy, Janeway entered Yale University, his father's and brother's school. In his subsequent application
to Cornell Medical School, he recalled,

> While at college my main intellectual interests were in history and
> the so-called cultural subjects, so that, although I took all the
> scientific work required for admission and enjoyed it a great deal, the
> courses which I remember most distinctly and which have meant
> most since college, were non scientific. My major was German [his
> overall mark was 91], but I also took four years of history and three
> years of English besides the required premedical work. So much of
> your education at college is outside the actual curriculum—lectures,
> discussions with friends, trips abroad—that it's hard to give an accu-
> rate picture, and I've had more than my share of these.[62]

His personal files at home included his marks at Yale, which were all
high, and these in an era before grade inflation: general biology, 93;
zoology, 88; elementary chemistry, 95 (he received the New York Yale
prize in chemistry in his freshman year); qualitative chemistry, 88;
quantitative chemistry, 80; organic chemistry, 90; physics, 85. He went
on to remember, "My interests focused on history, economics, social
problems and the paths of philosophy and religion. Two of my most
exciting teachers, Professor Schreiber, whose fourth year German
course on Goethe was language, culture and philosophy taught at its

best, and Professor Allison, whose lectures on medieval history, especially his traditional Good Friday lecture, when he described the origins and meaning of the Mass, were among the most dramatic I've ever heard."[63]

Charles Janeway was an avid student of history: "I was trying to learn what life was about and to see where I could fit into a satisfying career in modern America."[64] His was no narrow scientific education, so much in vogue today for premedical students. Janeway's files contain a hand-written notebook of over 100 pages with a detailed outline of world history with special focus on religion. The meticulous outline is in his clear handwriting and resembles his later notes in patients' charts: clear, concise, essential facts with occasional personal interpretations.

In his junior year, Charles received a prestigious oration appointment, and also was elected a member of Phi Beta Kappa. His high intelligence and outstanding achievements as a student were forecasts of the great achievements to come. He also recalled,

> In actual extracurricular activities, I was actively connected with the University Christian Association and an officer my senior year, and since college I've kept up contacts with liberal student groups in Europe as an officer of the American Committee of International Student Service . . . As for athletics, I played on the soccer squad freshman and senior year, rowed on a class crew sophomore and junior years, and got an insignia for playing on an informal university Rugby team my last year at college.[65]

This statement gives a very good example of his broad interests and commitment to service and international activities from an early age.

A former classmate, Sol Liptzin, wrote Janeway to say that he was "reminiscing recently about our young days with the International Student Service in Europe and America, we recalled that the youngest of the delegates to the conferences we attended, 1929–1931, were David Lewis and C.A. Janeway. Both were interested in making this a better world. Lewis went on to a career as the leader of a Canadian political party, and you were then entering medical school, hoping to make your contribution to mankind as a physician."[66] Liptzin then told of his subsequent career as a theologian. He had just completed his seventeenth book, *Biblical Themes in World Literature*. A letter from another Yale colleague, Elmore McKee, (Class of 1929) reflects on the activities of the religious group when they were at Yale together from 1927 to 1931 and influenced the Yale administration to institute a campus chaplaincy in spite of an "anti chapel insurrection."[67] Such were young Janeway's friends: cultured, worldly, scholarly, and possessing religious traits that Janeway shared with them. Charles certainly was intimately involved with international service and with a prestigious religious group while at Yale. Some of his commitment to international activity and a high moral code likely had their origins there.

John Whitcomb, Janeway's roommate at Milton, also was a classmate at Yale. Whitcomb recalled that Charles joined Dwight Hall, a Christian liberal group dedicated to the underserved; he served on their council, which was led at that time by Martyn Keeler, who later became Charles's brother-in-law. Charles was a deacon of the University Church. As a demonstration of his efforts to help the oppressed, Whitcomb recalled that Charles tried to get the son of the laundry lady at the college to help her carry the laundry. During the first year, Whitcomb also recalled, Charles was "besieged by efforts of his close friends to join a fraternity, Alpha Delta Phi." He refused, using the rubic "unchristian" because of the minority classmates who were excluded from fraternity life. This was an important aspect since the fraternities had their own eating facilities; the alternative choice was to take meals at "Commons" or eat nearby. Charles must have done one of the latter, for he never joined a fraternity, although Whitcomb noted that "Fellows who went to Sheffield Scientific School [had] their own eating facilities," and Janeway was in that school.[68] Whitcomb said that this religious association, (Dwight Hall and the University Christian Association at Yale) was a fairly radical, pacifist, pro-labor, pro-Soviet group. Whitcomb also recalled that, while at Yale, Janeway demonstrated in support of the necktie workers strike; he and his fellow students distributed brochures throughout New Haven and were ultimately apprehended by local authorities. At a hearing he was let off, however.[69]

Charles early showed his support for minorities and for others that many were wont to look down upon. In one instance, according to Whitcomb, when a member of the "Dwight Hall Cabinet" got a New Haven girl pregnant, "Charlie managed to arrange for a secret abortion, with adequate care for the mother of the child." In another instance, there was one black student in the class, a man named Kern; Janeway befriended him and escorted him to a football game in the Yale Bowl. Both of these acts called for some personal courage at that time. Whitcomb further recollected that, after rooming together for their freshman year, in the spring Charles "announced that Kern would join us along with Rigoux (to room together)." The foursome applied for a four-man suite. "We lost out on that application," Whitcomb recalled, "and Charlie put us down for two adjoining suites and I was assigned Kern as my roommate by Charlie's action and choice (rather than continue to room with him as I desired). This is where Mrs. Janeway and Agnes came in as a pressure group; they feared Charlie would be recruited as a potential missionary and go to China . . . this would deflect Charlie from getting to be a great physician."[70] Eleanor Janeway apparently was concerned that Whitcomb would influence her son to become a missionary. It is clear that Charles Janeway was committed to serve the underprivileged, especially abroad, although, as it turned out, he did so through his medical career and not as a religious missionary.

Little is known of Janeway's romantic life during this period. The first girl he mentioned in any papers was his wife-to-be, Elizabeth Bradley. His marriage at the age of twenty-three, between his second and third year of medical school was an uncharacteristically defiant— although characteristically courageous—act, for it was not expected at that time that medical students would be married. What his mother thought of this is not recorded. Charles's judgment of Betty as his future wife was excellent, as were most of his later selections of faculty to serve in the department while at Harvard.

Charles Janeway was a pacifist until World War II, when he changed his views, much to the unhappiness of some other pacifists such as his Yale friend, George Brooks, a labor leader. (Brooks later became head of the School of Industrial and Labor Relations at Cornell.) Whitcomb told us that at Yale Charles became more individualistic, although ultimately he did join Skull and Bones, the prestigious and conservative senior society. He defended this choice because, as Whitcomb recalled it, "since a tiny minority were solicited for membership, hence no exclusionary aspect."[71] At Charles's wedding most of the ushers were Skull and Bones men, which, in Whitcomb's terms, meant that he had become more conservative by then. Whitcomb felt that there was tension in Janeway's mind over joining Skull and Bones, since he had argued against fraternities and societies as elitist during most of his time at Yale. Charles's son told of taking his father to his fiftieth Yale reunion and being asked to drop him off at a corner a block or two from Skull and Bones, referred to as the Tombs by Yale graduates. It was tradition that no outsider should know where the senior society home was, not even Janeway's son, who was by then a Professor at Yale (even though Janeway admitted that everyone knew where it was)![72]

Charles Janeway had catholic interests all his life, a trait that was apparent in his Yale years. He coached a basketball team at a settlement house in New Haven, and sang in both the Freshman Glee Club and the University Glee Club. His intellectual accomplishments included the New York Yale Club prize in chemistry his freshman year, first rank standing that year and second rank in his sophomore and junior years. He was a member of Phi Beta Kappa and served as secretary until his resignation in October 1929;[73] we wonder whether the latter action was a demonstration against elitism.

During Janeway's years at Yale, many of his father's friends advised him to consider other pursuits than medicine and to "become a doctor only if I felt I couldn't do anything else."[74] He ultimately chose medicine and applied to both Cornell and Columbia medical schools. He entered Cornell in September 1930, having chosen that school in part because of the influence of professor Graham Lusk, who had been a close friend of his father's, as well as because a "group of outstanding people, many of whom had known his father well," were professors there.[75] The school was also convenient, being only a short ride on the elevated from the Janeway apartment in New York City. He continued his exemplary academic performance at Cornell and later at Hopkins, where he completed his medical education. Thus, Eleanor, it might be said, got her way: her son was going to be a doctor. One suspects that many others who had known his father were similarly pleased, despite Janeway's recollection that he should become a doctor if he "couldn't do anything else." One of those people likely was his father's old boss, William Welch, dean of the Johns Hopkins School of Medicine. The Janeways had a long close relationship to the legendary dean of Hopkins, who had praised Charles's work at Yale and had presented a portrait of Theodore to Hopkins in 1925. In 1930 Eleanor wrote to him, passing on the most recent news of her son. "I thought you would be interested to know that Charlie, who has a fine memory, has done well . . . I hope he will carry on the family tradition. He graduated from Yale, has gone to medical school at Cornell . . . I left the decision to him . . . I rather favored Hopkins. He preferred to be here in New York and the fact that we would be together. He is very like Theodore, a clever and devoted student."[76] As we shall see, Charles Janeway did transfer to Hopkins for his third and fourth year. Both of Eleanor's wishes were satisfied.

One notes a remarkable similarity in the obituaries offered in memory of Gamaliel, Theodore, and Charles. At the time of Charles's death in 1981, the Boston *Globe* reported that "His word was as good as anything in the world. He never did a dishonest thing in his life. He was a decent, compassionate man of total integrity."[77] The same words could have been written about his father and grandfather. Indeed, very similar words were. How very alike were the attributes of three generations of Janeway physicians: keen knowledge, skilled clinicians, commitment to duty, sensitivity to others, and commitment to public service. Indeed, that tradition of medicine continued and still continues. CAJ's late son, Charles Jr., was a graduate of Harvard Medical School, a pathology professor at Yale Medical School, and a distinguished immunologist; Charles Jr.'s daughter, Katherine, carries on the tradition, a sixth-generation physician, not only as a Harvard Medical School graduate but as a resident pediatrician at Children's Hospital Boston and as Chief Resident in Medicine (*i.e.* Pediatrics) there in 2003–2004, where her grandfather served for so long. (One of us commented recently, "It is so nice to have a Janeway back at the Children's.") Another granddaughter, Elizabeth Gold, the daughter of Janeway's daughter,

Elizabeth, also became a pediatrician; at this writing she is in pediatric residency at Toronto Sick Children's Hospital.

We believe it is difficult to find another family with such a long history in so many collateral branches, which also has had so many members with such distinguished careers in medicine.

2 MEDICAL SCHOOL, MARRIAGE, RESIDENCY, FIRST FACULTY POSITION

WHEN CHARLES Janeway entered medical school at Cornell in New York City in the autumn of 1930, that institution was located in downtown New York but was in the process of building a new medical school facility, the one that is still at 68th Street and York Avenue, joined to the then new twenty-seven-story white edifice of New York Hospital. It was here that Janeway received his pre-clinical medical education and got a foretaste of the medical world that he was to enter. He transferred to Johns Hopkins medical school in 1932 for his third and fourth clinical years. He once told one of us (RJH) that he transferred because he was concerned that, with the new hospital just opening, there would be start-up problems, and he thought that he would get a better clinical education at Hopkins. Perhaps a more important influence on the decision was that he had just been married in the summer between his second and third year, and his bride, Elizabeth (Betty) Bradley, had accepted a job as a social worker at the Harriet Lane Home for Invalid Children (as the pediatric service was then known at Hopkins). They also wished to "start their lives independently," according to Betty.[1] A further reason likely to draw them to Baltimore was that Charles's good friend, Dr. Barry Wood, had married Lee Hutchins, the daughter of a Johns Hopkins graduate, and was now a medical student at Hopkins. Janeway also was returning to the institution where his father had been chair of medicine and to the locale where he had spent his early childhood days.

The meeting of Charles and Betty was the essence of romance: they first encountered one another on an ocean voyage to Europe. Betty kept among her memorabilia the passenger list for "Student Third Cabin" on the "Twin Screw Steamer *Rotterdam*" that sailed from New York on June 15, 1929 for Plymouth, Boulougne-sur-mer, and Rotterdam. She disembarked at Plymouth. Among the passengers listed were "Miss Elizabeth Bradley" and "Mr. C.A. Janeway," who disembarked at Rotterdam. Betty's list reveals that she checked off a number of other passengers and put stars by the names of only a few—Charles Janeway was one of them. Betty remembered that a "lady pediatrician" introduced them. On their return they announced their engagement. He was only twenty years old; she was twenty-one. Janeway wrote Betty every day after they returned. Betty kept these letters but was reluctant to share them. The authors speculate that the letters probably were too intimate and revealed an especially romantic side of Janeway that was different from the somewhat austere demeanor he presented to the professional world.

Betty recalled that at first her mother was opposed to the marriage because she, herself, had not married until she was thirty-seven and thought Betty should wait as well. They did wait, in fact, until Betty had graduated from college. But Charles and Betty were still young when they wed in the garden of Betty's family summer home at Annisquam, on the North Shore of Massachusetts on July 9, 1932. As Betty described it, "Everyone stood in the arbor and my friends from school and college held white ribbons to make an aisle through the 150 or so people." The best man was John Musser: he and the ushers were all Yale men, members of Skull and Bones. That was the last time Betty saw her father, who died suddenly while Charles and Betty were on their honeymoon in Bermuda. The wedding was "the last gala event in the garden," Betty told us. Not long after her father's burial, in Lowell, Massachusetts, her mother sold the garden. Charles Janeway still had two years of medical school to finish. His marriage was an unusually courageous act at the time, for in those days married students and residents were frowned upon and sometimes were even dismissed from residency if the marriage became known.

Betty was born November 28, 1908 at her parents' home on Beacon Hill in Boston. She was graduated from Vassar, Phi Beta Kappa, in 1931. She was president and valedictorian of her class, and became a medical social worker after one year at the Simmons School of Social Work in Boston. She then worked at Johns Hopkins Hospital, in the Harriet Lane Home for Invalid Children to support the couple during Charles's last two years of medical school. She worked with mothers on welfare and adoption placement, a field she would return to later in life. Charles's transfer to Hopkins from Cornell Medical School after his second year would seem to owe as much to his marriage to Betty and her job in Baltimore, and their desire to start life anew, away from the family, as it did to any desire he had to return to his father's school.

The Bradley family did not have as many illustrious physicians and clerics in its background as the Janeway family did, but it too was an old, distinguished family of English heritage.[2] Betty's father, Charles Frederick Bradley (called Fred), after graduation from Dartmouth College, was a minister in Chicago and taught classics there before poor health forced him to return to Boston in 1900 with his first wife, Susan, to whom he was married for twenty-five years. When Susan died, childless, in 1905, Fred was devastated and was persuaded to take a trip around the world with Mr. and Mrs. Henry Marquand in 1906–07. In 1907 he remarried, to Betty's mother, Mary Emery, his first cousin once removed. He was fifty-eight; she was thirty-seven. Betty was born the following year. Another child, a boy, was born in 1909 but died of pneumonia at an early age. In 1914 Betty's sister, Mary Adelaide, was born. Mary Emery's father, Alfred Eastman Emery, was a physician in Wilton, Connecticut. After college, Mary Emery taught school in Concord, New Hampshire; she frequently visited Betty's father and first wife in Boston and corresponded with Fred Bradley on his round-the-world trip, thereby beginning the romance that led to their marriage.

The Bradley family has ancient English origins; it is mentioned in records as early as 1185.[2] The first Bradleys to come to America arrived on the ship *Elizabeth* in 1635. The Emerys were mentioned in the battle of Hastings in 1066, and the first Emery arrived in America the same year as the Bradleys. Both families settled in Concord, New Hampshire. Eventually the Bradley family moved to Chicago. In an appendix to Betty's account of her life there is a speech by Aunt Ella Bradley Ward (her father's sister) about life in Chicago in the late nineteenth century. Aunt Ella recorded that the Bradley family moved west in 1839 and suffered through the great Chicago fire of late 1871. Both parents and a sister died early, leaving Betty's father, Fred, a sister, and a brother, Frank. Fred and Frank attended Dartmouth College together, although they were two years apart in age; they were graduated in 1873. Fred taught classics at a Chicago Baptist seminary that later became Northwestern Theological School.

Betty's life-long liberal view of the need for equality seemed to be a familial trait, for her father told her that his father had helped runaway slaves and was grief-stricken at President Lincoln's death. The family apparently had some wealth, perhaps from land they bought in Chicago; in any event, Betty's father was able to spend the summer of 1889 in Europe and a year in Heidelberg and Berlin in 1890–91, followed by trips abroad in 1895 and in 1900–01 to the French Riviera. In his own words, added as an appendix to the Bradley family history, Fred remarks, "My wife, an invalid at the time, was greatly benefited by the winter in the Riviera." Further trips occurred in 1902 and 1903. By the time Betty sailed to Europe with her parents in the summer of 1914, when she was five years old, her father told her that he had "crossed the Atlantic seventeen times," an unusual travel history for that era. (The 1914 trip was interrupted by the outbreak of war, forcing the family to return home.)

Betty's father suffered from trigeminal neuralgia (perhaps migraine, as it was present in several family members, including Betty) that became so severe he had to retire from his job in Chicago and return to Boston, where Betty was born. Charles Janeway noted that he only knew his father-in-law when he was an old man but even then he (Fred) was forced to retire for a day or two with severe headaches every so often.[3] Fred and his brother Frank purchased and renovated a home on 90 Mount Vernon Street, facing Louisburg Square on Beacon Hill, and he and his brother built the family's summer home at Annisquam in 1902. Betty's father did not work at an income-producing job after returning to Boston; rather, he devoted the rest of his life to volunteer activities. That lifestyle, his home on Beacon Hill with several servants, and his ability to educate his children in private schools suggest that he must have had a substantial private income. He devoted much of his time to issues of family welfare and child labor legislation, and was treasurer for twenty-four years of the Child Labor Committee in Boston. Betty's commitment to the underserved likely had its roots in her father's volunteer work. Upon Fred's death he willed over $100,000 to his widow. The remainder passed to the two daughters when Mary died. She survived her husband by thirteen years. Betty recounted that her mother lived on in widowhood, doting on the grandchildren and dying soon after the end of World War II from a stroke. Charles wrote his mother about Mrs. Bradley's death. He was happy that Betty had had a good talk with her mother a few days before. He reported that the funeral was nice and simple and, "I think Mrs. Bradley would have liked it."[4]

The Bradleys, then, were that combination, not uncommon in the Boston of those days, of a liberal family in terms of their political views, yet had enough money to have live-in help and many other luxuries of the upper classes. Although Betty remembered that her father had many wealthy friends, she also said, "He would tell me that [having money] was one way of being successful, but he thought there were others, concerned with your inner life, your ability to learn, to create." Betty recalled her family life as warm and loving. Her mother's two most prominent characteristics, she wrote, were love and humor. "One of the lasting memories of my parents," she wrote, "is of their talking in the night. Whenever I woke up, I heard soft friendly voices . . . I never recall angry words . . . It gave me a secure, comfortable feeling to hear them." Betty went on to write, "There was quite a lot of emphasis on being good in my family. I was taught table manners, to curtsy, to look at people when I spoke to them and to think of the feelings of others . . . Our meals were fairly formal and always started with daddy saying grace . . . We had finger bowls at dinner . . . Mother had a buzzer under her feet . . . with which she summoned the uniformed maids"

In 1931, after Betty was graduated from Vassar, the family faced financial difficulties (presumably, like so many other Americans, owing to the stock market crash) and rented out the home on Mt. Vernon Street while living in a smaller house at Annisquam. Betty was enrolled as a social work student at Simmons College that year and needed to commute daily from Annisquam to Boston. Betty's sister, Mary Bradley (referred to as Mare in the family history), married Dr. Eugene (Bill) Meyer, son of the owner of the *Washington Post* and brother to Katherine Meyer Graham, more recently the owner of the *Post*. Meyer was a psychiatrist in Washington and was on the faculty of the Johns Hopkins medical school. Mary worked for Charles Janeway in his Boston laboratory in the 1940s while her husband was a medical officer overseas. After World War II she took a degree in Public Health at Hopkins and became an epidemiologist, being one of the early investigators who demonstrated the relationship between smoking and cancer of the lung. In Charles's files are a copy of one of Mary's papers and an editorial in *The Lancet* in 1977, unsigned but with a handwritten note from Mary indicating that she wrote it. Mary and Bill Meyer had four children and later were divorced. Both Betty and Mary were very intelligent, ambitious, and possessed of a strong social conscience.

The archives at Johns Hopkins contain a hand-written letter from Charles to Dr. Andrus, the assistant dean, after Charles had been accepted as a third-year student. The letter apparently was in response to a request for a photograph of himself, for he says he would send a photograph "as soon as I get enough time off to have one taken." He thanked Andrus for the privilege of coming to Hopkins, and went on, "Even though I may not have looked it in your office last Saturday, I was excited enough to let out a cheer when you told me I was accepted."[5] That was a revealing comment: Charles, apparently, was not always the restrained, austere person he displayed to most of us who knew him in later life. Still, he did not let out the cheer in Andrus's presence. That was the Charles Janeway the authors knew. An unsigned report of the interview, presumably with Dean Andrus, reads: "Mr. Janeway called at this office for an interview. He is a very keen, pleasant young man with a delightful personality, son of Dr. T. C. Janeway. He will have completed the work of the first two years at Cornell Medical School in New York. He has made an outstanding record there and his record at Yale would place him well up in his class."[6]

Teachers at Cornell had recognized Janeway's talent and must have been sorry to have him leave. In the spirit of honesty and generosity, Dean Graham Lusk of Cornell informed Dean Andrus at Hopkins:

> I write to commend to you Mr. Charles A. Janeway, who desires for several reasons to transfer to the third year class at Johns Hopkins . . . Young Janeway has had remarkable high standing in school, college, and during the last two years in our medical college. I think it is gen-

erally conceded that he is the best all round student at Cornell Medical College at the present time. Besides this, he is a young man of excellent stability of character and of judicial temperament. I am confident that he will be as great an ornament to the medical profession as time goes on as were his father and his grandfather.[7]

Lusk died not long after writing the letter. When sending condolences to his widow, Janeway expressed his special loss, "for in these last two years at Cornell, Dr. Lusk has really been my father-in-medicine and has filled the gap for me that Father's death made . . . it was as if he were trying to repay his love for Father by helping me start my medical career." (In his letter to the dean's widow, Charles recounts how Lusk encouraged him to transfer to Hopkins because he—Lusk—felt that some were "running rough shod" over so much of what he had labored for all his life to achieve at Cornell.)[8] Janeway's decision to transfer may have been motivated by what he perceived as a chaotic situation at Cornell as much as from a desire to go to Hopkins with Betty. Most probably, she could have found work in New York as well as in Baltimore.

Professor Stockard, chair of the anatomy department at Cornell, also wrote to Dr. Andrus. "At the end of the 1st year he [Janeway] was rated the best student in his class. This was not entirely on the basis of grades any more than on account of his very capable and discreet method of work and study. He is a most superior student and any medical school would be fortunate to have him among their students."[9] Janeway thus had acquired a sterling reputation at Cornell. Characteristically, he never appeared conceited nor driven, even though his record at Cornell was impressive. In the first two years, in every course he received a grade of 92 or above, mostly 95s and 98s, except in bacteriology, his later field of specialization, where his grade was only 89! Perhaps most telling for the future of his pacifism was his mark in a course called Military Science: 75![10] In his subsequent clinical courses at Hopkins, where no numerical grades were given, he received "very good" except in obstetrics and psychiatry, where he received a grade of "good."[11]

During the two years that Charles and Betty Janeway spent in Baltimore while Charles was completing his medical school training the

Janeways and the Woods were very close. They spent two pleasant years living on adjoining floors in a building across from the hospital. The couples' plan for living involved "sharing meals and letting wives take alternative months in running the catering department . . . [it] was a happy environment with medical school surrounding us in the hospital neighborhood and with the wards, laboratories and library all within one or two blocks of where we slept and ate."[12] Charles's prior association with Barry Wood at Milton Academy was not the only cement in the Janeway's relationship with the Woods in Baltimore. Betty had known Mary Lee (familiarly called Leal) Hutchins, Wood's wife, since Windsor School days in Boston, where Betty spent her high school years. Later, at Vassar, Betty would room together with Leal, Polly Bunting and Blanchette Hooker, who later married John D. Rockefeller, Jr. The closeness of Wood and Janeway is illustrated by a folder in the latter's files labeled "W.B. Wood, Jr., M.D." In it are found letters from Janeway to Wood and Wood to Janeway over a period of many years, often recommending people for fellowships to Wood at Hopkins or at Boston with Janeway. In one such letter, Janeway was responding to a query from Wood as to whether he would be interested in the chair of pediatrics at Washington University, where Wood was then chief of medicine.

When Charles was a freshman at Yale he knew and often saw Dr. Edwards Park, who had been professor of pediatrics in New Haven before leaving in 1927 to chair the pediatrics department at Johns Hopkins. John Whitcomb remembered that during their Yale days Park would invite Janeway and friends to his home, and that "Park's sister was Marion Park, later president of Bryn Mawr College."[13] At Hopkins Charles came increasingly under Dr. Park's influence. He had known Park when he was a young boy growing up in New York, at which time Park served as a younger colleague in Theodore Janeway's practice, especially helping Theodore with his studies of hypertension. After Theodore's death, Park befriended Charles even more and became a father figure.

Park followed Howland as chief of pediatrics at Hopkins and was probably another of the reasons that Charles was attracted to Hopkins for his third and fourth years of medical school. Park's research was on rickets, one of the major diseases of children in the early twentieth century. He was president of the American Pediatric Society in 1942 and the first recipient of its John Howland award, in 1952. Charles Janeway often recalled the happy days in Baltimore with the Park family: the Janeways would join them Sunday evening for supper, where they would listen to Dr. Park read aloud and describe the campaigns of the Confederate armies in the bordering regions of Maryland. They would also join the Parks for Sunday afternoon bird walks, again listening to his recollections of vivid stories of the charge of General Pickett's gallant men in grey up the slopes of Cemetery Ridge at Gettysburg. Dr. Park also had a special love for fly fishing and, as noted before, taught Charles the art of casting the fly for trout in Adirondack streams.

A number of other individuals left a lasting impression on Charles during those Hopkins years, including Dr. Read Ellsworth, who had studied under Dr. Fuller Albright at Massachusetts General Hospital. Ellsworth was a role model for many "aspiring young clinical investigators" as well as for Charles. Other important influences included T. Campbell Goodwin, who had been a chief resident in pediatrics at the Harriet Lane Home and who was a warm personal friend and later became chief of pediatrics at Mary Imogene Bassett Hospital in Cooperstown, New York; Warfield T. Longcope, who followed Charles's father as Bard Professor of Medicine at Columbia and later as chairman of the Department of Internal Medicine at Johns Hopkins; and Louis Hammon, who had been his father's physician during Theodore's final illness. However, none meant more to Janeway than Ned Park.

Charles's devotion to Dr. Park is most evident in a folder he kept at home, labeled "Dr. Edwards Park." The folder contains letters from Clement Smith, suggesting that Janeway write a biography of Park, and the number of letters and reprints in the folder demonstrate that he was planning to do so. (As was the case with Charles's autobiography, which he once started, his serious chronic illness after retirement also prohibited him from writing the story of Dr. Park.) The folder contains letters from and to Park (affectionately called Punk) from 1939 through 1969, the year of Park's death. In the early years Charles asks Park for advice, especially in the 1939–1941 period, as to whether he should join a volunteer overseas group from Harvard to take over a field station to treat communicable diseases among some of the evacuated children in the countryside in England. In these letters Charles expresses his sympathy with England but gives his arguments that have convinced Betty and him not to go. Most telling is his second reason. "I have just embarked on a big research problem here, working with the Department of Physical Chemistry . . . to develop readily available supplies of purified proteins solutions for the treatment of shock."[14] Almost every letter to Park ends with a discussion about trout fishing and the details of Janeway's family. Park was indeed the father figure Charles had lost so many years before.

In 1934 Charles and Betty returned to Betty's home town in order that he might intern at Boston City Hospital in internal medicine. Boston City Hospital's fine reputation as a teaching hospital, the excellence of the affiliated Harvard Medical School, and the opportunity to live on Beacon Hill with Betty's mother and aunt all helped steer their decision. Charles's son recalled, "he was interviewed by a trio of famous physicians at the City Hospital, Castle, Minot, and Weiss. Castle and Minot both asked questions about hematologic problems, for which he had no answer; Soma Weiss then asked him, "Well, since you do not know the answer to these questions, why don't you tell us something about the common cold? . . . [Charles] claimed to know little about that as well."[15] Nevertheless, Janeway must have been persuasive. He was accepted.

Boston City Hospital was then in its halcyon days. Among the attending physicians were Dr. Soma Weiss, expert in the pathophysiology and treatment of cardiovascular disease and an extraordinary teacher;[16] Dr. George Minot, who only that year (1934) had won the Nobel Prize for demonstrating that raw liver would bring about remission in patients with pernicious anemia; Dr. William Castle, who demonstrated the importance of the extrinsic factor in the liver and the intrinsic factor in the upper gastrointestinal tract in accomplishing remission of this disease; Dr. Chester Keefer, who was studying infectious diseases and their pathogenesis, as modified by malnutrition, liver disease and other rampant chronic illnesses; and Dr. Maxwell Finland, who was studying the treatment of lobar pneumonia with type-specific anti-pneumococcal serum. The creation of this marvelous service and the Thorndike Laboratory was the genius of Dr. Francis Peabody. The Laboratory served as an unparalleled experience for young, aspiring clinical research-oriented physicians. Charles's appointment ended in April 1936, but he stayed on at the Thorndike in Dr. Keefer's laboratory for the summer of that year.[17]

At the end of two stimulating years, Charles returned to Baltimore in September 1936 for a final clinical year as an assistant resident in medicine. He was, in a sense, coming home again. After all, after he and Betty were married they went to Baltimore to finish his remaining two years of medical school. The subsequent two years as a house officer at Boston City Hospital had been highly stimulating, and Betty recalled that she and Charles took long walks toward the end of this period as they tried to decide whether to go back to Baltimore, his roots, or remain in Boston, her roots. They decided to return to Johns Hopkins for Janeway's residency in internal medicine, along with Barry Wood. Despite the fact that it was forbidden for house staff to be married because they were supposed to be at the hospital every night, on duty, the Janeways chose Hopkins anyway. The Woods and Janeways again shared an apartment, on North Wolf Street in Baltimore; this apartment had a common dining room, living room, and kitchen. The two families contrived a method of signaling each other's home, so that one resident could cover for the other while one was at home, but still be able to get back to the hospital quickly if needed. In spite of what sounds like crowded conditions and sometimes hectic scheduling, life was not too Spartan for the newlyweds. Charles, in fact, described it as a "rather idyllic student life."[18] The Janeways and the Woods were welcomed by the Longcopes—(Dr. Longcope was then chief of medicine)—the Parks, and the Knoxes, all former colleagues of Theodore Janeway. These families would invite the couples to Sunday dinner; Betty recalled that they frequently had two invitations for each Sunday. Who covered the hospital then is not clear.

At the time the Janeways returned to Hopkins, Dr. Longcope was remembered by Charles as "splendid." Associations with fellow house officers such as Drs. Barry Wood, A. McGee Harvey, Joseph Lillienthal, and Robert Austrian, all of whom became medical leaders, were particularly important. Of special note at that time was early evidence of Janeway's proclivity for scholarship. His first paper, written with Dr. Harvey, was a description of three patients who developed acute hemolytic anemia during the administration of sulfanilamide.[19] A second paper was written with Barry Wood.[20] Harvey would later become chairman of the department of medicine at Johns Hopkins, and Wood later chaired the department of medicine at Washington University in St. Louis and subsequently was dean and vice president of medical institutions at Hopkins.

In August 1938 the Janeways again returned to Boston. Charles reflected later that his life might be thought of as "a tale of two cities–Boston and Baltimore," a reference to his close association with these two cities during his personal and professional life.[21] He left Johns Hopkins with considerable regret, having learned much from such teachers as Dr. Charles Austrian and Dr. Sam Wolman, who were senior outpatient instructors, Dr. Edwards Park in pediatrics, Drs. Longcope, Hamman, and Howard in medicine, and Drs. Adolf Meyer and Ester Richards in psychiatry. Since, however, his career had now turned to a more basic understanding of the scientific principles involved in laboratory medicine and their application in the clinical arena, he decided to spend his time in the Department of Bacteriology and Immunology at Harvard. Janeway's son told us of an interesting anecdote that must have been a part of family lore: "At the end of his Hopkins residency, he applied to the Rockefeller Institute for Medical Research but was turned down. At the last minute, Hans Zinsser offered him a job in bacteriology at Harvard."[22] The department was headed by this brilliant scientist, who had gathered in his department Dr. John Enders, in microbiology; Dr. Howard Mueller, in metabolism of bacteria; Dr. Roy Fothergill, who studied *hemophilus influenzae* infections; and Zinsser himself, who had extensive experience with rickettsial disease. Zinsser's days were divided between laboratory work and lecture and teaching time with medical and graduate students.

Janeway's investigations resulted in a number of papers published with colleagues in Zinsser's laboratory, as well as with physicians working at the Peter Bent Brigham, as today's Brigham and Women's Hospital was then known. Two notable papers were written with Dr. C.A. Chandler[23] from experience in the obstetrical hospital. His expertise in bacteriology was being used in settings other than the Brigham. Janeway's personal laboratory work book, labeled "Harvard Med. School, Dept. Bacteriology, 1938–1939, Miscellaneous Ideas and Experiments," has several pages of "Fundamentals of Antigen-antibody Reactions" with lists of possible experiments: "Sulfanilamide and Chemotherapy," listing possible experiments to demonstrate loss of virulence among streptococci exposed to sulfanilamide; and the beginnings of a paper, "Sulfanilamide, Summary." He reviews the evidence that sulfanilamide is bacteriostatic and that the organisms are only killed when antibody is present. The work book illustrates the origin of his lifelong interest in the role of antibodies, whether as necessary adjuvants to therapy or as in preventive vaccines. Each part of the book is a joy to read; Dr. Janeway's handwriting, so clear then, remained neat and legible all his life.

Charles's interest in infection and infectious diseases is evident in papers that he published with other colleagues, including Dr. Paul Beeson,[24] Drs. Fox and German, from Zinsser's laboratory,[25] and Drs. Williams and Longcope.[26] His work not only led him to understand the basic mechanisms underlying antimicrobial therapy in bacteriological disease but also its associated adverse effects. He undertook further studies of illness based on experimental hypersensitivity, including nephritis and the nephrotic syndrome. His work with the side effects of antimicrobials led him to believe that in the face of complicated and unclear medical dilemmas it was often better to "discontinue all treatment," which was often followed by improvement of the patient; early, then, he displayed a degree of therapeutic nihilism he articulated often throughout his career.

Life in the Zinsser laboratory was described by Charles Janeway in his Thayer Lecture. He related that he wanted to "learn laboratory and clinical methods for use in studying patients and for their responses to disease and for attempts to develop more effective methods of treatment."[27] He was always interested in the ultimate application of science for the benefit of patients, and saw modern science as the way to get there. The life of Zinsser and those in the laboratory sounds today like the ideal academic career, but one so difficult to achieve, "Zinsser, a brilliant lecturer whose day was often divided into an early horse back ride before breakfast, then work in the laboratory or conferences in his office with other staff members or fellows . . . The lunch hour frequently became an informal staff meeting with critical discussion of the research being done here and elsewhere, and challenging scientific

problems and achievements. Every lunch hour was a liberal education."[28]

In Janeway's library at home was a copy of the autobiography by
Zinsser, *RS, His Romantic Self,* inscribed by Zinsser, "To Charlie Janeway: Your father taught me; I taught you; I hope you have a chance to
teach my son." Janeway's papers also included a hand-written, undated
note in pencil, from Zinsser to Janeway, apparently written soon after
the birth of Janeway's daughter, Elizabeth, noting that he (Zinsser) was
a member of the American Birth Control League, which favored restriction of family size. The exact quote from Zinsser raises eyebrows
now, and probably did then; one doubts that Janeway approved of the
sentiment underlying the praise: "as a member of the Advisory Committee of the American Birth Control League this applies only to the
proletariat. May your own family line flourish. *Vivat-Florat Crescat genus
Janeway.* Affectionate congratulations to the growth of this also."[29]

Among the young staffers in Zinsser's laboratory were John Enders,
J. Howard Mueller, and Morris Shaffer. Shaffer recollects that

> Charlie was a welcome addition to the Dept. family and he made a
> very favorable impression on me by his quiet, self-possessed manner.
> I don't remember his ever referring to his family antecedents, al-
> though I later learned that his grandfather and father were distin-
> guished physicians . . . Charlie's initial work (1937–1938) had been
> concerned with sulfonamides; by 1942 he was deeply engaged in the
> study of immuno globulins, derived from the fractions of Cohn and
> Oncley.

Shaffer later recalled that "I took my mother to see him for medical
help when she developed a severe case of herpes zoster; he struck me
as a skillful internist and a "very parfait gentilhomme" . . . It was a surprise to me when he accepted appointment . . . at Children's Hospital
but I anticipated that he would be as successful in the new arena as he
had been in adult medicine—and this proved to be the case."[30] Impressions such as Shaffer's, recollecting Dr. Janeway when he was in his
early thirties, ring so true to those of us who got to know him later,
when he was our chief. He was humble, quiet, gentlemanly, a skillful
clinician, confident, and a competent human being.

In 1939 Janeway was offered a teaching job under Dr. Soma Weiss at the Peter Bent Brigham Hospital. Weiss had assumed chairmanship of the department of medicine at the Brigham and was the Hersey Professor of the Theory and Practice of Physics at Harvard upon the retirement of Henry Christian in 1938. Charles's duties included the organization of the bacteriology and immunology laboratories of the hospital and the development of research and teaching in infectious diseases for students and house officers. Weiss placed great confidence in his "young men." He put Janeway in charge of the bacteriology laboratory to supervise tasks that had previously been done by interns in laboratories scattered throughout the hospital. In this newly equipped and reorganized bacteriology laboratory, "Janeway examined culture plates himself each day."[31] He continued this practice throughout his career, often taking students and residents to the bacteriology laboratory to examine the cultures personally.

It was during this period of time that Janeway worked closely with Dr. Gustav Dammin, who later became the Brigham's pathologist and chairman of the Army's Epidemiologic Board, and Paul Beeson, who later held professorships at Emory University, Yale, and Oxford. Beeson was Weiss's chief resident at the time.[32] Another of Weiss's residents was Dr. Eugene Stead, who was later chair of medicine at Emory and then Duke University, and Dr. John Romano, later chair of psychiatry at the University of Rochester School of Medicine. These were stimulating times, involving "a small, active, enthusiastic Department of Medicine with a very congenial blend of younger men with ambition and older men with experience, working under the dynamic, but tragically brief leadership of Soma Weiss."[33] It was well that the group was so stimulating, because salaries for full-time physicians were low: in Janeway's personal folder containing all of his hospital and medical school appointments over the years, there is a note from the Bursar (of Harvard) that Janeway's salary for 1941–42 would be $2,100;[34] a year later this was raised to $2,175,[35] presumably for Charles's work in the bacteriology laboratory and teaching, since the same year, 1942, there is an announcement that Janeway had been appointed Senior Associate in Medicine at the Peter Bent Brigham Hospital, "without salary."[36]

In 1939, the approaching war, coupled with his desire to contribute to the defense effort, led Janeway to gravitate to the department of physical chemistry at Harvard, upon the advice of Weiss. The driving force in this department was Dr. Edwin J. Cohn. Other scientists included Drs. J. L. Oncley, John Edsall, Walter Hughes, Douglas Surgenor, George Scatchard, John Enders, and Otto Krayer. The physicians, including Drs. Soma Weiss, Janeway, and George Thorne, were all members of the Peter Bent Brigham Hospital staff. Additional individuals who became involved later included James Tullis and, from the University of Pennsylvania, Drs. Joseph Stokes and Sydney Gellis. The focus of the group initially was the study of the use of serum albumin in the treatment of shock. The ultracentrifuge was critical in allowing these studies to proceed. The work received the support of a major National Research Council grant. The Committee on Medical Research at the Office of Scientific Research and Development funded many of Dr. Cohn's subsequent projects. Cohn also wished to pursue the fractionation of the globulin components of blood, but never convinced the military to fund the effort. For this he turned to support from the Rockefeller Foundation.[37]

Charles Janeway was actively involved in both albumin and gamma globulin work. This early work on behalf of the military and for the purposes of treating shock led to later studies of albumin in nephrotic syndrome, which Janeway pursued with Drs. Metcoff and Gitlin at Boston's Children's Hospital. He became involved with Dr. Enders and others in the use of gamma globulin at the Brigham as well as at the Boston Lying-in Hospital and the Children's. This interest in immunology and gamma globulin would lead, after World War II, to Janeway's discovery of agammaglobulinemia simultaneously with Dr. Bruton and his subsequent work with Drs. Gitlin and Rosen on immunodeficiency diseases at the Children's. Many papers originated from these endeavors, including the use of albumin from plasma fractionation in the treatment of shock and hypoprotinemia, gamma globulin in the treatment of measles, and the uses of blood derivatives in the clinical setting. Most of these papers were written by Janeway alone. Cohn never co-authored a paper with him, although he supported all his activities. From these endeavors Harvard was able to develop a number of patents, but with the stipulation that they would be "royalty free and on a non-exclusive basis." This view of the use of medical discoveries for the general good and without personal profit became basic to

Janeway's views of medicine's responsibility to the public, and are a far cry from the situation today, when most universities are keen to develop patents in order to reap the financial rewards.

Dr. Janeway served on two important committees as a result of his work with Edwin Cohn. The first was a commission to control the quality of blood fractionation, the predecessor of the U.S. Division of Biologic Standards. Members, besides Janeway, included Drs. Edwin Cohn, John Enders, Roger I. Lee, Ross McIntyre, George Scatchard, and Norman Toping. Janeway also served on the Committee on Blood and Blood Derivitives of the National Research Council and the American National Red Cross; he chaired the committee and was joined by Drs. Louis Diamond, John Gibson, Edward Buckley, Carl Walter, Robert Pennell, and Charles Emerson.

Following Cohn's death in 1953, the department of physical chemistry at Harvard Medical School was discontinued. The Protein Foundation was formed to continue certain components of the work, and Dr. Janeway became director of this new entity in 1954, its president in 1955–1960, and its scientific director until 1968. The Protein Foundation eventually evolved into the Center for Blood Research, led until 2005 by Dr. Fred Rosen. Its presidents have included Janeway and Drs. Diamond, Douglas Surgenor, and Rosen. Janeway later reflected that Cohn was an "outstanding chemist with energy, drive and [the] organizing ability of a captain of industry."[38] Dr. Tullis, a later member of this group, noted that Janeway took it upon himself to secure funding for the Protein Foundation after the war by obtaining a grant from the Hartford Foundation that led to support from the National Institutes of Health (NIH).[39]

During World War II, Charles Janeway felt, like many, that he should serve in the military. He made some enquiries and word got back to his brother-in-law, Dr. Robert Wise, who was then chief of surgery at a U.S. Army general hospital; Wise thought that Janeway could be appointed chief of medicine at the 98th General Hospital, a unit being developed for overseas assignment, with the rank of Major. Janeway was tempted, but wrote to Wise that, "nothing would be more fun . . . than to be chief of the medical service . . . unfortunately . . . I am not a free agent . . . being designated 'essential' am unable to leave . . . I am afraid I probably am still more useful here than I would be elsewhere. At least, that is what those who are above me seem to think."[40] And so he remained at Harvard, doing the clinical work with plasma proteins for the duration of the war.

The relationship between Drs. Janeway and Cohn was not intimate, but was sufficiently close that Janeway served as Cohn's personal physician. This remained true even though by the time Cohn died, Charles was chairing a pediatrics department. He was also Mrs. Cohn's physician. Tullis commented that the interdisciplinary working of the Cohn group, involving basic scientists and clinicians, probably was a factor in Janeway's later support of this model at the Children's. Tullis also thought that Janeway's interests in international issues were stimulated by the Cohn group, which included several foreign scientists.[41]

Cohn's research group would meet weekly in his office for an hour and half to discuss the projects to be carried out: "the goal was to develop a safe and effective blood substitute for stable storage, ease in shipment and clinical use in all conditions and climates." Janeway noted further that the program was also important, "because it thrust my loyal colleague, Louis Diamond into national service as the first technical director of the Red Cross National Blood Program and ultimately made hematology, immunology and genetics central to our department's program under Drs. Diamond, Rosen, Nathan and Gerald."[42]

Janeway's deferral from military service was a wise move by the military because it resulted in the rapid development and deployment of human plasma albumin instead of whole blood or bovine albumin for use in battlefield injuries. Nevertheless, Janeway was ambivalent. In one letter to Park he wrote, "Silly that when you are home doing the most interesting work you could possibly be doing and able to live with your family, that you should want to go off somewhere and be bored for a long time, but I'm afraid that is inevitable at my age."[43] He probably felt guilty, considering his pacifist early years and his realization of the horrors of Nazism and Fascism, and with his brother and brother-in-law in service; perhaps he worried that he would be considered a service dodger. In several of his letters he expressed his deep commitment to Britain and to the United States entering the war. In World War II he was no pacifist.

Dr. John Romano was one of the young internists recruited by

Soma Weiss to the Brigham in September 1939. Romano described the anxiety in Boston on Monday, December 8, 1941, the day after the attack on Pearl Harbor, when warnings spread that planes were headed for Boston, "My wife and Charlie's wife came to our offices and I remember on the medical floors we were putting the patients under the beds, painting the windows black."[44] This traumatic feeling was exacerbated early the next year, when Soma Weiss died suddenly of a subarachnoid hemorrhage on January 31, 1942. Romano described the shock and disbelief of the interns and staff: "That evening, my wife, Miriam, and I held an open house for the staff and both Charlie and Gene [Stead] were there."[45] Weiss's unexpected death devastated the young faculty he had assembled. In a letter from Janeway to Barry Wood, who was then in the Army in Louisiana, Charles wrote, "Soma's loss has been a staggering blow to all of us, personally and professionally. It is almost impossible to get used to the idea that he isn't around to turn to for advice and help. . . . He had more gifts and more lines than anyone I think I have known . . . I am tremendously lucky to have had a chance to be so intimate with him. In the blood substitute work . . . we are now going forward at a good rate."[46]

Soon after Weiss's death, Janeway began gravitating to Boston Children's Hospital. He was appointed to supervise the microbiology laboratories at that institution because most of the staff there were away at war. In a long letter to the chief of the department at the Children's during the war, Janeway wrote, "After thinking very hard about your offer [for the development of a unit for the clinical study and teaching of infectious and contagious diseases at the Children's], and discussing it with a number of people whose judgement I trust, I have decided to accept, provided certain details can be worked out." He listed the conditions "which I feel must be imposed, if I am to do an adequate job." He then indicated his salary needs, "$5,000 a year," the privilege of seeing private patients, the ability, "In order to train myself in pediatrics, to have a visiting service, and especially to take charge of a newborn service at an obstetrical hospital, as this would teach me more about the peculiarities of pediatrics than any other opportunity."[47] Janeway was never really comfortable with the care of newborns but recognized this need early. He went on to ask that the hospital provide interns from the Children's and from the Brigham, and requested from the medical school a budget of $10,000 for a research fellow, two technicians, supplies, and equipment. He was not bashful about asking for the resources needed for setting up a program that he felt would be productive.

Boston Children's Hospital approved this arrangement. The appointment led Charles A. Janeway increasingly to be asked to see children with serious infectious diseases at the hospital, and set the stage for his appointment in 1946, surprising as it may have seemed to some, as chief of pediatrics there and the Thomas Morgan Rotch Professor of Pediatrics at Harvard Medical School. Janeway was prepared as few others in medicine were and as virtually no one in pediatrics at the time was to lead a department into a new era of clinical research based upon fundamental scientific advances. But his vision was broader than science alone. He saw pediatrics as a field that translated research into clinical care for all children. As he assumed the chair at the Children's, he applied his vision at first to those children who sought care there. He had not as yet articulated his role of doing that for all children everywhere, but the seeds had been planted for his world view. He would not be satisfied with remaking an academic pediatric department in Boston, important as that was; he was prepared to lead in building a modern pediatric department and at the same time to become the pediatrician to the world's children.

3 Tenure as Chief of Medicine at Children's Hospital Boston

Building a Department

THE APPOINTMENT of Charles Alderson Janeway as Chief of the Department of Medicine (as the pediatric department at the hospital was called)[1] at Boston's Children's Hospital must have caused surprise as well as satisfaction in the Harvard community. The Children's was to be the place where he spent his longest and most productive years. It was also the first instance of what, even today, is a rare occurrence: a Chair of Pediatrics who was appointed from internal medicine, having had no or very little prior experience in the discipline of children's health care.

How did an internist become the Thomas Morgan Rotch Professor of Pediatrics and Chief of Medicine at the Children's? As noted in the previous chapter, Janeway had been recruited by the new Chair of Medicine, Dr. Soma Weiss, at the adjacent Peter Bent Brigham Hospital in 1938 as head of its infectious disease section. A week before Pearl Harbor, Dr. Kenneth Blackfan, Chief of Pediatrics at the Children's, died unexpectedly at age fifty-eight.[2] Dr. Richard Smith, a senior practitioner in Boston and founding head of the Department of Maternal and Child Health at the Harvard School of Public Health, was temporarily appointed Physician-in-Chief until the end of the war. In 1942, with much of the Children's staff departed for the war, Smith invited Janeway to be a visiting physician and Assistant Professor of Pediatrics at the Children's. This was a part-time appointment, inasmuch as Janeway's full-time job was still in internal medicine at the Peter Bent Brigham Hospital. Smith felt that two candidates, Janeway and John

Dingle, were equally capable of being acting chief of infectious diseases. But he preferred Janeway, who was then appointed by the hospital's Staff Executive Committee.[3] In this role, Janeway cared for children with serious infectious diseases; these patients were housed in a
new, twenty-bed isolation infectious disease ward of the hospital.[4]

Dr. Janeway accepted the new appointment in September 1942.[5]
Even before the formal appointment, Janeway's interest in infections
had brought him as a consultant from the Brigham to the Children's to
see children with infectious diseases. He had earlier considered pediatrics as a career because of his long-time family and personal friendship
with Dr. Edwards Park. He may have chosen internal medicine instead
because of the example of his father and grandfather, although pediatrics probably had been in his mind for a long time. The chance occur-
rences of Blackfan's early death, the World War, which resulted in de-
pletion of staff at the hospital, and Dr. Richard Smith's initiative in
seeking him out, precipitated his change of specialties.

As noted in chapter 2, Janeway had agonized over whether to accept
an Army commission. He was deferred from military service because
he was part of the Protein Laboratory at Harvard that was doing high-
priority, war-related research. Family, and his research, kept him in
Boston for the duration. When Dr. George Thorne was appointed to
succeed Weiss at the Brigham and Weiss's old position was no longer a
possibility, this additional factor made a career shift appealing. Nonetheless, nothing was finalized until late 1945. After World War II
ended, Harvard was seeking a permanent Chair of Pediatrics. The institution settled on Dr. Janeway, in part, we suspect, to keep in the Harvard firmament one whom the search committee recognized as a rising star. He then was only thirty-seven years old; with the prize at the
Brigham closed to him, it was likely that he would have been wooed
away by another medical school. The appointment turned out to be
ideal.

At that time, infectious diseases were the most frequent medical
cause of illness and hospitalization among children. Infectious diseases
and immunology remained Janeway's primary research and clinical interest, but he became a complete pediatrician with time. Soon after Dr.
Janeway died, Dr. Clement Smith, director of research on newborns at
Boston Lying-in Hospital and a pioneer in the study of newborn physi-

ology, wrote, in his elegant way, that "some administrative genius had discovered that no one of appropriate age in pediatrics had anything like the training, experience, and scientific achievements which Charles Janeway had accumulated as a clinical investigator and probable future professor of internal medicine."[6] Alexander Nadas, in his inimical, humorous way, has written that "the appointment of Charles proved that [A] smoke-filled committee rooms inhabited by . . . knowledgeable people do have useful roles [while, B] the American system of open doors, or perhaps more importantly, open back doors, is a useful entrance to center stage."[7]

In the curious Harvard tradition, those who are appointed to a "chair" as, in the case of Charles Janeway to be the Thomas Morgan Rotch Professor of Pediatrics, and who do not have a Harvard degree (he having a B.A. from Yale and the M.D. from Johns Hopkins), are given a Master of Arts, *honoris causa,* "in order that you may enjoy all the rights and privileges in Harvard University" and in order to make them, in the language of a former president, "children of the house."[8] Such a degree was conferred on Dr. Janeway in July 1946. At the same time he was informed that "By vote of the Corporation your salary for the year ending June 30, 1947 will be ten thousand dollars."[9] While the Children's probably added to that amount, it is of interest that this was less than the $12,500 his father had received on appointment as Chief of Medicine at Hopkins thirty-four years before. In later years, Dr. Janeway developed a reputation as being positively parsimonious about faculty salaries. Given Harvard's parsimony to him, it may be small wonder that he was reluctant to start junior faculty members at more than this, and that he kept them at low levels for a long time.

After Janeway's appointment as chief, he worked hard to learn traditional pediatrics. He sought out Drs. McKay, Berenberg, and others for their knowledge. Berenberg wrote to us about Janeway's formal initiation into pediatrics:

Unlike other Department Chairmen who had non-pediatric backgrounds, and refused to take the Boards in Pediatrics and who were voted into the Academy [of Pediatrics] by virtue of their position, he insisted on taking the Boards and studied vigorously and effectively. The one place where he had a good deal of trouble was with methods and calculation of infant feeding during the era when formulae were written on a percentile basis . . . and predicated on dogma rather than pathophysiology. I recall tutoring him only in that aspect of the anticipated examination and, at his request, helped him with a cram course right up to the last minute before the exam. Both of us took it the same time. On the day we entered the room, [we were] greeted by jeers and affectionate boos from the assembled candidates, who were rather startled to see the chief . . . their reaction was one of affection and respect.[10]

Dr. Janeway worked hard at anything he undertook. After six months at the Children's as a consultant in infectious diseases, he wrote Dr. Park, "Incidentally, now that I have been in pediatrics for six months, have had a turn at both ward and outpatient work, I find myself very happy in my new corner of the profession. I don't know whether I can qualify as an adequate pediatrician or not but at least I enjoy it."[11]

It is important to understand the state of the Children's, and pediatrics departments throughout the United States, in 1946. The era of subspecialization in pediatrics was just beginning. Dr. Howland, at Hopkins, the first full-time professor of pediatrics in the United States, had developed the first department in the country that had a quantitative chemical research laboratory, but he adamantly refused to establish specialty clinics. Dr. Park, his successor, began a few subspecialty clinics, notably those for children with tuberculosis, cardiac problems, and psychiatric disorders, but these clinics were based upon clinical interests of faculty members and a collection of patients rather than on organized laboratory research. Dr. Janeway began to build the department in Boston at about the same time that programs with subspecialist clinics were being started at the Babies Hospital at Columbia University's School of Physicians and Surgeons in New York, at Cincinnati's Children's Hospital, Montreal's Children's Hospital, and at Washington University in St. Louis. Thus, a few pediatric departments in the country then had just begun to develop subspecialties and divisions, but none had such a complete roster of what nearly every school has today, and as the Children's developed at Boston under Janeway.

We do not claim that Janeway developed the first specialized units in pediatric departments in the United States, but his view that basic laboratory research should undergird most new specialty units was more evident at the Children's than in most departments elsewhere until well into the 1960s. He was wary of building divisions on single organ system diseases, however, because he did not want to erect barriers between disciplines. As an example, immunology, infectious diseases, and renal diseases shared some basic research models. Dr. Janeway's own research, producing experimental nephritis by immunologic means,[12] was an example of why he did not want to erect "silos" between disciplines. Later, in the new Enders Research Building, he fostered interdisciplinary research by clustering research instruments on one floor to stimulate interaction among different scientists. Even so, Janeway, who was trained in the latest research methods in infectious diseases in Zinsser's department of bacteriology and immunology in the medical school, tended to replicate the model of appointing clinicians who were or could be trained in research methods in basic science departments relevant to a given subspecialty.

When Dr. Janeway arrived at the Children's, a pediatric neurology unit existed. Years earlier, Dr. Bronson Crothers had persuaded Dr. Blackfan to set up a separate children's neurology unit with its own ward. It was the first specialized and separate physical unit at the Children's for medical problems (various surgical specialties did exist, however), and, prior to 1946, the only one. However, it did not become a separate department until the arrival of Dr. Barlow as chief in 1962. In the 1940s, when Dr. Richard Smith was chief, there were three major lieutenants in the department: Drs. Louis Diamond, Clement Smith, and James Gamble. Diamond had begun his pioneering work in hematology and leukemia and the elucidation of the various manifestations of erythroblastosis and its treatment with exchange transfusion. Smith had a small general pediatric practice at 319 Longwood Avenue but increasingly focused his time in neonatology, studying newborn physiology at the Boston Lying-in Hospital. Dr. Oscar Schloss, Blackfan's predecessor, had recruited Gamble from Johns Hopkins and had built a small metabolic laboratory for him. Gamble's research had laid the scientific basis for the parenteral fluid therapy that was to become world famous with the "Gamble-gram," the graphic presentation of the mineral components of the extra- and intracellular spaces. Gamble rarely went to the wards or saw patients, however.

The other faculty were all part-time, supporting themselves in practice. Dr. Stewart Clifford, a private practitioner, provided clinical care for newborn infants at the Lying-in Hospital, and Dr. John Davies, also in private practice, was responsible for the clinical infectious disease laboratories.[13] In the mid 1940s, Dr. Harold Stuart, based at the Harvard School of Public Health, had inaugurated his classic study of physical growth in normal children (resulting in the first growth charts to assess height and weight of an individual child compared to a cross sectional norm), and another group, also in collaboration with the Harvard School of Public Health, was developing the Drinker respirator for patients with poliomyelitis. Dr. Edwin Wyman, another practitioner, had rebuilt the dome of the main building at the hospital, the Hunnewell Building, with "Vita-glass," which allowed transmission of ultraviolet rays, and the resultant production of vitamin D in the children, to treat those with rickets. None of these practitioners had a separate unit or a designated subspecialty division, and all continued to see general pediatric patients. Only Dr. Gamble and, after 1943, Dr. Diamond were full-time in the hospital, and Diamond continued to see patients throughout his career. All of the other faculty earned their living by doing general pediatric practice.

Other departments of the hospital (besides medicine) at the end of World War II included pathology, under Burt Wolbach and later Sidney Farber; surgery, under William Ladd and later Robert Gross; orthopedics, under Frank Ober and then William Green; and neurosurgery, under Franc Ingraham. Similar to most children's hospitals, the Boston facility arose more from the need for specialty surgical skills than from concern for the special care of children with medical diseases. As is told in Dr. Clement Smith's excellent historical work,[14] the Children's reflected this history; it had several departments of surgical specialties but only one medical department in 1946.

Those in the pediatric (i.e., medicine) department were supported by their own wealth or the patient care resources that they generated themselves. Charles Janeway never developed a strong, independent financial base for the department as a whole but rather relied on the quality of the people he appointed to generate their own resources, largely from federal research funds or private foundations, in contrast to earlier times, when the sources were largely patient care. The success in generating funds to support research in each division, in large part due to the research ability of those faculty he appointed, characterized CAJ's years as chair.[15] Dr. Diamond recalled how little money for research there was from the hospital in those earlier days, "When we wanted money we had to either suggest some way of getting it or go out and get it ourselves."[16] The only grants from extramural sources were Diamond's, Clement Smith's for neonatology, and Janeway's for infectious diseases. Diamond noted that the family of one of his patients continued to give money year after year for his research. The Children's Hospital Corporation (i.e., the Board of Trustees), which in later years developed a very successful general endowment fund, was not, in 1946, supporting faculty or research. Such support as existed then was for building and services. In this the corporation was being true to the Harvard tradition, "every tub on its own bottom." The Children's and the Department of Medicine, and the individual faculty, followed this tradition until larger service funds became available and there was some cross-subsidization of units and divisions.

In 1946 the main hospital building was the Hunnewell Building, the domed structure facing Longwood Avenue. Opening to the rear, on a large, grassy back yard, were eight scattered, small one- and two-story stucco-covered buildings that housed separate medical, surgical, and orthopedic wards and the then independent Infants Hospital that had relocated from the marble building on Shattuck Street (later to be the first home of the Harvard School of Public Health). Dr. Gamble's laboratory and the operating rooms were also in these buildings, and all this existed while "still leaving room for two excellent tennis courts."[17] By the time CAJ retired as chief in 1974, the physical face of the Children's had so changed as to be unrecognizable except for the domed edifice at 300 Longwood Avenue. All of the cottages, except the Ida C. Smith, which is now the Adolescent Medicine Division, were long gone. The departmental structure by then comprised nineteen specialized divisions and several hundred staff in many different disciplines.[18]

The classically styled Hunnewell edifice, facing the Fenway region of Boston, still represents "the Children's" to most Bostonians, as it did in 1946. Today, however, that building does not even house the front door of the hospital. At about the time CAJ took over as chair of the department, the Board of Trustees and other clinical chiefs were about to become involved in a massive building program. In 1946, James Farley, Chairman of the Board, announced plans to build a Children's Medical Center, the first vision of what was to become the largest children's medical facility in the United States. As an official report had it, "The Children's Medical Center was established in 1946 by affiliations of existing institutions engaged in various areas of service to children to achieve the complete care and treatment of children by broadening the scope of services available."[19] It was the beginning of decades of growth, part of which occurred during Janeway's tenure. Some of the expansion resulted from the modern business method of acquisitions. Eight other Boston institutions were amalgamated into the newly named Children's Hospital Medical Center, the House of the Good Samaritan (a hospital for the care of children with rheumatic fever) as well as social service institutions such as the Children's Mission to Children (an old Boston social service agency built with the donations of children). By 1955 these institutions had much to celebrate: one was the Nobel prize for medicine that went to Drs. Enders, Weller, and Robbins for their work that made polio vaccines possible; others were the Lasker, Passano, and E. Mead Johnson research awards to various faculty. National awards went to the hospital otolaryngologists; one went to Edward Neuhauser in radiology; the Moxon medal from the Royal College of Physicians of London was awarded to Dr. Gamble, and the highest nursing award from the National League of Nursing was awarded to the former Director of Nursing, Ms. Goostray. New physical buildings, as well as national and international awards, were evidence of remarkable growth in the first decade after World War II.

The visitor to Boston today can appreciate this growth by walking along Longwood Avenue and looking at the domed structure where the main entrance used to be. When Charles Janeway arrived, that was all there was, as viewed from the road. It could be taken in at a glance. Now, the pedestrian has to turn around to take it all in, or at least that which can be seen amidst the relentless urban mass of the modern city of Boston. Details about the building program are available in the files of the Medical Staff Executive Committee's "Minutes" at the

Children's, but a few facts are noteworthy. The physical plant reflected, to some degree, the changes Dr. Janeway was bringing to the Children's and, by extension, to pediatrics in the nation.

The Farley Inpatient Building was intended to replace the cottages. It was a major effort of the then President of the Board of Trustees, James Farley, who advanced the idea for the structure at the beginning of Janeway's tenure; the building was finally finished in 1956. The building was used as an inpatient facility until 1990, when it was replaced by the current inpatient building. The Farley building still stands and contains laboratories, an inpatient psychiatric unit, and various ambulatory procedure units. It was the first structure in the evolving Medical Center, and it seems fitting that it still serves. The Fagan Outpatient Building, completed in 1967, was designed to replace the very crowded ambulatory clinics that were in the Hunnewell Building. That building, thirteen stories high, still serves its designed function. It is a subspecialized structure in that the multiple departments and divisions are housed on various floors.

The Enders Research Building was the last structure completed while CAJ was chief. The research effort until that time was spread broadly around the hospital campus, but was mainly housed underground in proximity to the current Farley Building and under the current hospital library. Construction of the original Enders Building began in 1970. It contains a number of floors devoted to mental retardation research, as well as surgery, medicine, and other subspecialty research laboratories. The structure was erected in stages; the last addition, which increased the building's size by 50%, occurred in the 1990s. Thirty percent of the cost for that last expansion was funded by the Howard Hughes Medical Institute, providing space and support for a significant number of senior and junior Hughes Investigators.

The Enders Building might be considered the structure most linked to Charles Janeway. Its initial funding in 1971 was a result of the first special award from the Hood Foundation to him, and the eighth floor was named the Charles A. Janeway Laboratories for Pediatric Research. Even in retirement, CAJ continued his interest in this research building. A handwritten letter exists in which he thanked a hospital employee for keeping him updated about the balance of the Hood

Foundation monies, which amounted to over $100,000 and were to be used for expansion of the sixth and thirteenth floors. Dr. Janeway wanted the employee to let the trustees of the Hood Foundation know that the suggested use had "my full approval."[20]

Although the current burst of new construction was not done during Janeway's tenure, the base of visionary new buildings that were initiated while he was chief made the later additions possible. The process continues. A new research building was built across Longwood Avenue from the Enders Building and was occupied in November/ December 2003; it increased the research space of the Children's by 30%. In addition, a new clinical building on the location of the old Carnegie Building, between the Jimmy Fund and Bader Buildings, houses an intensive care unit and ten floors devoted to the care of critically ill infants and children. The Janeway era initiated this burst of growth, even though Janeway was not the major architect of the building program. The faculty he recruited, however, made necessary the expansion of research laboratories and specialized clinical services.

One part of the physical plant that changed relatively little during Dr. Janeway's tenure, however, was his office. That space is still the departmental chair's office today, although scheduled to be moved in 2007. It was a small space on the third floor of the Hunnewell Building that was always simple and furnished modestly. In CAJ's time it contained two large blackboards, one mounted on the wall and the other movable. The walls held pictures of famous physicians who had taught and influenced him (Hans Zinsser's photo was among them); in the small hallway leading to his office from the secretaries' desks and waiting room were other pictures of all the chief residents who had served while he was head of the department. Behind his desk were individual pictures of all his children. The stationary blackboard listed the tasks he had to do. Tasks completed or those he intended to fulfill were checked; tasks not checked or that contained notations on the side were those he was going to procrastinate about or pay no attention to. During periods when he had to be out of town, the movable blackboard listed directions to various members of the department.

Dr. Sherwin Kevy, a long-term chief resident and deputy chief, reported that

On any given day, when going into Dr. Janeway's office, you could
easily tell the mood he was in. If he sat and his eyebrows were furrowed, one knew that this was not a good time for discussion of any
important matters. The most notable trait that Dr. Janeway had during a discussion was to write a letter at the same time he was talking
to you. This was not a manifestation of being impolite but was one
of the best ways he could concentrate both on what he was writing
as well as the conversation. If you stopped talking he would keep on
writing and would say, "Don't worry, I'm listening," and would repeat the last sentence or two that you mentioned.[21]

There was usually a pile of papers on Dr. Janeway's desk. One of us
(RJH) learned that he worked from the top of that pile. When for several weeks I had not received a reply from him to my memo, I inquired
about this. He laughed and told me that he periodically threw away the
pile and said, "If it's really important they will write again! Most things
get solved by that time."

Charles Janeway brought the skills of the internist—careful history
and physical examination—to pediatrics, where he added the developmental and behavioral aspects of children and a passion for encouraging research in the basic sciences that underly clinical problems. His
ability to ask pertinent historical questions and carry out a meticulous
physical examination were traits imprinted on all who trained under
him. His legible, careful notes in the medical record of any patient he
saw impressed all of us. Most impressive was his ability to synthesize
complex information from many sources and use patho-physiologic
reasoning to arrive at clear conclusions.

In Janeway's Thayer Lecture[22] and in a report of the first 100 years of
the Children's,[23] he outlined his own career and what he believed was
needed for a faculty in a department of pediatrics, or in any clinical department. First was a need for sound clinical training. If one was to
pursue a career in academic medicine, he believed it was necessary that
a clinician learn a scientific discipline. This would include laboratory
and clinical methods for use in the study of patients and for evaluating
their response to disease and of staff efforts to develop more effective
treatment. The ideal of how a department should run was rarely
achieved in clinical departments, but Dr. Janeway's belief that a
scientific discipline should be in the background of every faculty mem-

ber was central to his idea of how to build a department. For pediatric departments such a philosophy was a relatively new focus. Nearly every new faculty member he appointed either had a scientific research discipline or was encouraged to develop one after appointment. This was not limited to the laboratory sciences, for he encouraged one of the authors (RJH) to secure training in the research methods of epidemiology, sociology, and anthropology and apply these methods to health services research. He encouraged the other author (FHL) to become skilled in the new field of biochemical pharmacology and toxicology. CAJ's focus on research for faculty did not mean that he denigrated clinical skills. He emphasized that faculty needed both: the ability to employ new research methods and clinical excellence.

After Janeway became chief, divisions created only because of a faculty member's clinical interest tended to be the exception. Instead, clinics were more often based on the development of a scientific base for investigation rather than a disease or organ system[24] He clearly believed in selecting physician-scientists who were well-trained investigators, or could be so trained, and who were also competent clinicians. This concept probably came from his experience in the internal medicine department at Boston City Hospital and from the manner in which Dr. Walter Bauer was building the department of medicine at Massachusetts General Hospital as well as his own experience in Zinsser's laboratory. Dr. Janeway did not have a strong structural view of the development of divisions; at times he called a group a unit, at other times a division. There did not seem to be a hospital-wide organizational chart to decide the label for a group until the end of CAJ's tenure. At the major children's hospitals of the era, from 1946 to 1960, there was also considerable variation in the names of groups. Janeway's contribution was to develop these groups around talented clinician/researchers. He was not interested in formal organizational charts or reporting lines.

Dr. Janeway also had a strong inclination to select his subspecialty leaders from within the institution. No search committees selected these chiefs. He believed in placing highly talented individuals whom he knew and trusted in important roles. Examples are Alexander Nadas in cardiology, Dane Prugh in child psychiatry, Ross Gallagher in adolescent medicine, David Gitlin and Fred Rosen in immunology, David Nathan in hematology, Park Gerald in genetics, and Samuel Katz and David Smith in infectious diseases. In addition, the authors and Richard Grand (gastroenterology) were physicians who had either trained at the Children's or had collaborated with Dr. Janeway in research. If a person had strong intellectual skills based on science and good clinical medicine, CAJ was inclined to put him at the helm and allow a division to develop rather than to go outside to try and recruit someone he did not know. If Janeway was sure about someone, he appointed the person. If not, he assembled a few of his close associates to help him decide. He had an intrinsic capacity to recognize talent. On at least one occasion he tried, unsuccessfully, to recruit from the outside for the Gamble Professorship. After three unsuccessful efforts he appointed Dr. Fred Rosen from within.[25] This was a most distinguished appointment, equal or better than any he could have recruited from without. He appointed very few women until near the end of his tenure, but was a leader in recruiting what were then a minority at Harvard, Jewish pediatricians.

The availability of research methods and his intellectual curiosity were the driving force in Janeway's own research and in the building of the department, but he also had an underlying concern for applying this research to treatment of patients. As time went on, he broadened his interests within the context of historical and cultural issues in medicine, in an orchestrated effort to improve the health of all children in the community, especially for populations that were not receiving care, including those in developing countries as well as those who came to tertiary-care children's hospitals. These concerns symbolized his professional life and the type of scientifically oriented department he proceeded to build when he became chief. The concept that the responsibilities of a department of pediatrics extended from the "benches to the trenches" and from the individual patients to families and the community was quite new when he took over at the Children's, and still tends to be talked about more than accomplished by many pediatric departments. Janeway's approach was in sharp contrast to John Howland's view at Hopkins, where Howland did not develop new clinics or community programs and urged academic pediatricians to avoid policy activities.

Dr. Janeway's early development of the Department of Medicine (pediatrics department) was slow. As noted, he liked to "grow his own;" the first new members of the expanding faculty were drawn largely from former residents. Among the residents in 1941, when Janeway was about to become involved with the Children's, were four who would subsequently play large roles at the hospital and in U.S. pediatrics: Fred Robbins, Thomas Weller, Alexander Nadas, who, as we will see, developed pediatric cardiology, and William Berenberg, who was to spend his entire career at the Children's in general pediatrics and was a local and national leader in the field of cerebral palsy and handicapped children. Among the residents was Lillian Frances, the first woman intern there.[26]

For much of Janeway's tenure, only he, Louis Diamond, and Clement Smith held professorial rank. When the first author (RJH) was recruited, he asked Dr. Janeway as to the future opportunities for faculty advancement. CAJ replied that there were only the aforementioned three permanent positions but that there would be many good offers to go elsewhere. At that stage, in the mid-1950s, he did not see building a larger, more permanent faculty but saw his role as developing young people and populating other medical schools, while of course having enough young staff, most of whom would eventually leave, to provide the best and the latest advances in therapy and to do good research. Dr. Jack Metcoff is a case in point. Metcoff said that Janeway built the first scientific pediatric department by identifying important emerging areas, finding the right people, often from within his resident staff, and frequently sending them elsewhere for further training, but he did not build the department entirely on his own personal interest or expertise. As Metcoff expressed it, the combination of perceptiveness to new developments that required new faculty and organization of the department, together with humility and support of young faculty, placed Janeway, in Eric Erikson's terms, truly in the "generativity cycle" of his life.[27]

Dr. Janeway had known Metcoff when the latter was an intern in medicine at the Brigham and Janeway was a young attending physician. When Metcoff was on assignment in Algiers during World War II, he treated some children who had smallpox and sent Dr. Janeway pictures of the patients he saw. This led Janeway to reply promptly with the suggestion that Metcoff consider pediatrics as a career. Metcoff agreed. When Metcoff returned, Janeway organized a special training program, half-time at the School of Public Health with Dr. Frederick Stare (a leading nutritionist) and half-time as a resident in pediatrics. Metcoff's initial work with Janeway after finishing this training was testing the Cohn fraction of albumin in patients with nephrotic syndrome. This led ultimately to CAJ's suggestion that Metcoff work with Dr. Gamble and develop (and later lead) the metabolism and renal program at the Children's.

Later, when job offers came to Metcoff, Janeway advised against considering them until the offer of chief of pediatrics at Michael Reese Hospital in Chicago came. Then he counseled Metcoff to take it. Recalling this, Metcoff noted that Dr. Janeway believed that "a good department does not keep people, it trains them."[28] He encouraged his junior faculty to pursue suitable opportunities as they arose. One of us (RJH) had a similar experience: Dr. Janeway advised against some early offers, but when the chair at the University of Rochester was offered he said, "This is the one for you." Metcoff felt that one of Janeway's most important attributes was his role as a people developer. He helped young faculty members to define their roles as academicians as well as clinicians. Once, when Metcoff discussed his concern over a faculty member leaving, Janeway reassured him that it was the function of the Children's (and, he might have said, himself) to develop faculty for the United States and the world.

Dr. R. James McKay, Janeway's second chief resident and the first chair of pediatrics at the University of Vermont (a position he held for many years), was a Harvard Medical School graduate who knew Dr. Janeway as an internist at the Brigham while McKay was a student. He decided to take his residency at Columbia University (Babies Hospital, New York) to experience another approach to pediatrics, and planned to return to Boston and take a fellowship in pediatric endocrinology with Dr. Allan Butler at Massachusetts General Hospital. Janeway, however, asked him to return to the Children's as chief resident in 1948–49. While McKay was chief resident, he thought the residents should have one three-day weekend off each month, this at a time when residents had no official days off. He approached the chief with the idea. Janeway agreed, on the condition that McKay find coverage.

McKay ended up providing most of the coverage himself, but he told the incident to demonstrate Dr. Janeway's sensitivity to the needs of the house staff.[29] Perhaps CAJ remembered his days at Hopkins, when there also were no official days off!

Dr. Janeway's sensitivity and concern were highest for his patients. McKay recalled a time when he was concerned that patients with cancer were very upset with the then limits on parental visiting (only one hour a week). He took Janeway to the wards to see such a patient, who was disturbed by the lack of contact with his parents; subsequently, at Janeway's insistence, the visiting hours were increased to every afternoon.[30] Janeway's concern for children was echoed by Dr. Berenberg:

> He had a genuine affection for children and, although he was not one to demonstrate it physically, his devotion to the welfare of children and patient care was indeed legendary. I seldom saw him demonstrate anger, but on one or two occasions when there was near abuse or unnecessary use of children for research, he came close to erupting . . . In the years before one had clinical research committees . . . he took on the role of the child's advocate here at the hospital and blocked some efforts at clinical research that were ill conceived.[31]

In the minutes of one of his first meetings of the Staff Executive Committee of the hospital (August 10, 1945), Dr. Janeway spoke of the need for parents to be able to talk directly to the attending physician. At a later meeting he advocated that parents be given a card with the attending physician's name, to increase this communication. Dr. Thomas Weller commented that when Janeway first arrived as chief, he spent much time with the residents and made rounds regularly, in part, Weller speculated, to learn more about pediatrics. Weller noted that, in those days, CAJ often cracked jokes and was not the austere, quiet, aloof person some thought he later became.[32]

Life in the clinical divisions at the Children's did have some negative aspects. One that disturbed faculty was the lack of opportunity for promotion within Harvard. This probably reduced competition between faculty for the limited number of tenured positions, but those who stayed on were concerned about Janeway's reticence to put up individuals for tenure. He was chief for more than twenty years before he nominated the first such person. In 1968, Park Gerald was about to leave; even then, Dr. Nadas had to intervene to convince CAJ to offer him tenure, which was achieved in 1969.[33] Drs. Rosen and Nathan were granted tenure shortly thereafter.

Dr. Berenberg also commented on Dr. Janeway's statesmanship, whereby he kept the interest of the whole hospital paramount:

> He was frequently willing to give space to another department for their welfare. On the other hand, when there were matters of principle to be considered, he was a tower of unyielding strength and commitment. He acted without fear in matters relating to ethics, principle and integrity. He was totally without prejudice from the ethnic and racial viewpoint and, if anything, leaned over backwards to try to make room for those groups who had been faced with prejudice in the past. He did more to break down the existing "quotas" at the admissions level in the medical school than any other individual or group.[34]

4 Tenure as Chief of Medicine at Children's Hospital Boston

Developing Subspecialty Divisions

In the prior chapter we observed that Dr. Janeway played an important role in pioneering and fostering the establishment of subspecialities in pediatric medicine at Harvard and elsewhere, basing them on available research methods to solve problems of health and disease. His background in general internal medicine and scientific research enabled him to supply a new perspective and approach to the field of pediatrics. Further, the methods and solutions he introduced or helped to introduce were carried out by physicians who went to other hospitals throughout North America and abroad. They had a large impact on revolutionizing and modernizing the diagnosis and treatment of childhood diseases and injuries worldwide. The focus of the current chapter will be to review and detail the innovations Janeway effected at the Children's during his tenure as chief of medicine there. Much that is done today in the medical treatment of childhood disorders took root during the time that Charles A. Janeway was an important and novel presence on that early scene.

Pediatric Hematology

Louis K. Diamond, after his internship at the Children's in 1928, had been on its staff since 1929 and had, as a colleague of Blackfan, the earlier chief, become interested in hematology. Diamond had of necessity practiced general pediatrics, however, there being no source of funds for salary with an academic appointment. Diamond described the clinical syndromes of several blood disorders, including the one bearing his name, the Diamond-Blackfan Syndrome. In the early 1930s, he and others recognized that the underlying common cause of what had been, till that time, thought of as four separate diseases of the newborn—jaundice of the newborn, anemia, kernicterus, and hydrops fetalis—were all associated with incompatibility of Rh factor between the mother and her baby. These syndromes came collectively to be known as erythroblastosis fetalis. In 1943, Diamond was finally able to devote himself fully to academic pediatrics with the development of the Blood Grouping Laboratory, an affiliation of four hospital programs with a grant of what seemed then like a generous award of $10,000 for five years from the Hood Foundation to exploit the recent discoveries of Rh disease. In 1946, Diamond was the first to develop the treatment of exchange transfusion therapy for that condition.[1] From this modest beginning Diamond became one of the first to develop the specialty of pediatric hematology in the United States; he was able to train new faculty, many of whom went on to lead divisions of pediatric hematology in the United States and overseas.

When Diamond approached retirement in 1969, Janeway reached into the department of medicine at Harvard to recruit David Nathan, an internist and one of the new breed of molecular biologists, as well as a superb clinician, to replace him. This appointment was to be one of Janeway's last, but it demonstrated his pursuit of excellence in faculty as well as his recognition of the new fields of biology and research methods that were to contribute so much to medical progress. The brilliance of this appointment was confirmed later, when Nathan assumed CAJ's leadership position as chief of the department of medicine at the Children's.

We digress now to explore a special relationship that led to considerable controversy and concern for many. In the mid 1940s Diamond, working with the hospital's chief pathologist Dr. Sidney Farber, noted that folic acid increased the rate of proliferation of leukemic cells and reasoned that folic acid antagonists might be used to treat children with leukemia. In 1948 Diamond and Farber "launched the modern field of cancer chemotherapy by successfully testing the folic acid antagonist aminopterin to treat children with leukemia."[2] The treatment did, in fact, produce complete, albeit transitory, remission of the disease. For reasons that are unclear, Farber then developed his own clinical unit, the Children's Cancer Research Center at the Children's, which became a part of the Division of Laboratories and Research under Farber. In 1953 Farber encouraged the Variety Club of Boston to join with numerous other organizations in New England, including first the Boston Braves and subsequently the Boston Red Sox baseball clubs, to support the Children's Cancer Research Foundation and labeled its efforts the "Jimmy Fund," after the name of an anonymous twelve-year-old cancer patient. With the enormous increase in funding that resulted, the Farber program for children's cancer and the Diamond program for children's hematologic diseases became separate; it appeared, from a distance, that these two strong personalities had difficulty working together thereafter. The Cancer Research Foundation, with its enormous fund-raising ability, as well as with support from the National Cancer Institute of the U.S. Public Health Service, provided needed resources to build a separate building, closely tied to the Children's Hospital but relatively separate from the rest of the medical department. Consequently, there was often conflict. Diamond did not see patients there.

For most of us assigned to Farber's program as house staff, the experience was not always happy. Its building and funding and trustee organizations were separate, and although the clinic outpatient care and faculty interactions are in fact very close and active with the department of medicine, we had little say in the care of patients but had to deal with very sick children and their distraught parents. For example, we would be told to give a patient a new cancer chemotherapy that we knew only by its experimental number and did not know its mechanism of action nor its side effects. We learned little and felt like technicians; we had little contact with Dr. Farber. The contrasting experience with patients on Diamond's hematology service, where there were rarely cancer patients, was striking. Although Diamond was known as a demanding teacher, he was always willing to spend time teaching students and residents. The separation of the hematology from the oncology service made no sense to us and we suspected that there must be strong antagonism between Diamond and Farber, although we never heard either express this openly. Farber, however, played a very important role in expert committees in Washington; his status resulted in increased resources for study and care of patients with cancer and the building of research facilities. With these contacts and his fund-raising abilities, he was a major force in the new building programs at the Children's.

A few years after Nathan came to the Children's as successor to Diamond, he became concerned that oncology patients were not receiving optimal care at the Jimmy Fund because Farber was opposed to combination chemotherapy. Nathan talked to Dr. Janeway about this; Janeway asked him, what was the evidence? Nathan suggested that they bring in the leaders of the National Cancer Institute of the National Institutes of Health to review the program.[3] The subsequent investigation reported the same findings. Janeway solved the dilemma by allowing the Jimmy Fund to continue to care for oncology patients but for Nathan to care for those on NIH protocol studies. This compromise was rather typical for Janeway. Nathan felt that Berenberg often tried to maintain peace between Drs. Janeway and Farber and that, while the relation with Farber was not close, Janeway respected Farber greatly as a remarkable builder at the Children's. (The relationship between Drs. Farber and Janeway will be discussed in a later chapter.)

When we interviewed Diamond for his impressions of Dr. Janeway, we thought that he might have been resentful about Janeway's position as chief, a position for which he, Diamond, seemed likely to have been the inside candidate. But Diamond said that he had no such ambitions and that Janeway's appointment was a brilliant one, as it brought new science into pediatrics. Diamond thought, however, that CAJ's greatest contribution to the Children's was to keep peace between Robert Gross, the dynamic chief of surgery, and Farber, each of whom would have liked to have broken off and created his own hospital, with himself as head. Both Farber and Gross developed very important services in Boston; their contributions were of national importance and were identified with the Children's.[4]

Diamond raised an interesting point. Many of us felt that Dr. Janeway was too passive in this contest. He never uttered a word publicly against Gross or Farber, and often seemed to defer to them when we would protest about the lack of teaching while on the Jimmy Fund service. One of the few complaints that some of us made about CAJ was that he was "too nice a guy to tangle with these strong men."

Berenberg noted, however, that Janeway "related extremely well to Dr. Gross."[5] In retrospect, we can see through Diamond's eyes that this was Janeway's way to maintain the Children's as a single institution. If the price he had to pay for such maintenance was to appear less strong, he was willing to do it for the good of the institution. The wisdom of this approach became clear when, after the death of Farber in 1973, the new head of hematology, Nathan, was able to integrate the two services and later to forge a combined division of hematology and oncology within the vastly expanded, nearby pediatric and adult Dana-Farber Cancer Center.

Nathan cited the beginning of bone marrow transplantation at the Children's as an example of Dr. Janeway's style of decision making. He and Dr. Rosen had decided that such transplantation should be done, but Farber was opposed. Nathan described their meeting with Janeway concerning the matter thus:

> We needed Charlie's permission to start. Into the office we went, I bubbling with a speech, Fred all the while watching me with savage looks to remain silent. We sat there. No one said a single word. I was literally bursting with poorly suppressed anger at Dr. Farber and brilliant lines about bone marrow transplantation. Fred kept looking at me venomously, his lips tightly pursed. I got the message. After five absolutely impossible minutes, Dr. Janeway got to his feet. "Well," he said, "I think we understand each other completely." I was stunned. With a sidelong look, Rosen motioned me toward the door. "Fred," I said, "What in God's name happened in that room?" "David," said Fred, "Don't be stupid. You don't have to talk to Dr. Janeway for him to listen. He heard you and he heard me. You got your instructions. Let's go do transplants."[6]

Dr. Diamond saw early the contributions that genetics would make to pediatrics, since many of the hematological disorders were genetic in origin. Accordingly, he effectively began the clinical cytogenetics program at the Children's. He encouraged Dr. Park Gerald, one of his young faculty, to go abroad to receive training in this new field and, upon his return, to head a new division of clinical genetics and cytogenetics at the hospital. Gerald was one of the young faculty who were being recruited actively for other institutions, and whom Nadas strongly urged Janeway to promote to tenure in order to keep him in Boston. He obtained support from several sources for the program and proceeded to map the genes on human chromosomes in children with inherited conditions; his work fostered improved counseling of parents. The hematology division under Diamond and Nathan expanded as new research methods became available. Its achievements were Diamond's legacy.[7] The division attracted patients from all over the world and trained many of the leaders of pediatric hematology today.[8]

Immunology and Infectious Diseases

Charles Janeway was at home with infections of children, in spite of his lack of formal training in pediatrics. His work during World War II with Cohn on plasma proteins had opened up the world of immunology to him; during that period his publications included several on the role of one of the plasma proteins, gamma globulin in treating and preventing measles and hepatitis. He saw across the now separate specialties of infectious diseases, immunology, and renal disease, recognizing the interrelation of all of human physiology, especially in those three areas. His colleagues, recognizing this broad vision, wrote after his death that human health and disease for Dr. Janeway was a "seamless whole" from biology to behavior. For him there were no disciplinary boundaries in science, only problems to be attacked with appropriate scientific methods.[9]

With the arrival of David Gitlin, who had been trained in protein chemistry and was a pediatric resident at the Children's in 1949, there began a fruitful collaboration to study a number of diseases of plasma proteins and the use of these substances therapeutically. Among these was the use of serum albumin to produce diuresis in patients with nephrotic syndrome. This led the group, joined by Jack Metcoff, to study renal diseases before the subspeciality of nephrology existed. The story of the first description of the condition known as agammaglobulinemia, which manifests clinically with recurrent, severe bacterial infections, reveals much about Dr. Janeway and his approach to research. He thought of the good that research might do for understanding disease, not the recognition he might receive from it. As Dr. Fred Rosen remembers it,[10] the finding of absent gamma globulin in a young man at Walter Reed Army Medical Center, a patient of Dr. Ogden Bruton, led to the discovery. Bruton and his colleagues at Walter Reed had acquired an electrophoresis apparatus and were testing blood samples for gamma globulin. Bruton did not understand the finding in that patient, and sought out Dr. Janeway for clarification. Janeway told him that there were four such patients at the Children's. Bruton, Dr. Leonard Apt, Dr. David Gitlin and Janeway submitted a single abstract on these cases to the Society for Pediatric Research.[11] Janeway suggested to Bruton that he report his case, and he did so.[12]

Apt, who was a resident at the Children's at the time, recalled[13] the story somewhat differently. The essentials are the same, however: the four investigators submitted an abstract to the Society for Pediatric Research, and Bruton published his case. In 1953 the team from the Children's reported nine cases,[14] a finding that was reported in the *New York Times*.[15] The condition is today known as Bruton's agammaglobulinemia. There has always been some controversy about priority of publication, but such priority, and the naming of the disease after the discoverer, was not high on Charles Janeway's agenda. Over the next decade, he, Gitlin, and their colleagues, now joined by another former resident at the Children's, Fred Rosen, published over twenty-five papers delineating many other aspects of the role that various immune blood components, both in terms of the absence of and abnormalities in gamma globulin and complement, play in human health and disease. Although not technically the first to report the initial case of agammaglobulinemia in the medical literature, Janeway's team expanded the knowledge of the whole field of gamma globulins in health and disease, and the field is generally accepted as one of the major contributions that he and his colleagues made to science.

Although Dr. Janeway created several separate divisions within the Children's, separation or fractionation of clinical pediatrics was not his way of seeing the world. In his report on the history of the first 100 years of the Children's and the plan for the new Enders research building, Janeway and his colleagues called for joint use of equipment by scientists from all departments and for "collaboration between members of different clinical departments and basic scientists [that] should add a wholly new dimension to the research potentialities of this institution."[16] CAJ saw the study of the interrelation of the body's physiology as the centerpiece of the research effort rather than as separate bodies of knowledge based on organ systems, while at the same time realizing that in today's complex laboratory research no one can master all fields:

> As science comes to depend increasingly upon complex expensive and highly sophisticated techniques, team work becomes more important in medical research . . . the success [of the new research building], however, will depend upon the extent to which the clinical scientists who work there keep one foot in the hospital and one in the research building, or the basic scientists maintain close contact with clinical investigators and other scientists in the building as well as with professional colleagues in the academic departments of the Medical School and neighboring institutions. The building was planned to promote just this type of communication.[17]

It was in immunology that Charles Janeway contributed his own research, although, as chief, much of it was done with colleagues. These contributions are detailed in a later chapter.

In the early days there was little of the separateness between divisions seen today in the organization of pediatrics departments. Indeed, when I (RJH) was a young faculty member, informal monthly meetings occurred in faculty members' homes; one person attended from each division, including orthopedics as well as most of the traditional medical divisions. Participants would present their research, usually in its early conceptual phase, to colleagues in the different divisions and get interdisciplinary feedback that often opened up a new approach to the research. Although Dr. Janeway did not participate in these meetings, he passionately fostered this interdisciplinary exchange. Though I was a young faculty member at the time, I felt that I was part of the whole Children's Hospital and of the intellectual ferment of different disciplines rather than being confined to my own area of expertise.

When Dr. Janeway arrived as chief, the research laboratory (primarily working on viral infections) was run by Dr. Enders in the Carnegie Building, in space given by Dr. Farber. Later, a series of outstanding pediatricians headed this division. Dr. Sidney Kibrick succeeded Enders. He was followed by Dr. Samuel Katz, who later left to chair the department of pediatrics at Duke, followed by Dr. David Smith before Smith became chair of pediatrics at Rochester. David Carver was an active member of the team before becoming chair at Toronto Hospital for Sick Children and later chair of pediatrics at The Robert Wood Johnson School of Medicine in New Brunswick, New Jersey. Every one of these individuals was an example of Janeway's success at training future pediatric leaders.

The divisions of infectious diseases and immunology were separate during most of Dr. Janeway's tenure, although they interacted closely, in part due to his close involvement in both. A formal division of immunology was created with Fred Rosen as chief in 1968, and was later combined with Allergy in 1974, when Dr. Harvey Colten was recruited. Ultimately, Raif Geha, a Janeway resident, took over from Rosen. If there is a helter-skelter quality to the foregoing, the impression is not altogether false. Dr. Janeway never was overly concerned with neat administrative organization. He was guided by the science and the caliber of the faculty he had.

The Division of Allergy

Allergic diseases are common; any children's hospital will have many patients with various diseases labeled allergic, especially asthma and eczema. Although there are immunological aspects to most allergies, and in some institutions the division is part of immunology, this did not happen at the Children's during the early years of Janeway's administration, perhaps because there was, at the time he took the helm, a strong clinical program led by a charismatic physician who was in private practice but also ran the allergy clinic, Dr. Louis Webb Hill. Hill once was President John F. Kennedy's pediatrician. He used to tell the residents stories of his experiences, and one of them was that JFK had the worst case of colic he had ever cared for. When I (RJH) was caring for a number of Irish families in Boston, this story, told to exhausted parents of children with colic usually helped them to accept the problem, perhaps in the hope that their child, too, would grow up to be President. Hill also opined that anyone who had been a colicky baby should not be President! This opinion was, presumably, an example of his political views rather than an insight into the science of allergy.

When Hill retired, Janeway recruited another skilled clinician to become full-time head of this division, Dr. Harry Mueller. When Mueller retired, CAJ recruited Dr. Harvey Colten to head a new division of allergy. Colten was a rare outside recruit; his selection illustrates that Janeway could be a formidable recruiter, albeit he did it rarely. Colten tells that he was about to accept a position at Johns Hopkins, but after an hour with CAJ, accepted his offer. Since leaving the Children's Colten has gone on to an extraordinary career as chair at two medical schools and dean at two others. He is yet another example of Janeway's ability to recognize talent.

Metabolism and Renal Disease Division

Dr. James Gamble headed a "Metabolism" unit when Charles Janeway arrived at the Children's. Its work in the 1930s and 1940s was concentrated on body composition and related disorders, dehydration, and acid-base and electrolyte disorders, and the data defined in Dr. Gamble's special laboratory (which became known as "Gamble-grams") were published as a handbook that was used by generations of pediatricians. The research done there led to the successful treatment of diarrhea, one of the most prevalent and fatal diseases of childhood at that time. Several other leading pediatric research teams in the country made major contributions to this field. William Wallace briefly assumed directorship of this division at the Children's in 1952 before leaving to become chair of pediatrics at Case Western Reserve University in Cleveland in 1953. He was followed by Jack Metcoff, and then by Robert Schwartz in 1968.

Dr. Janeway's long research interest in kidney disease began with his landmark study producing experimental glomerulonephritis in rabbits. His interest in a different kidney disorder, the nephrotic syndrome, began with a review of a large series of patients with Dr. Lewis Barness, owing to the fact that one major manifestation of the disease is hypoalbuminemia, a condition he was familiar with from his work in Cohn's plasma fractionation laboratory and in the treatment of shock. From these experiences, Janeway developed a program to care for patients with nephrotic syndrome and other kidney diseases; that program began under Dr. Jack Metcoff, and later a full renal division was developed under Dr. Francis Fellers (The renal division currently is headed by Dr. Harmon, a resident under Janeway). The metabolism unit was headed by Dr. Schwartz. After Schwartz left, the "metabolism" designation was dropped. The interest of both Metcoff and Janeway in hypoproteinemia led them to collaborate with a pioneer Mexican pediatrician, Dr. Joaquin Cravioto, on the hypoproteinemia of malnutrion in developing countries; that collaboration was an example of the lack of traditional boundaries to CAJ's scientific interests.

Endocrinology

Dr. Berenberg felt that endocrinology and cardiology were top priorities for Janeway when he assumed the chair in medicine.[18] Endocrinology as a discipline at Children's had originally been part of metabolism, but emerged as a separate division with the recruitment of John Crigler, Jr. to head the division. Drs. Nathan Talbot and Allan Butler, who earlier had developed the area of metabolism and endocrinology at the Children's, had left to go to Massachusetts General Hospital to join Dr. Fuller Albright's group. Dr. Edna Sobel, an endocrinologist, was for a time in the laboratory division of Dr. Farber's group and provided clinical services at the Children's before she went to Albert Einstein School of Medicine in New York City.

Dr. John Crigler was one of the few senior faculty recruited by Dr. Janeway who had not been trained at Children's. After residency at Johns Hopkins (1946–1950), then as a fellow with the pioneer pediatric endocrinologist, Lawson Wilkins (1950–1951), Crigler spent three and half years at Massachusetts Institute of Technology in the biology department, learning basic science techniques. He was recruited by CAJ in the first or second year of his fellowship at MIT but felt that he needed to finish his work there before coming to the Children's. In his interview with the authors, Crigler noted that Janeway "was very understanding and agreed to an additional six months of my extended fellowship."[19] Crigler arrived at the Children's on January 1, 1955. His laboratories were located initially in the House of the Good Samaritan, which was on Binney Street next to the Jimmy Fund building. At that time, the Good Samaritan Hospital was admitting fewer patients with rheumatic fever, owing to the decline of the disease. In 1965, Crigler was asked by Farber to apply for one of the new NIH-funded General

Clinical Research Centers. When that was approved, Crigler became director and principal investigator, positions he continued to hold for many years. Several other divisions used this resource. In 1976, Dr. Fred Rosen became director and utilized the research center for bone marrow transplantation.

In his interviews Crigler noted, with his usual modesty, that the extensive program in endocrinology at the Children's had been made possible by the outstanding fellows and staff that he recruited. Even so, Dr. Janeway clearly had recruited well in picking Crigler, who over the years established one of the outstanding endocrinology divisions in the world; his fellows have gone on to great distinction elsewhere. Crigler noted that he shared with Janeway a vision that the endocrine division would not only serve the clinical needs of the hospital but also "establish a competitive research and training program."[20] The first fellows were appointed in 1956; in the same year, Crigler received his first NIH research grant to study the isolation and characterization of thyrotropin. In 1959, he added a Ph.D. research scientist to his staff, establishing the pattern that most of the divisions have followed: to have basic scientists as well as clinicians, thus accomplishing one of Janeway's most cherished goals, that divisions do basic science as well as clinical work. Crigler was especially effective in interdepartmental and interinstitutional collaboration on research projects. He collaborated with neurosurgery, orthopedics, and adolescent medicine at the Children's, as well as with the endocrine units at the Peter Bent Brigham Hospital, Massachusetts General Hospital, the Joslin Clinic, and several other institutions in Boston and elsewhere.

Crigler pointed out that Dr. Janeway's contributions included: (1) recognition of the need for clinical research as a science and initiation of the Clinical Research Center; (2) the ability to evaluate people critically but in a positive way; (3) support for the adolescent, family health, and international programs; (4) his willingness to edit everyone's papers; and (5) his immense integrity. In the latter regard he knew how not to talk down to people, but led by example, recognized diversity, and never tried to control people but rather built on their strengths.[21] Crigler later noted that CAJ

> was very strong on bringing the basic sciences into the clinical programs . . . [he] had great intellect and great integrity with an excel-

lent research and clinical background. These elements allowed him to pick outstanding division chiefs . . . he was wonderful to work with as division chief, but while one never felt close to him—he was very supportive. You always knew he was there . . . He didn't give a lot of praise but he recognized integrity, responsibility and commitment to the hospital.[22]

Division of Newborn Medicine

One of the problems facing any children's hospital at the time Charles Janeway became chair was caring for newborns who are born in an outside maternity hospital. This certainly was true at the Children's. The Boston Lying-in Hospital was across the street and a hundred yards down Longwood Avenue, not far away compared to some institutions, but a practical barrier nonetheless existed between it and the Children's. Until after World War II, most newborns were cared for by obstetricians; only if they needed surgery or complex medical treatment were they transferred to the pediatric hospital.

In the 1930s there was a separate hospital, the Infants' Hospital, for, as the term implies, the treatment of children under one or two years of age. It was located then on Shattuck Street. Later this building was to become the Harvard School of Public Health, but it has since returned to the Children's as its administrative offices. Infants who required hospital care after leaving the maternity hospital were cared for here. Neonatology, the science of and care of babies in the first month of life and for a few additional months beyond, including those born prematurely as well as those with medically or surgically treated disorders, was in effect practiced in both the maternity hospital and the Infants' Hospital. At this earlier time there was little that could be done medically for these small premature infants other than to keep them warm, protect them from infection, and feed them. The major controversy in pediatrics at that time concerned the optimal formula to feed these small babies. At the Infants' Hospital Dr. Blackfan, in collaboration with colleagues from the School of Public Health, studied and developed environmentally controlled incubators for the care of prematurely born infants to provide warmth and isolation. In the 1930s, a new nursery for babies born prematurely was built at the Lying-in Hospital; Dr. Stewart Clifford, a practitioner in Boston, was appointed director. In 1935 Dr. Clement Smith was asked to join that group to do research on the physiology of newborns, thus initiating the field of scientific neonatology. A number of talented young pediatricians took fellowships with Dr. Smith, including Dr. Janeway's successor, Dr. Mary Ellen Avery.

Janeway did little to change this productive division during his tenure, in part because "if it ain't broke, don't fix it," which he may have thought was the case given the presence of an internationally recognized scholar-investigator in Clement Smith, and in part because it was the one field of pediatrics in which the internist-turned-pediatrician, Charles Janeway, remained less skilled. Nonetheless, several major research efforts came from the unit during his time, including Dr. Avery's elucidation of the importance of deficiency of surfactant as the cause of respiratory distress syndrome of the newborn, and the National Collaborative Study (*i.e.*, collaborative with several other institutions) of a large sample of women from early pregnancy through to the follow-up of their babies for many years later.

Neonatology now dominates most pediatric departments and is no less strong at Children's. Dr. Nathan suggested that in his later years of his tenure Dr. Janeway did not recognize sufficiently that neonatology in the department was in trouble and had not advanced with the times.[23] It took Dr. Avery to remedy this. With the building of the new Brigham and Women's Hospital across Francis Street, connected by a bridge to the Children's, the physical separation was reduced and a joint collaborative program between the Children's Hospital, the Brigham and Women's Hospital and the Beth Israel Hopital was begun. The neonatology program in Boston now is a model of regional coordinated care of the newborn.

Child Psychiatry

Child psychiatry had a difficult time entering the Children's Hospital. Many pediatricians were skeptical of child psychiatry; witness the well-known polemic of the famous pediatrician, Joseph Brenneman, "The Menace of Psychiatry."[24] Although the substance of his argument was less provocative than its title, Brenneman was against what he felt was the unscientific psychological advice that psychologists (who were more the focus of Brennerman's ire than psychiatrists) were giving parents about child rearing. More reasoned was the paper given by the chief of neurology at the Children's, Bronson Crothers, who was concerned that if pediatricians turned over the psychological aspects of children to others, they would be less effective.[25] Crothers was a seasoned clinician who cared for seriously handicapped children and recognized the seamless whole of children and the difficulty of separating physical from psychological problems. As a result, when Janeway arrived at Children's there was no child psychiatry program. For whatever reason, he decided to change this.

Dr. Janeway's decision may have been influenced by his wife, Betty, and her medical social worker training, and it probably stemmed as well from his own sensitivity and clinical skills. Whatever the inspiration, he set about to add the first child psychiatrist to the staff. Janeway selected wisely, appointing Dr. Dane Prugh in 1949. Prugh had been trained as a pediatrician at the Children's, following a pattern for many of his appointments, wherein he would select people after he had gotten to know them as residents. Prugh was committed to the care of children with chronic physical and mental illnesses. He was known as a good pediatrician, which helped to make him more acceptable to the skeptical staff of the hospital. Prugh modeled his role on the liaison concepts of Dr. George Engel, under whom he had trained in psychiatry at the University of Rochester, and provided consultation to pediatricians who were concerned with problems of behavior in their patients, especially those in the hospital.

Because of his keen interest in having all divisions do research, Dr. Janeway supported Prugh's research efforts. One of them began shortly after Prugh arrived. At that time visiting hours for parents were limited to two hours a week on Sunday, and there was little or no effort to provide play time for children in hospital, although some other children's hospitals had by then implemented "play programs." At that time also, however, a growing literature, especially in Britain,[26] described the harmful effects of hospitalization on children, in part owing to separation from their mothers. Programs of ward management had been organized in a few hospitals in the United States to mitigate this adverse effect of hospitalization. These programs included preparation for hospitalization when possible, arranging for the mother to visit frequently or stay in hospital with her child, the presence of a nursery-school teacher to provide a safe haven where no medical treatments would be done, and education of the nurses to be sensitive to each child's psychological needs. Little research had been done to evaluate the efficacy of such measures, however; Prugh decided to carry out such a trial at Children's. Prugh realized, as did Janeway, that such a inquiry, organized according to a rigorous research design, was especially important in order to effect changes there as well as in other hospitals

The results demonstrated "a significant lowering of the incidence and severity of reactions at all age levels." In addition, the study showed the inaccuracy of many shibboleths, such as the myth that children whose parents visited more would cry more or have more cross infections.[27] While there was at the time a general movement to humanize the care of children in hospital, this study lent experimental justification to the movement. The fact that it came from the Children's, known to be somewhat antagonistic to psychological aspects of child care, gave the results greater impact. Janeway was solidly behind the study and implemented the program. Today it all seems like common sense: all children's hospitals have open visiting, a play program (now generally called a child life program), preparation for admission, and all the other parts of the intervention made more than fifty years ago; but such "common sense" was not in evidence then. CAJ, the bench scientist, recognized this need and acted upon it.

Ms. Brooks Barnes, head nurse on the infants' ward at the Children's during much of Dr. Janeway's tenure, felt that much of his interest in parents staying with their children in hospital stemmed from his experiences abroad, where he saw mothers living in hospital and noted the calming influence that their presence had on their children.[28] In an interview with us, Prugh told another anecdote about Dr. Janeway that characterized his behavior. Sally Staub, the nursery school teacher Prugh had brought in to direct the child life program, had a rule that no physician could examine a child in the nursery school area. One day, Janeway came and started to examine a child there. Staub immediately walked up to him and reminded him of the rule. CAJ accepted it immediately, showing that even the chief was not above the rules.[29]

In 1953, Dr. Prugh left to head the child psychiatry program at Rochester; Dr. George Gardner, Director of the Judge Baker Guidance Center, was appointed chief of child psychiatry at the Children's. He brought with him to the Children's money for a new building that was erected across Longwood Avenue, and a large staff. The new building was connected by tunnel to the Children's, and the resulting collaborative service, training, and research capabilities enhanced the hospital's psychiatric endeavors.[30]

In 1958, Dr. Janeway was invited to give the Margaret S. Brogden Memorial Lecture on the fiftieth anniversary of the Social Service Department at Johns Hopkins. He chose the title, "The Child, the Parent and the Hospital," and elaborated on the theme of how the hospital should manage children and families to mitigate the trauma of hospitalization.[31] The choice of Janeway to give this lecture was itself unusual, for he was known at that time primarily for his work in immunology and infectious disease, not social work. One might speculate that Betty's former role as a social worker at Johns Hopkins influenced his selection, but that was not the case. A letter from Miss Helen Woods, Chief of Social Work at Hopkins, which thanked him for agreeing to lecture, apologized for the fact that she had not known that Betty had been a social worker there.[32] In his acceptance letter Janeway wrote, "Whether or not I am capable of speaking effectively on this subject, I am not sure, but it is one in which I am much interested. As a result of this lecture, I look forward to filling in a lot of gaps in my own personal knowledge."[33] (That he prepared diligently is apparent, for the folder for the lecture contains many reprints and hand-written notes from his reading of the literature, an outline of the lecture, and a handwritten, full text of his talk.)

What caused this apparent change from the scientist-clinician to the pediatrician sensitive to children's emotional needs? Certainly a factor was Prugh's research. In Janeway's folder for the Hopkins lecture are two of Prugh's papers, including Prugh's research study. The text of the speech indicates that CAJ did his homework. Janeway acknowledged that in earlier days, death from infectious diseases had required restriction of parental visiting, but now, "pediatricians, freed by the advances in the treatment and prevention of infectious diseases . . . have been able to turn their attention to the emotional and social problems of hospitalization." He believed that the answer to the question, "Does hospitalization have a deleterious effect on the child?", lies in a series of related questions such as, "What kind of hospitalization?", "For how long?", and "What kind of child?" He noted that studies in child development had now provided "practical yardsticks by which progress of the child in intellectual and social maturation could be measured with an accuracy approaching physiological measurements." He concluded by talking about hospital construction, since Hopkins was planning a new children's unit: "hospitals for children ought to free themselves from the shackles of conventional adult hospitals. Play space, sound-proof treatment rooms, companionship unless individual isolation is essential . . . mother or nurse should be with the child as much as possible and decoration and use of colors which stress a homelike atmosphere are all important."[34] It is a wonder where these ideas came from. Janeway learned from those around him. His mind was prepared for new ideas and he was able to massage them and incorporate them into his own articulate vision of the world.

In 1971 Dr Julius Richmond, then Chair of Pediatrics and Dean at Syracuse University Medical School, and former Director of Project Head Start, was appointed successor to Gardner. Dr. Janeway pushed very hard to accomplish this appointment of a pediatric colleague whom he knew would foster integration of pediatrics and psychiatry. Janeway's initiation of the Adolescent Program and the Family Health Care Program at the Children's also fit this mold, and these, together with the initiation of the child psychiatry program, demonstrated his commitment to the social-psychological aspect of pediatrics.

Dr. Janeway's interest in mental health problems did not end with those services at the Children's. Dr. John Houpis, a pediatrician from Vermont, told us how helpful Janeway was in establishing the first mental health clinic in that state. After the tragic death of a young man by suicide had succeeded in mobilizing the community, Janeway helped Houpis to obtain the necessary data to support such a clinic. At that time CAJ was Chairman of the Hood Foundation, which supported initiatives in child health in New England, and suggested that the Hood Foundation might support the work, "since they received their milk from the cows of Vermont and thus had an important reason to support the effort."[35] Hood took the hint; they awarded a grant of $25,000 to start the clinic. In addition, Janeway knew the Commissioner of Mental Health for the state of Vermont, and his brother, Edward, was a state senator. The two of them mobilized the necessary support for a child guidance program in the state.

Pediatric Cardiology

One of Charles Janeway's first appointments in 1949 was the first full-time chief of pediatric cardiology, then a nascent subspecialty of pediatrics. Probably only the Johns Hopkins pediatrics department had an academic leader in this field, which was at that time new, largely descriptive, and offered few therapies. Janeway selected a most improbable person, Alexander Nadas, a Hungarian-born refugee, who was then practicing general pediatrics in Greenfield, Massachusetts, to head this new division. Nadas had received a short training in adult cardiology in London, but it is difficult to know why Janeway settled on him, albeit Nadas had spent a year as a resident at the Children's during the war and CAJ knew him personally. After that residency, Nadas went with Clement Smith to the University of Michigan at Ann Arbor for a brief period and, when Smith returned to Boston, he subsequently went into private practice in Greenfield. Undoubtedly, Smith played a role in "selling" Nadas to Janeway. Nadas recalled for us that Dr. Janeway told him simply that "he wanted me to do for Children's what Sam Levine had done for adult cardiology at the Brigham."[36] What marching orders! Both Levine and Nadas put cardiology on the map at their respective hospitals.

In his contribution to the 1969 annual report, which celebrated the one-hundredth anniversary of the hospital, Janeway noted that he had been able to obtain funds for construction of a cardiovascular unit at the Children's from the Sharon Sanatorium and the trustees of the Children's.[37] Nadas noted that "Sharon supplied the seed that enabled Dr. Janeway to establish an integrated cardiology program at Children's."[38] The unit was an integration of medical and surgical cardiology services for children, an unusual and essential partnership. The Sharon Sanatorium, founded in 1891, was originally designed for care of patients with pulmonary diseases (largely tuberculosis) and later for children with rheumatic fever (by the 1970s both diminishing diseases). For many years the Sharon Board kept control of the endowment and supplied annual support for the cardiac unit at the Children's, but in 1988, during a large campaign drive at the hospital, the board of the Sharon sanatorium merged its assets of over $3,000,000 with the Children's, of which a portion was to be used for the support of an Alexander Nadas professorship in pediatric cardiology.[39] In this report

Janeway's long-term planning is evident, for, "In 1948 Charles A. Janeway, M.D. spoke to the Sharon Board about the work in cardiology that was going on at Children's Hospital . . . and relayed the urgent need for updated facilities . . . In 1949, the Sharon Board of Directors approved a plan to use $160,000, money that enabled Dr. Janeway to establish an integrated cardiology program at Children's."[40] Thus, twenty years after Janeway had planted the seed, it came to fruition when the assets of the Sharon Sanatorium merged with the cardiology division at the Children's.

The cardiology unit benefited from still another hospital merger. A formerly separate hospital, the House of the Good Samaritan, located adjacent to the Children's, played an important role in its cardiology program. The House of the Good Samaritan was originally intended for patients with rheumatic fever, until the 1950s the major cause of heart disease in children. With the decline of that disease, the problems of congenital heart disease became more apparent. The House of the Good Samaritan joined the Children's in 1949 as one of the affiliated institutions comprising the Children's Hospital Medical Center. Benedict Massell, who spent his entire career at the Good Samaritan, became chief in 1952 and served that unit until his retirement in 1973.[41] Although it would have been intellectually appropriate to combine the Good Samaritan with the cardiology division, Dr. Janeway did not do this at first. We suspect that his action (or inaction) was taken so as not to create tension between the two directors. He opted to keep each somewhat independent, although the Good Samaritan (and its endowment) was amalgamated with the Children's. Dr. Janeway did not flinch from a fight, but generally was a peacemaker who tried to avoid conflict if he could. Perhaps he had learned the lesson that his father had not: that it is foolish to try to change things that cannot be changed or for which the price is too great. After the natural further decline of the incidence of rheumatic heart disease, and Massell's retirement, the Good Samaritan building became, for a time, the research laboratories for Crigler's endocrinology division and later a long-term care facility for the Children's. The building subsequently was sold to permit use of the land for part of the new Brigham and Women's Hospital.

Another of Dr. Janeway's decisions, one that is still debated as to its wisdom, was to establish a separate department of cardiology at the Children's in 1969, making it independent and equal organizationally to the department of medicine. In many ways this has allowed cardiology to grow and flourish, but removed it from the financial and oversight role that the department of medicine might have provided. Nadas recalled that it was done on Janeway's initiative; he recalled him saying, "Cardiology is too big. Do you want to split it off as a separate department?"[42] Nadas recalled that he said no, but he had expressed in a letter to Janeway that cardiology then accounted for about 25% of the department's caseload, planting the seed, perhaps, for ultimate separation.[43] When the Enders building was built, no space was allocated for cardiology. When Nadas asked Janeway about this, CAJ replied, "you are not a squeaky wheel"[44] That said, Nadas then felt it advisable to accept Janeway's offer that cardiology be a separate department. Another argument in favor of a separate department was that the clinical inpatient unit was a combined medical-surgical one; having independent departmental status made this relation with surgery easier; a balance of power, each a department.

With Nadas as chief, there was no doubt that cardiology was integrated into the department of medicine, while its independence allowed it to expand and become the pre-eminent cardiology center in the nation. The actions of some of Nadas's successors, however, rendered it unclear whether a separate cardiology department was best for the entire pediatric service. In most medical school departments there are only a few "money makers"—cardiology and neonatology especially—and in order for a department to offer the supporting services that have difficulty making money—infectious diseases, genetics, endocrinology, and general academic pediatrics—there needs to be support from the money makers, a sharing of the wealth. At the Children's there probably were sufficient resources for most divisions, but in most institutions it would be a mistake to separate cardiology from pediatrics. Nathan expressed this view in his interview that one of Janeway's weaknesses was "dismemberment of the department of medicine."[45]

Cardiac surgery at the Children's had achieved national prominence with Dr. Gross's first successful ligation of a patent ductus arteriosus in a patient in 1938. A group at Los Angeles Children's Hospital and other places soon were doing the same operation successfully. In Dr. Donald Fyler's history of cardiology at the Children's, he notes one aspect of CAJ's chauvinism: Janeway was critical of many institutions outside the East Coast. When Fyler went to Los Angeles in 1957, Dr. Janeway told him, "someone had to go out there and help those poor people."[46] Today his view might be called Eastern nearsightedness, or snobbery by some.

Gross developed many new techniques for repairing the hearts of children with congenital defects. He was the national leader and for some time did not perceive the need for pediatric cardiologists. Fyler noted that "it was several years before Gross became comfortable with the input from clinical cardiologists." Eventually, however, a combined medical and surgical cardiology unit functioned well. Receipt of a large program-project grant from the National Institutes of Health in 1966 enabled the Children's to add a large research unit to this department, under Dr. Abraham Rudolph. The success of the cardiology department at Children's is indisputable. It is the largest pediatric cardiology unit in the world, owing in great part to the leadership of Nadas and his successors. Fyler's history documents the contributions of the department and acknowledges the contributions of Nadas and his staff. Dr. Janeway participated in major decisions with this unit, but, as was his style, did not interfere with faculty who were doing well. His contribution was to recruit the genius, Nadas, obtain the initial resources, and give him room to excel. This Nadas did.

The Adolescent and Young Adult Medicine Division

The Children's Hospital was the first pediatric hospital to develop a special clinic for adolescents. It did so in 1951.[47] Charles Janeway considered this to be one of his most important contributions to pediatrics. Janeway's background as an internist probably gave him experience with this age group and prompted him to see the gap in services for adolescents in both pediatrics and internal medicine. In 1951, Dr. J. Roswell (Ross) Gallagher agreed to begin an adolescent unit at the Children's. From 1935 to 1949, Gallagher had been head of student health at Phillips Academy in Andover, a well-known preparatory school; he was, therefore, experienced as a clinician who had dealt with the health and socio-psychological problems of adolescents. During that period he wrote a number of scientific papers on sports injuries, appendicitis, and primary atypical pneumonia, and after that, while he was a school health physician in Connecticut, he participated with Janeway in a study of the prophylaxis of measles with gamma globulin. Gallagher's appointment, then, continued Janeway's pattern of appointing people he knew were talented and up to the job for which they were chosen.

As clinic chief at the Children's, Gallagher collected a number of specialists from the Harvard hospitals to be available on a consulting basis. The clinic was open to "boys and girls aged twelve to twenty-one, regardless of their ailments."[48] Gallagher obtained funding from both the William T. Grant Foundation and the Commonwealth Fund. Dr. Robert Masland, successor to Gallagher, noted that when he became chief in 1967, funds from the Grant Foundation were not being made available for the program. The president of the hospital said it was not possible to provide funds since they were being used to support the physical space of the unit. As Masland reported, "I went to Charlie and told him I would like to get a lawyer to look into this matter. Charlie supported me completely and [subsequently was told that] the monies from the endowment fund have been turned over to the adolescent program for educational purposes, especially to support fellows."[49]

The adolescent unit was originally located in a lower floor of the Hunnewell building, but in 1974 the old Ida C. Smith Ward, built in 1930 for the surgical service, was "elevated fourteen feet above its original level, and thus made accessible to the Fagan Building and the Prouty garden [and] . . . became a unique, historic and 'special home' for the adolescent program."[50] In a 1953 letter to the Commonwealth Fund, Gallagher reported on the clinic after two years of operation. The focus was on the training of physicians in the "care of this age group, rather than in a specialty or disease[-oriented hospital or clinic], and [in] a place where young people would receive the best care, if they could be seen in a clinic exclusively theirs, not one where they would sit side by side with either infants or mature adults . . . the emphasis must be on the boy or girl, not the ailment."[51] Young people made their own appointments. Gallagher "advocated sitting next to the patient or on the same side of the desk as the teen patient to make them feel less intimidated and more at ease."

Because the clinic had from the beginning a multi-disciplinary staff, including psychologists and psychiatrists, it was an expensive service. Gallagher noted that the hospital agreed to "underwrite the deficit during the first two years of operation." He went on to say that "since the care which we give is very time-consuming it makes me doubt that . . . it can be self supporting . . . through fees alone. For this reason a group known as the Associates of the Adolescent Unit is being formed . . . and within a year or two this group will be able to raise sufficient funds so that our program will not further increase the hospital's deficit."[52] It is unlikely that such a group could have been able to supply the necessary funds for very long. For many of the faculty, and to some degree, for Charles Janeway, the realities of medical care financing were not high priorities.

Congruent with Dr. Janeway's vision that research was central to all the activities of the department, research was begun in the adolescent clinic, initially with physicians from the Peter Bent Brigham hospital on such topics as dysmenorrhea, methods to diagnose hypothyroidism, studies of hypertension, and growth and development of adolescents. Gallagher was a pioneer and an articulate advocate for adolescent clinics; he made the unit at the Children's a very visible innovation. With Dr. Jean Emans's arrival in 1975 as a resident under CAJ, adolescent gynecology became a major focus and has resulted in the major textbook in the field being published and edited by Emans and Dr. Donald Goldstein. In the unit, many future leaders of adolescent medicine were trained. Week-long continuing medical education courses by the faculty in adolescent medicine have proven popular with practicing physicians for many years.

The clinic's similarity to the programs in child psychiatry and family health did not always make it popular with the pediatric residents at the hospital, many of whom preferred to work with patients with traditional medical diseases. In all of these cases, however, Janeway let it be known that he supported the programs and believed that it was important for pediatricians to have such training. He recognized, before many other leaders of pediatrics did, that bio-psycho-social medicine was becoming more important in the general milieu of medicine, as traditional medical diseases were being prevented or treated successfully. In his letter asking for funding for the expansion of the adolescent program to include more teaching and research, he emphasized that this was "one of several allied efforts to relate the student's medical experience to the community and to a more comprehensive view of the patient he serves."[53] He pointed out the department's programs with the Harvard School of Public Health and a student-health service affiliation with the Judge Baker Guidance Center, and wrote, "We hope that the development of a family medical care program, as an integrated effort of all those concerned . . . the Medical, Dental, and Public Health Schools . . . may be a natural sequel."[54]

Dr. Masland, who succeeded Gallagher, tells of the way in which the transfer was effected:

> I can recall my visit with Charlie, when he asked me to be the acting chief until a permanent chief could be named. He was very open and honest with me and told me that he thought it might be useful to consider an endocrinologist or a research person for the position. For a year I was acting chief, and then one day a letter arrived from the president's office, naming me as the chief. I called Charlie to make certain that the announcement was appropriate and he confirmed that he wanted me to be chief. I still do not know . . . whether or not other candidates were interviewed . . . or offered the position. Charlie never discussed this with me.[55]

Masland's experience was somewhat typical of Dr. Janeway's manner of dealing with faculty. He was straightforward when in direct conversation, but not too forthcoming about one's future. And he rarely discussed salary. Masland recalled later that CAJ wanted the adolescent unit to become more scholarly and told Masland, "You must do more research."[56] Scholarship, research, and high-quality clinical care were all part of one piece to Janeway. He would be proud of the current state of the adolescent medicine in this country, a field he helped to create.

Another facet of the unit's program involved it in one of the most controversial issues of our day: abortion. The adolescent clinic's staff were not immune to the controversy; they were caring for a number of teenage girls who had become pregnant. If they were to offer truly comprehensive services, this must include abortion when necessary. Masland recalled:

> Can you imagine the turmoil over this matter, to carry out abortions for teenage girls at the Children's Hospital! Charlie Janeway got this through the executive committee and trustees, feeling as I do that to be discriminatory against women is uncalled for and that Children's Hospital must set an example for all of pediatrics as to what comprehensive care for children and adolescents really means.[57]

Dr. Janeway could be very courageous when he felt it was necessary. In his files at home there is a large folder with over 100 letters, almost all of them condemning this new service in the inflammatory terms that have become so prominent in the abortion debate. The fact that he kept this folder at home must have meant that he wanted to protect it from public scrutiny. It is clear that he was solidly behind the service, however.

Similar to most of the divisions at the Children's, the Adolescent Fellowship Program trained health professionals for leadership positions in many other medical school and hospitals.[58] Masland recalled that, of all the things Janeway had accomplished during his time as Physician in Chief at Children's Hospital, he thought that history might remember him as the one who brought adolescent medicine into being as a legitimate interest for pediatricians.[59] Dr. Janeway's legacy in adolescent medicine was carried on in the Charles Alderson Janeway Medical Service at the hospital, one of three medical-pediatric inpatient services at the Children's (later reduced to two). During Dr. David Nathan's tenure as physician-in-chief at Children's, he created three inpatient units on the principle of a full-time permanent staff rather than the more usual rotating attending staff (more recently changed to semi-permanent attending physicians). The adolescent unit was appropriately named the "Janeway" service; it included a multi-disciplinary staff of physicians, nurses, social workers, a dietician, a physical therapist, a pastoral care staff, and, more recently, hospitalists. This service was a fitting tribute to CAJ's promotion of adolescent medicine at the Children's. However, changes continued, and today the Janeway Service no longer exists.

Another example of Dr. Janeway's effort to humanize the care of adolescents in the hospital was the establishment of a "Teen Center" for hospitalized adolescents in the early 1970s. He tapped Dr Sprague Hazard, who had been in private practice for many years, and one of the authors (FHL) to accomplish this. He mobilized a small amount of money to collect data documenting the effectiveness of the center and convinced the hospital to build the teen center on the adolescent ward. It demonstrated his belief that every innovation should be studied and reported, as was this one.[60]

Division of Child Health and The Family Health Care Program

In 1948 a new Child Health Division was established with Dr. Harold Stuart as director. The division provided well-child services and did research on growth and development of "Normal and Under-par Children."[61] Dr. Stuart was responsible for developing the first growth charts, based on his longitudinal study of normal children, which have since been used by generations of pediatricians to assess growth of their patients. The division was housed in a three-story wooden building on the corner of Longwood Avenue and Blackfan Street. Here well-child clinics were held, staffed by Harvard School of Public Health pediatricians and Boston City Public Health nurses. A multi-disciplinary faculty of pediatricians, psychologists, dietitions, and nurses was developed. It served young families from nearby areas, predominantly Irish Catholic families from Roxbury, and was the place where residents from Children's learned the care of the well child and preventive pediatrics.

When I (RJH) was finishing my chief residency in the spring of 1955, and had arranged to have a fellowship in cardiology with Dr. Nadas, Dr. Janeway called me into his office one day in May to ask if I would take over direction of the Division of Child Health upon Dr. Stuart's upcoming retirement and develop a program funded by the Commonwealth Fund for a home care program. The grant had been obtained by Dr. Prugh, the chief of child psychiatry, prior to his departure, as a vehicle to study and teach the social aspects of child health, as well as to provide care at home for children who would otherwise be in hospital for chronic illness. I reminded Dr. Janeway that I was committed to Dr. Nadas. He said, "I'll take care of that." It was a fortunate career shift for me, since I had been aiming at a generalist practice career before going to the Children's, and I suspect that CAJ, in his incisive way of fitting young people into careers that best suited them, saw that I would be better in this role than as a cardiologist.

I spent the first few months learning about well-child care and public health from the wonderful staff, and visiting several programs in "comprehensive care" in the eastern United States. With the reduction of need for long-term care of children with infectious diseases, I felt that a purely home care program to provide services for the convalescent child was no longer necessary, but a program to provide preventive and curative care to families was needed in order to teach general pediatrics and continuity of care to students and residents. Janeway never questioned my decision to change direction and always supported the program. Many residents were ambivalent about the idea of taking time away from the hospital to provide continuity of care to mainly physically well families who had common illnesses, largely infectious and behavioral problems. To overcome this, I also recruited children with chronic physical diseases from the specialty clinics of the hospital as well as well children, and had the residents provide most of the care, even for the children with chronic illnesses. To help residents feel committed to these patients, most were recruited from the inpatient services; the resident who had cared for them in hospital became their continuing care physician. CAJ always supported this as well, even against some opposition from other faculty, who were not happy about my taking patients from their clinics. We served as the medical home for these children while still maintaining their contacts with the specialty clinics as consultants. A supplemental grant from the Hood Foundation allowed the recruitment of a social worker, and a Children's Bureau grant supported fellowships in general pediatrics.

In conjunction with a similar program at Massachusetts General Hospital, we conducted a random controlled trial of medical education by assigning thirty-two third-year students to one of the two programs; their charge was to follow and care for a family with children and a pregnant woman for the last two years of medical school.[62] There was some opposition by faculty to taking students out of clinical rotations when the time of delivery came or an emergency illness arose. Once again, Janeway and Dean George Packer Berry supported

our efforts fully. This characteristic was typical of CAJ's behavior toward all the other division chiefs; once he picked people to lead divisions, he was behind them 100% and would do all he could to help
them succeed.

By 1960 I realized that I needed to develop research skills if I was going to succeed in academic medicine. Dr. Janeway stepped in to help
me obtain a Commonwealth Fund Fellowship for a year in England,
starting in August 1961. During my year in England I was concerned
about leaving a new program with a small staff, and I must have written Janeway about my concerns. He wrote, "I'm afraid I have not been
as close to the Family Health Program as I should be, but I will make it
a point of getting in there."[63] With a million other things to do, this
was his way of reassuring me. I am not sure how much he got "in
there," but I was reassured. Late in October, Dr. Janeway wrote to ask
if I would be willing to be Harvard's nominee for a Markle scholar
award.[64] What an honor! The fact that Dr. Janeway had convinced the
Dean that I should be Harvard's candidate that year was evidence of
his support and guidance to me, as he was to all of his faculty.

When I returned from England, I applied to the Commonwealth
Fund for a grant of $169,176 to evaluate the Family Health Care Pro-
gram. In his supporting letter, CAJ wrote:

> From the time that I became head of this department, I have felt that
> it was essential that we not only explore in depth the major problems
> of disease in childhood with the tools of the basic sciences, which are
> of course derived from the natural sciences, but also that we study
> the means of applying such knowledge, as well. The problems of
> medical care, for children especially, are to a large extent the prob-
> lems of the families in which they live and grow. To study these
> problems, one must combine the research tools and concepts of the
> basic medical sciences with the newer methods and ideas from the
> behavioral sciences.[65]

This is a succinct statement of Janeway's philosophy about academic
pediatrics: integration of biology and behavior, and the application of
knowledge obtained from research in order to improve the health of
children.

When I left the program, Dr. Joel Alpert, who had been a fellow in
the division and was then a junior faculty member, was appointed di-

rector. In 1966, Alpert proposed that the Family Health Care Program (FHCP) develop a Family Medicine residency program. This was the beginning of the national resurgence of general practice as the re-named "family practice." Most programs required a separate department of Family Medicine. There being none at Harvard, Alpert proposed a four-year program wherein the resident would spend three years at the Peter Bent Brigham Hospital and the Children's, and a year at the FHCP. The residents were to have some experience delivering babies at the Boston Hospital for Women. The chairs of medicine and obstetrics agreed, according to Alpert, "because of Charlie,"[66] and the FHCP received a grant from the Family Health Foundation of America. The program also had fellows in family medicine, practitioners who wished to become teachers of family medicine. The program went on for four years, until the Board of Family Medicine required more experience in obstetrics and gynecology to qualify for the federal support.

When Alpert left to become chair of pediatrics at Boston University, Dr. Richard Feinbloom became chief of the division. Support from the hospital administration declined and, after Janeway retired, the clinical program was transferred to Cambridge for a time, but ultimately it was discontinued and even the Division of Child Health was dropped, to be incorporated later into the ambulatory services of the Children's and the Martha Eliot Community Health Center in Roxbury. In the preface to a monograph written about the experiment, CAJ wrote, "The work specifically demonstrates that family health care or primary care . . . is as legitimate and important a field for academic medical endeavor as [are] clinical teaching and research based on modern molecular and cellular biology."[67] He ended the preface with ringing support for the flexible public/private collaboration for funding "That is a far cry from the inherently rigid and monolithic nature of the governmental organizations that control educational programs and research activities in many other countries."

As we will see in chapters concerning Dr. Janeway's many international activities, although he was a strong supporter of universal access to medical care in the United States, he was leery of monolithic governmental support of research and teaching. In Dr. Janeway's report in 1969 he declared,

We need to approach the problems of health care as we would any other problem—by analysis, experimentation and evaluation. . . . we need research on health care . . . But where is the laboratory? Fortunately it is already here, since one purpose in organizing the Family Health Care Program in 1955 was to provide a laboratory for the study of health problems in the community as opposed to the hospital . . . We feel that the Medical Care Research Unit of the Family Health Care Program should become an essential component of our hospital.[68]

Toward the end of his career, Dr. Janeway became an eloquent champion of Family Medicine. Changes in leadership of the program at the Children's, the development of a Harvard Medical School support of a Center for Research in Medical Care, and an alternative clinical primary care unit, the Martha Eliot Center, led to elimination of the Family Health Care Program and its research, and the incorporation of some of its activities into the general ambulatory division of the Children's.

The Boston Poison Information Center

When Dr. Lendon Snedeker, Assistant Director of the Children's in the 1950s and 1960s, was active in the American Academy of Pediatrics, the first poison information center was developed in 1953 in Chicago. The American Academy of Pediatrics established a Poison Control Committee and advocated that other institutions establish such centers. With this knowledge and under the auspices of the Massachusetts Chapter of the Academy, Snedeker proposed organizing such a center at Children's and asked one of the authors (RJH) if he would develop it. The Boston center became one of the earliest such centers in the United States.

Development was very basic. Most children who poison themselves at home ingest either household cleaners or other common and available substances or medicines. At the time our program began there were no files of the ingredients of common household products; accordingly, during the first summer we employed a medical student to go to several stores and record the trade names of products that were being ingested by children, together with the addresses of the companies that manufactured them. We then wrote the companies and asked for the ingredients so that we could more rationally treat children who ingested them. From this initial survey grew the information center that took telephone calls about ingestions, at first only from doctors but ultimately from patients (*i.e.*, parents) as well. Emergency-room pediatric residents answered such calls at that time. This education of residents about common emergency problems and the prevention of poisonings fit naturally in the Family Health Care Program's emphasis on educating pediatricians about common disorders and their prevention. RJH's successor as chief of the division, Dr Alpert, also assumed directorship of the Poison Center, and in 1972 the other author (FHL) succeeded Alpert as director.

I (FHL) assumed leadership of the Poison Information Cener in 1972. In 1976, the Commissioner of the Massachusetts Department of Public Health formally appointed a state-wide committee to create a Poison Control System for the Commonwealth. The committee was charged with developing a staff trained to disseminate information to the public and professionals twenty-four hours a day, seven days a week. Staff also were to promote dependable public and professional education, carry out toxicology research, and obtain public and private support to fund the system. A request for proposal for the new home of the Massachusetts Poison Control System was distributed in 1976; Children's Hospital/Harvard Medical School, Boston City Hospital/Boston University School of Medicine, and the University of Massachusetts Medical School all applied. An outside committee of experts ultimately chose the Children's as the site of the newly created system, with FHL as director. The budget to cover the increased activities of a single Center and system of care for the Commonwealth was increased significantly by the state and by contributions to the Center through the Massachusetts Department of Public Health.

The new information center for the Massachusetts system was housed at the Children's. It enlisted the majority of the teaching hospitals and community hospitals in the Commonwealth in helping to support the center financially and use it to manage serious overdoses. The center carried out active public education, as well as professional education for physicians, pharmacists, and nurses throughout Massachusetts. A fellowship training program in medical toxicology was developed; its trainees subsequently assumed leadership positions in toxicology and poison control work throughout the United States and conducted research in collaboration with the pharmacology department at Harvard Medical School. Finally, the center used the state system to carry out clinical studies on drugs in children and adults. The Poison Control Center, although housed at Children's, is now truly a Commonwealth-wide system. It comprises the acute-care hospitals in the Commonwealth and is run by an advisory committee appointed by the governor of Massachusetts and responsible to the Department of Public Health for the quality of information that it dispenses.

Dr. Janeway did not play an active role in this development but approved of it as a community service and as a facet for teaching residents about one of the common pediatric emergencies. My (FHL) relationship to Janeway and the toxicology program is illustrative of the way he developed people and programs. After completing my chief residency, I was grappling with my future: I wanted to pursue academic medicine and was trying to decide between infectious diseases and toxicology. I talked to CAJ about my dilemma. He listened carefully and then outlined the advantages and disadvantages of pursuing the road more traveled (infectious disease) and the road less traveled (clinical pharmacology). Relative to the latter, I remember quite clearly his saying that I would need to be trained in the new pharmacology; there would be more opportunities in the less crowded and new field. He never told me which course to pursue, but left the decision up to me. I left the meeting the beneficiary of wisdom that helped me make the wisest and best decision. Dr. Janeway dispensed his wisdom gently and persuasively, but always in his recommendations was the underlying advice to become trained in the newest research skills if one was to pursue a career in academic medicine. That advice was followed, and helped me to move the poison information program into the new fields of clinical toxicology and pharmacology.[69]

The Nutrition Division, Cystic Fibrosis, and the Pulmonary Division

This group grew out of the interest of one faculty member, Dr. Harry Shwachman, and the diseases in which he was clinically involved. Shwachman was director of the clinical laboratories at the hospital and had training in pathology. His training and interests led him to care for patients with the newly recognized disease, cystic fibrosis. Much of the research that differentiated the two diseases—cystic fibrosis and celiac disease—was done in the department of pathology under Dr. Farber. Children with either of these disorders have difficulty metabolizing food and their differentiation was, in the early days, difficult. Both conditions produced malnutrition. Together with Dr. Charles May, Shwachman and his colleagues developed in 1943 a model comprehensive program to care for these children, including their pulmonary problems. The Nutrition Division, led by Shwachman, thus included GI diseases, now usually cared for by gastroenterologists, and patients with cystic fibrosis. Only later would patients with cystic fibrosis be subsumed by the pulmonary division—its current home.

The beginnings of the pulmonary division started from a different clinical base. Dr. Berenberg recalls that in the pre-antibiotic, days patients with bronchiectasis comprised a large population at the Children's. A clinic was developed, staffed by Berenberg, Dr. Robert Smith, a pediatric anesthesiologist, and Dr. Charles D. Cook as a fellow.[70] Another strand in the development of the pulmonary division was the link to the pulmonary physiology laboratory of the Harvard School of Public Health, where Philip Drinker had invented the "Iron Lung" together with Dr. James L. Wilson at the Children's[71] for patients with acute bulbar poliomyelitis, and care of chronically lung-impaired patients from the Mary MacArthur Convalescent Hospital in Wellesley. Dr. Benjamin Ferris was a link between the Children's, where he had trained as a pediatrician, and the School of Public Health, for the application of this technology to patients with poliomyelitis as well as his later studies of the epidemiology of other pulmonary disorders.

Dr. Charles Cook, who was trained as a neonatologist and in pulmonary physiology as well as working in the clinic for patients with bronchiectasis, reported to the authors that "Charlie encouraged me to do research in that area [i.e., pulmonary neonatology] and let me work more than half time for several years with Jere Mead and others at the Harvard School of Public Health," and at that time the pulmonary group at the School of Public Health was one of the outstanding groups of pulmonary physiologists in the world. Like most "divisions," pulmonology survived without any hospital funds. We did pulmonary function tests without any charge . . . equipment came from tiny grants and [by] begging for cast-off equipment. Fellows [I usually had one plus a technician] were paid by tiny grants or via a fund I fortunately had from a grateful well child care patient."[72] Still another strand in the development of the pulmonary division was the work of Dr. Clement Smith and his colleagues on respiratory physiology of the newborn. Dr. Mary Ellen Avery, while a fellow with Drs. Smith and Mead of the School of Public Health, made one of the most important discoveries of newborn diseases with her research showing the role of lung surfactant in the etiology of what was then called hyaline membrane disease. This research led to today's effective treatment.

In 1964, laboratory studies of pulmonary function in children were developed by Dr. Mary Ellen Wohl with strong support from the School of Public Health and with the recruitment of Dr. Warren Gold, who had trained with Dr. Julius Comroe at the University of California, San Francisco.[73] This development, and the overall history of pulmonology at the Children's is typical of many of the subspecialty areas: it emerged from patients' needs and changed with the changing prevalence of diseases and evolution of new research methods; it was developed in its early days by someone on the spot with an interest in the area, and was funded by small and irregular sources. But Charles Janeway stimulated those in charge to develop a research program linking the division (pulmonology, in this instance) with other Harvard resources when necessary. After Cook left to become chair of pediatrics at Yale, Warren Gold continued to provide pulmonary function laboratory tests but the unit was not recreated as a division until Janeway's successor, Avery, appointed Dr. Denise Streider as chief in 1976. It appeared that pulmonology was not one of Janeway's high-priority areas. Under Streider and Wohl, the pulmonary division cared for children with pulmonary diseases, including tuberculosis, cystic fibrosis, and some with asthma. Studies and care of children with asthma, reflecting the disease ubiquity in the pediatric population, also were conducted by researchers in immunology and general pediatrics.

Gastroenterology and Nutrition

Nowhere was Dr. Janeway's development of specialty units more dependent on people and their interests, rather than on traditional organ systems, than in this division. During most of his tenure, gastroenterology was practiced in the division of nutrition and pulmonology under Dr. Shwachman, as noted above. With Shwachman's retirement and the sophisticated developments in diagnostic procedures in gastroenterology, a new and separate division was necessary. Dr. Richard Grand recalls that he asked Dr. Janeway for career guidance and told him that he wanted to go into gastroenterology. Janeway, in Grand's words, "Picked up the phone and talked to Kurt Isselbacher [chief of gastroenterology in the department of medicine] at the Massachusetts General Hospital. At the end of the conversation he said, 'Isselbacher has accepted you at the MGH, now we need to find support'."[74]

This was often typical of CAJ—betting on someone he knew and trusted (Grand had been a house officer at the Children's) and then sending him off for training, often in a department of internal medicine. Grand returned to head the division in 1976, after Janeway had stepped down as chair. Among the research achievements of this division was its laboratory work on the development and control of intestinal and exocrine gland function. Investigators studied the development, synthesis, and intracellular processing of intestinal disaccharidases and the development of mechanisms of synthesis and secretion of macromolecules in exocrine glands, with special importance assigned to the study of intestinal sucrase using animal models. Other major research interests included studies of the development of bile acid metabolism, growth failure in inflammatory bowel disease, and nutrition and trace element balance in chronic renal insufficiency.

Division of Child Development

Child Development was another division that Charles Janeway developed based upon the people available. The Child Health Division and the Family Health Program had emphasized education of students and residents in child development, but with the departure of the first two directors of the Child Health Division and the division's closing, he went to the famous local pediatrician, Dr. T. Berry Brazelton, and asked him to become a full-time faculty member to head a new division of child development. Brazelton's appointment occurred in 1972, near the end of Janeway's tenure but after Brazelton had served as Patient Coordinator since 1967, following Dr. Helen Glaser.[75] CAJ's vision of a future department of pediatrics included a strong child development unit, however. He spelled this out in the 1969 annual report:

> Just as basic medical sciences are an essential foundation for the diagnosis and treatment of organic disease, knowledge of the behavioral sciences is required if the physician is to meet his patient's needs for support in the areas of emotions, behavior and social adaption . . . To this end, I believe that a center for the Study of Child Development, based at the Children's Hospital, should be created . . . Such a Center would tap the resources of the entire University.[76]

Janeway recognized the need for infusion of psychological principles with the highly specialized technical aspect of the clinical services. This led him to appoint Helen Glaser first, and, with her departure in 1967, Brazelton, who had written extensively for parents on developmental and behavioral problems in children as Coordinator of Patient Care Services. Both of these appointments were, in part, reactions to opportunities. Glaser had moved to Boston with her husband, who was director of the Peter Bent Brigham Hospital. When the Glasers left Boston, Brazelton, who was anxious to become a full-time faculty member in order to teach and do more research on the psychological development of children, became available. Janeway had the vision to appoint them. Much of the story of this division belongs to a later time; the division flowered under successor chairs of the department.

Ambulatory Services

In the early days of Janeway's tenure, all of the specialty groups and division faculty cared for their own ambulatory patients in an area called the Outpatient Department, which was located in the Hunnewell building. In this area, children referred from physicians throughout New England were seen for consultations or for continuing care of their chronic diseases. The clinic was directed by a succession of pediatric faculty. The first director during Janeway's tenure as chief was Dr. Charles May, who became editor of *Pediatrics,* the official journal of the American Academy of Pediatrics. May was followed by Dr. Sidney Gellis, who later had a spectacular career as chief of pediatrics at Beth

Israel Hospital in Boston and as chair of pediatrics at both Boston University (Boston City Hospital) and, still later, Tufts Medical School. John Tuthill, who later left to head health services at Exeter Academy, succeeded Gellis, and was in turn succeeded by Charles D. Cook, who directed the clinics in addition to his pulmonary work until he left to chair pediatrics at Yale. Cook noted that he took on the administration of the outpatient division partly to secure a more stable funding source for his salary, since that position was funded by the hospital rather than the department.[77] For most of these physicians, the position of chief of the ambulatory service was a secondary one, with their primary academic role in another area.

In 1964 a new ambulatory building was completed, resulting in a need for an overall director, including a director of the growing emergency clinic. Thomas Cone, who had recently retired from the U.S. Navy and was a well-known general pediatrician, was recruited in 1963 to work in the adolescent unit but, upon Cook's departure, became head of the new ambulatory division. Cone was known to Dr. Janeway, for he had been stationed at Portsmouth Naval Base for part of his career and had done some teaching at the Children's. Cone was not only a brilliant general diagnostician, he was the leading pediatric historian of his time.

A leader was needed. There had been a tremendous increase in the number of patients seeking care in the clinics. As Janeway noted in his 1964 report, medical emergency clinic visits had increased from 17,324 in 1962 to 27,640 only two years later, and the demand for general medical clinics and especially specialty clinics, such as those for children with cerebral palsy, mental retardation, arthritis, hemophilia, and numerous other conditions, had increased.[78] This was in part a result of demand by parents, the increasingly high reputation of the hospital, and the desire of staff to see patients with diseases in which they were interested. All these emergency, general, and specialty clinics were, for the first time, coordinated ably, thanks to Cone. CAJ's report noted that many of these specialty clinics were "supported by special voluntary groups such as Massachusetts Heart Association, The New England Kidney Disease Foundation, and the National Cystic Fibrosis Foundation."

Funding of clinic services then, as now, was derived from a patchwork of sources, altogether insufficient to meet costs. They were underwritten by faculty who were supported from other sources, often from research grants. Cone began to train and give increasing responsibility to a younger generation of talented pediatricians. Dr. Melvin Levine, after serving as resident, developed a remarkable understanding of ambulatory care issues and developmental-behavioral disorders. He helped Cone mature the education programs for students and residents. Cone also fostered the development of Dr. John Graef, another former resident, to direct the care and teaching in the emergency room. After Cone retired, Levine succeeded him as chief of the ambulatory services.

Handicapped Children's Program

The care of the complex chronic disorders of children is one of the success stories of twentieth-century pediatrics. In previous centuries, few children with such disorders survived for long. Many of these children have problems that cross traditional specialty boundaries; for example, children with a myelomenigocoele, who require care by a pediatrician, a urologist, an orthopedist, a neurosurgeon, a psychologist, a physiotherapist, and perhaps other specialists. Children with cerebral palsy comprise another large group of multiply handicapped individuals who require complex services. Mentally retarded children comprise still another example; Dr. Alan Crocker developed a model care program for such children, especially those with complex metabolic genetic disorders.

With advances in care, such children required life-long multi-disciplinary services. When Dr. Bronson Crothers was alive, he and the pediatric neurologists led the effort to care for such children at the Children's, since so many of their patients had neurological needs. Dr. Berenberg later worked with Crothers and developed an interest in children with such handicaps, now referred to as children with special needs. Berenberg rose to national prominence as president of the National Cerebral Palsy Association and developed special services for these children at the Children's. Although this was never a separate division of the department of medicine, in part because it included physicians from many other departments, Berenberg was picked by Dr.

Janeway to coordinate such multi-disciplinary services over many of the other specialty physicians, in part because of his extraordinary general clinical experience. The Children's Hospital has become an international leader in providing the model for the care of such children.

Despite what may seem to be Janeway's relatively low interest in the outpatient department as a research laboratory, he paid attention to teaching and personnel services in that department as few chairs do. He regularly taught third-year medical students there, and occasionally saw patients. Dr. Jeffrey Maisels recalled a wonderful incident:

> Dr. Janeway had a habit of coming down to the clinic on occasion to see how things were going and happened on a patient who was assigned to a room but had not yet been seen by a resident. He asked me if I would mind if he saw the patient . . . he proceeded to take a history and examine the patient, and he advised me of the findings and recommendations. He also dictated a letter to the referring physician [as was the custom for residents; the letter was then signed by the chief resident in the clinic, Maisels] . . . I have kept this letter, which may be unique.[79]

The letter was signed by Maisels but "dictated by Charles A. Janeway, M.D." Maisels went on to comment that this incident "illustrates his willingness to undertake a task normally done by a resident, right down to dictating the letter to the referring physician. These are examples of his personal characteristics of integrity, compassion and lack of pretension." The letter to the referring physician itself is interesting. It is two paragraphs long, only outlining the findings: "recurrent urinary infections which, because of their persistence and tendency to recur despite gantrisin treatment, require further study . . . She is to have an intravenous pyelogram and urine cultures were done today. She will be seen for a return visit and you will receive a full report at a later date."

Dr. Melvin Levine noted that many perceived the outpatient department as a place where Janeway could place residents from foreign countries until they improved their communication and clinical skills. Some eventually became "regular" residents, but when Levine questioned CAJ about the merits of this, he replied that "when they return to their native lands, these pediatricians will have far greater impact on the health of children than any of those American house officers whose skills we were embellishing on the wards."[80] Levine also reported that when he remarked to CAJ that he questioned why a resident from Bangladesh should work up a patient with obesity who was addicted to sweets, fried foods and starches, hardly a problem in Bangladesh, Janeway pointed out, "you are not really teaching the physician about obesity. We are teaching him how to take people's concerns seriously and how to be extremely systematic and thorough in evaluating the needs of a patient." Levine went on to say that "Several years later I served in the USAF in the Philippines . . . and had opportunity to travel to Thailand, Taiwan and India . . . Wherever I went, pediatricians who had trained at Children's . . . were all major leaders of child health in their own countries. They had an enormous impact on international child care."

Levine, who has become a leader in development and learning problems of children, further noted that

> Janeway taught me about the importance of developmental-behavioral pediatrics. He reinforced my interest during times when I seriously wondered whether the function of children was a legitimate segment of pediatrics. I was frustrated by the lack of interest and responsiveness on the part of the Children's residents. The ambulatory rotation was barely tolerated by them . . . During that time Dr. Janeway was especially sensitive to my plight. He pointed out that many residents were not really "ready" to deal with these complex, elusive and clinically frustrating problems. He stressed that we needed to be doing most of our teaching [of this area] to senior residents and to physicians already in practice . . . [These] should be advanced courses taught after residents had dealt with very sick patients. Such wisdom has been endlessly helpful and supportive to me."[81]

Dr. John Graef, on the other hand, felt that Dr. Janeway never fostered research in the outpatient department as he did in other areas; Graef thought that Janeway saw specialties as the core of the Children's Hospital mission. According to Graef, he appeared to support an academic role for special parts of the outpatient department, such as the Family Health Care Program or the work that Dr. Levine was doing with children with learning disabilities, rather than for the outpatient department as a whole.[82] Graef may have a point. As an example, when I (RJH) asked CAJ if I might become director of the outpatient department when Cook was leaving (in part for the same reason given by Cook; that it provided a more secure financial source of income than dependence on grants), Janeway responded that it was more important that I stay where I could devote more of my time to research, and not be burdened by administrative needs.

Dr. Janeway had his own style and methods as he went about developing special areas, most of which are now called divisions. In most cases he wanted faculty to do clinical research in these units, although he always emphasized that good clinical care was the bedrock of all services. He was not always consistent in the way he built, taking advantage of opportunities (both availability of funds and people) and needs of patients. He was concerned about the barriers that develop when divisions are created. After all, the word "division" means to divide, but he recognized that in today's world specialized knowledge and skills prevent faculty from working in many areas. We are sure that he would be a leading advocate for some of the efforts today to integrate research scientists from different disciplines and to foster cross-disciplinary research. (It is noteworthy that the current chair, Dr. Gary Fleisher, has had five vice chairs, all trained under Janeway, supporting the continuing influence of Janeway on the department.)

5 AFTER 1966— THE LAST FIFTEEN YEARS

By 1966 CHARLES JANEWAY had led his department for over two decades. During the second half of that tenure, he became more and more involved with international pediatrics, to which subject four chapters will afterwards be devoted. In the opinion of some, his increasing international focus led to a crisis in the department after 1966. But was there really a crisis?

After 1966, when Janeway returned from his sabbatical in the Far East, he faced a different department. Twenty years at the helm had probably diminished his enthusiasm for new programs and appointments. Several people had left and the demands on those remaining were accelerating. Dr. Nadas presented this state of affairs frankly in a letter he wrote to CAJ before the latter returned from his sabbatical: "This leads me into the most important thing, I believe, you should think about before you get back. How and whom are you going to keep or bring in. I don't think we can afford to lose any more people and we badly need some new blood."[1] Having reviewed all the needs in the department, Nadas was more blunt than most were with Dr. Janeway: "In other words, *you* will have to cut outside commitments quite brutally." Nadas was very concerned that the Children's was "sinking" and told Charles that "the only way we can reverse this feeling is to have *you* give all your time to the CHMC." Nadas was one of few—perhaps the only one—who was close enough to be so frank with Janeway, but at that time the feeling was general that the chief had become more involved with the children of the world than with the Children's. Nadas acknowledged this, saying, "I am sure you have thought many times about the same things and may have come to the same conclusions."

Having created the many divisions of the Children's and recruited the original chiefs, by 1966 Janeway was faced with recruiting new ones and expanding the numbers in each division (most still had only one or two faculty members). CAJ certainly did not cease his international activities after this warning, although it may have played a role in his resigning from the chairmanship of the executive council of the International Pediatric Association in 1968. After twenty years as chief at the Children's, was Dr. Janeway losing his creativity and energy? It would be natural if he were, as most chairs of departments are less vigorous after one decade, to say nothing of two. But in our opinion, Janeway had not lost much of his creativity. After his return from this sabbatical he created the Division of Genetics, with Park Gerald as chief, whom he promptly sent abroad for a year to learn genetic counseling and research methods; he promoted Masland to Chief of Adolescent Medicine in 1967; in 1968 he brought in David Nathan as successor to Diamond in Hematology; he made Fred Rosen Chief of Immunology; and he appointed David Smith as Chief of Infectious Diseases when Samuel Katz went to Duke. He also assigned several existing faculty to more permanent appointments.

Until this time, most faculty were limited to the rank of Assistant Professor or (a few) Associate Professor, without tenure. But a flurry of activity followed Janeway's return. In 1969 he made thirty promotions, a record number; this was followed by twenty-one in 1970.[2] Promotions occurred at all ranks, with five individuals achieving professorial status (Shwachman, Nadas, Berenberg, Cone, and Fyler) and Gerald achieving tenure at the Associate Professor level. During Dr. Janeway's last five or six years as chair, a large number of appointments and promotions continued to be made, including some from outside the institution. It would seem, then, that there was little if any diminution of his activity, at least insofar as creating new divisions and appointments is concerned. Most department chairs do not make major appointments in their last years, in part to allow their successors to put their own stamp on the department. Nevertheless, CAJ, even with his generous nature, did appoint several new faculty in his last two years of active service. Compared to earlier years, there were fourteen new appointments and promotions in both 1973 and 1974, his final years as chair. It does not appear, therefore, that Nadas's fears in 1965 were entirely justified; these appointments were made despite Dr. Janeway's continued interest in international activities.

Individual divisions grew by securing their own funding, mainly by securing research grants and expansion of fellowship training grants. Planning for the new Enders research building occupied a good deal of time for Janeway and his key staff. When he retired as chair in 1975, he left the department with a weak financial base. As noted elsewhere, money was not a high priority with CAJ; he did not build the clinical financial stream, a clinical practice plan that is now so essential for pediatric departments. His reputation was so good, however, that his support with a letter of recommendation concerning a grant submission to a foundation or the National Institutes of Health by any of his faculty often was the key to its success. It must be emphasized, however, that the base upon which he built the department was creative people, not secure financing.

To some degree this continued building of the department may have been due to the vigor of the new hospital director, Dr. Leonard Cronkhite, who, arriving in 1962, was able to add new resources and stimulate the building of a new main part of the hospital. CAJ wrote in his annual report for 1969 that "Under Mr. Wolbach's Presidency [of the Board of Trustees], backed by Dr. Cronkhite's extraordinary executive ability and stimulated by Dr. Farber's broad vision, the institution has surged forward again . . . We are now recruiting people . . . needed to make us capable of using the opportunities provided by our new facility."[3] CAJ's ability to appoint good people over the years is testified to by the number of Mead Johnson Research Award winners, among those appointees: Frederick Robbins, Thomas Weller, David Gitlin, Park Gerald, Carlton Gajdusek, Fred Rosen, Sam Lux, Jan Breslow, and Raif Geha. CAJ also mentored a remarkable number of pediatric department chairs.[4] Janeway saw his role as recruiting good people, guiding and mentoring them, and then sending them elsewhere to carry the banner of pediatrics that he espoused. He did this as he built a stable cadre of faculty at the Children's.

Charles Janeway was very happy at Children's Hospital, but it was

natural for other schools to try to woo him away. We think the only serious effort that he considered was to return to Johns Hopkins as Chair
of Pediatrics. It must have been a soul-searching process, for one of
those urging him to come to Hopkins was his mentor, Edwards Park.
In response to a letter that Janeway had written to him in 1955, Park
had written, in his fatherly way, that the department at Hopkins was
much smaller, with the "load of administration far less . . . I have feared
that you were spending too much of your time traveling around the
country . . . which do not represent fundamental contributions to
knowledge of which you are capable . . . Your finest development in
my opinion would depend on your ability to devote yourself to scholarship . . . I think that now you have your chance to change the course
of your life to that of scholarship."[5]

Dr. Park went on to add one more argument that has persisted to
this day, whether or not separate children's hospitals were better than
pediatric services integrated within a general hospital setting:

> I believe that the Children's Hospital is founded on incorrect princi-
> ples . . . to make pediatrics complete and independent and to make it
> stand out as an entity is an error. Here Harvey [Chair of Medicine] is
> prepared to make pediatrics with internal medicine on a parity with
> a view to making the study of the human being from birth to death
> continuous . . . I personally do not believe that the great progress in
> pediatrics is going to come from children's hospitals . . . you have the
> chance here to develop a different kind of a pediatric department
> than exists anywhere else in the country . . . Nothing could give me
> greater delight than to have you come and be my successor.

Park added what must have been a heartbreaker: "I should get great
satisfaction in the thought that a son of your father, to whom I owe my
start in life and whom I have venerated as no other man, were to take
my place here."

It must have taken a great deal of courage for Janeway to reject this
plea. There is no record of Janeway's immediate response to Park, but
he likely was torn by his loyalty to his and his father's alma mater. He
later formally declined the offer and noted that he was enthusiastic
about the appointment of Dr. Robert Cooke as chair at Hopkins.[6] CAJ
also complimented his old friend, Barry Wood, on Cooke's appoint-

ment. "I note that . . . Bob Cooke has accepted the invitation to come to Hopkins as Professor of Pediatrics. I just want to give you three cheers, because I think he is a very fine person, who is broad gauged, a good doctor, keenly aware of the social impact of pediatrics and medicine and yet a very good scholar in his own right."[7]

It is instructive that even here, as Dr. Janeway complemented Cooke, he reiterated the qualities he thought chairs should have, which he himself possessed, and which he sought to inculcate at the Children's, where he saw part of the department's mission as training leaders in the field of pediatrics. Sad to say, that constellation of capabilities—a fine person, a broad gauge, a good doctor, and being aware of the social impact of medicine—is one that chairs today often do not have. It is not clear why CAJ did not go to his alma mater and the school where his father had been Chair of Medicine, but Betty probably played a role in the decision. She was a Bostonian and felt that Harvard was more prestigious. And, perhaps Janeway did too, by that time. Most probably, it all came down to a simple case of liking where he was. CAJ told Thomas Cone that the Children's "had been so good to him and that he enjoyed it so greatly."[8] We doubt that he ever considered other opportunities seriously.

However, we do think that Dr. Janeway was prestige minded. Frederick Robbins noted that CAJ looked on the institutions of the east coast as the only ones of great significance. As Dr. Robbins reported,

> I was offered a position at Western Reserve as a full professor . . . At the time I was an associate [not an associate professor but only one rank above an assistant and one below assistant professor, a very low faculty rank] . . . which was not even on the tenure track. I went to see Charlie . . . he was very friendly and suggested that they might be able to offer me an assistant professorship. I reminded him that Reserve was offering me a full professorship. His reply was that that was about equivalent to an assistant professor at Harvard.[9]

It seems a bit jarring, even at this remote time, to think that the egalitarian, flexible Janeway had a touch of chauvinism. Perhaps by then he had come to believe that Boston, or Harvard, really was the hub of the universe.

The Children's was not always perceived as friendly to community pediatricians and community hospitals. There was a certain sense of superiority among the residents at the hospital, who referred to the practicing pediatricians by the pejorative term, "LMD"—local medical doctor. Dr. Janeway took pains to overcome this myopic attitude. In addition, during his tenure he arranged affiliations with several community hospitals. In the 1950s and 1960s, the Beth Israel Hospital, next door, had a small pediatric service. This became a full partner with full-time staff assigned by CAJ and a house staff rotation. Several distinguished pediatricians served as chief there, among them Sidney Gellis, Samuel Katz, and William Cochrane. Further afield, affiliations were developed with North Shore Children's Hospital in Salem, the Rhode Island and Roger Williams General Hospital in Providence, the Springfield Hospital in Springfield, and the Martha Eliot Community Health Center in nearby Roxbury. Janeway had the same commitment to the underserved in the Boston area as he did to those in the developing world. Not all of these outreaches were popular with residents who were assigned to them, and the administration of the Children's made little commitment to these hospitals. Most were looked upon as sources of referral and, over time, relations have fluctuated from cordial to cold. The department continues in its efforts and deep commitment to the broader Boston community. It all began with Charles Janeway.

In one sense, the entire experience at the Children's was an exercise in education. We discuss Dr. Janeway's educational legacy in a later chapter, but it should be noted here that he viewed education in a holistic manner, as something built in to all activities at the hospital. His view was quite advanced for his time. Undergraduate medical education, residency training, fellowships, postgraduate education were all based on the notion that a background in science and a scientific approach to problem solving must underlie everything else, that education is never finished but continues throughout one's lifetime and that, in medicine, the welfare of the patient inspires all that one learns. Janeway's own career unfolded that way; he was ever curious, always willing to learn. He tried to pass that spirit on throughout his tenure at Children's Hospital.

What were Charles Janeway's legacies at the Children's? What were his major contributions? What principles guided his building of the Department of Medicine? It does not appear that he ever discussed his vision with any of the people we interviewed. In his writings he articulated the need to build on people who were excellent clinicians and had developed research skills in the underlying sciences basic to their fields. The model first developed by Howland at Hopkins, in which faculty did laboratory research relevant to the clinical problems in which they were interested, was one basis, but he recognized, as had his mentor, Park, that clinical specialization was now necessary; accordingly, he developed specialty divisions. He wanted the faculty to have a deep grounding in the sciences basic to clinical fields, but with the training not tied directly to patients' problems but more generically so as to allow more crossover between disciplines. He was, in today's terms, anxious to avoid intellectual silos. He saw the interconnectedness of human biology.

In some areas he was willing to develop needed services without a laboratory science base; this was true of adolescent medicine at the beginning, for example. Even here, as Masland noted, Janeway urged more research. He saw the Children's as becoming a mecca for patients and, as such, the institution needed to have the latest specialty services available. But Janeway's emphasis upon the quality of the person as the basis for his building suggests that he did not have a grand vision of where he wanted the department to be, except for the underlying principles of high-quality service, high integrity of the faculty, and a scientific base for research where possible. That constellation might be considered his guiding philosophy. Janeway appears to have been an opportunist in building the department, responding to faculty and personnel who were available, providing the clinical services patients were demanding, pursuing the research developments that appeared promising, and taking advantage of whatever funding was available.

In instances when Dr. Janeway launched into new areas, it was his simultaneous commitment to working for community and social services at the Children's, and especially his deep commitment to and involvement in international child health, that made his tenure so different from any other chair of pediatrics. In these two areas he departed strikingly from Howland, who was not interested in such involvement and in fact argued against any involvement outside the hospital. CAJ even rejected Park's advice that he should spend more time in the laboratory and less as an educator and international pediatrician.[10] In our view, the remarkable thing about Dr. Janeway was that he did all of these simultaneously. His vision extended to the world. He advocated high-quality service and research at home (*i.e*, in hospital), to be sure, but he did not think that service and research should be limited to this setting. That breadth of his vision, in our opinion, is his greatest contribution. Beecher and Altschule, in their recent review of 300 years of medicine at Harvard, observed that Janeway's

> major efforts . . . have been devoted to focusing the development of the Department [of Pediatrics] on the health needs of children throughout the world—by the creation of highly specialized clinical units based on advances in biomedical research, the training of men and women from this country and abroad for positions of pediatric leadership, and efforts to study and improve not only the diagnosis and treatment of diseases in children, but also the practice and delivery of primary health and medical care. Thus his group has emphasized two apparently opposite trends—increasing specialization within pediatrics, on the one hand, and attempts to make pediatrics more comprehensive, on the other.[11]

Few leaders of pediatrics in the twentieth century could make that claim.

Throughout his long tenure and continuing through his final years as chief, one of Dr. Janeway's major concerns was that referring pediatricians have the ability to get their patients admitted to the Children's. This concern was not merely academic; residents often treated referring pediatricians with some disdain. Residents were accustomed to seeing very sick patients and often a patient was admitted who was said to be very ill, but turned out not to be. This was partly because the referring physician saw the child in an early stage and, as with many childhood illnesses, there could be rapid recovery. As a result, residents were liable to try to talk the referring physician out of admitting the child. Dr. Janeway was aware of this and sent a memo to all residents, stating, in effect:

> If doctor refers a case saying it needs to be admitted; A) If he says it's very sick, accept it instantly, unless there are no beds—then offer to

find one. B) if he says it's moderately sick, accept it gladly, unless there are no beds. C) If there are no beds accept one for an emergency, tell him the situation and ask how you can help. Motto: the doctor is right, and you are there to help him and his patient.[12]

He went on to describe the policy of calling the doctor back when the child had been seen and ended with three principles: "1) The doctor has a tough job—we're here to help him. Be polite and fair to him. 2) If in doubt, err on the side of admission or ask for help. 3) Don't let the ward staff beat you down." This last admonition was to counter the ward staff's tendency to try to keep patients in the emergency room from being admitted; it required more work for them. But Janeway would have none of it. He institutionalized his concern with passionate directives. Patients and referring doctors came first at the Children's.

Janeway was succeeded by Mary Ellen Avery as chair and chief of medicine. She noted how very nice he was, "his most negative comments were generally those of silence." She reflected on the seating of them together in the department's 1975 Christmas picture as his way of saying that he approved of her. She did find, however, that the financial status of the department was "out of step with the time."[13] His greatest failure was to be too frugal. He never asked for a pay raise himself; when he retired his salary was $37,000 a year, at a time when the going rate for chairs of pediatrics around the country was well over $50,000. He neglected to put the department on a sound financial basis as well, probably feeling that the faculty could get along as frugally as he. Even if faculty did so in the 1950s and 1960s, times had changed by 1974. Competition from other good schools made the Children's less competitive. Faculty were not willing to stay for the glory of being part of a distinguished institution and responded instead to potential future rewards by going elsewhere.

It appears that toward the end of his tenure Dr. Janeway did not spend as much time with the residents (they had a number of complaints when Avery arrived.)[14] Some were unhappy that decisions on rotations, especially to community hospitals, were made without consultation with the residents. Furthermore, the Children's was known for its parsimony to residents; it was one of the last hospitals in the country to pay salaries to residents. Old-timers justified this by saying that they had not been paid, so why should a new group be paid? Some in the hospital administration argued that, since they continued to receive many more good applicants then they could take, why pay them? Many house staff did not think Dr. Janeway was in favor of paying, since he rarely discussed the issue. The records, however, suggest that CAJ was an early advocate of paying residents. In a report of the Executive Committee of the hospital, which occurred only five years after he became chair of the department, "Dr. Janeway requested discussion at an earlier meeting of payment to house officers. From the discussion it was apparent that while as much support as possible was desirable, the subject of reimbursement must be handled at the trustee level."[15] At a meeting of this committee more than six years later, "Dr. Janeway continued a discussion of the subject of payments to house staff. He put into the minutes a resolution from the Staff Associates of the hospital that "urgently recommends the proposals contained in this report be transmitted to the Trustees . . . for action before the end of service of the present group of house officers in July 1958.[16] This report noted that only two hospitals in the United States did not pay house officers: Children's Hospital Medical Center and the Pennsylvania Hospital. Apparently no action was taken, for at the meeting of the committee the following January, "There was discussion [of house officers' pay] . . . Suggestion was made that funds of CMC be used . . . but it was pointed out that income on these funds were now being allocated toward the deficit."[17]

Later in 1958, at a subsequent meeting of the Executive Committee, it was recorded that,

> On a motion by Dr. Janeway, duly seconded, it was voted that the chiefs of staff: 1) Favor the payment of stipends to house officers and residents at this time; 2) Believe that every effort should be made to obtain agreements to a standard scale for the Boston teaching hospitals; 3) Believe that steps must be made now to find a way to capture Blue Shield and other professional insurance fees on ward service to pay the house staff.[18]

Two years later, at another meeting of the committee, there was discussion of the classification of house officer positions "so as to establish a schedule of positions to permit a decision about the coverage and range of stipends.[19] Finally, more than a year later, the committee recommended to the Trustees a schedule of House Officer stipends starting at $1,000 per year for interns, rising to $3,600 for chief residents.[20]

In June 1961, the Board of Trustees approved the recommendation for payment of house officers effective July 1, 1961, at the scale recommended by the Executive Committee. This was still about half what the other teaching hospitals in Boston were paying. At a subsequent Executive Committee meeting, a full discussion of resident staff salaries was initiated. Janeway's role continued as he, Dr. Gross, and Dr. Green "would form a committee to study the whole problem of house staff reimbursement."[21] The problem had shifted from whether to pay to how much. The issue, initiated in 1951 by CAJ, had taken twelve years to reach even that point. Residents' pay may not have been the highest priority for Janeway, but nonetheless, it seems clear that on this issue he favored and stimulated the Children's to join the rest of the academic hospitals in America in easing the burden of residents' period of training. Other problems occupied Charles's attention in his later years. Residents and faculty felt that he had not reinvigorated some of the divisions. This can be a problem whenever a chair stays a long time. Too, Janeway's health was beginning to fail, and his interests had shifted from the hospital and science to international pediatrics. Although he was revered, he probably stayed too long as chair. It would be left to his successors to rebuild some of the divisions he had originated.

By the mid 1970s, Charles Janeway was facing retirement. Since at that time the mandatory retirement age of a Harvard professor was set at his or her (there were few hers in that era) sixty-fifth birthday, a faculty search committee had been set up in early 1973 to find his successor. News of its decision came in the form of an announcement by Dean Robert Ebert in September, prompting Dr. Janeway to sit down and register his approval to the dean of the committee's choice:

> The appointment of Dr. Mary Ellen Avery as my successor . . . I can endorse . . . with great enthusiasm. I can't think of anybody I'd rather have succeed me, and I think she will have a very distinguished career here and bring the department strength in the one

area where we badly need it, because it is such a major and important part of pediatrics, namely the pediatrics of the fetus and newborn. She is perhaps the top person in the field in this country.[22]

In anticipation of Dr. Janeway's retirement, a dinner party was held at the Harvard Club in Boston on May 30, 1974, with many in attendance. At the time, Janeway had held his position for twenty-eight years, the longest tenure of any chief at the Children's and longer than any but a small group of chairs in the country. An official notice from the secretary of the Harvard Corporation in April 1975 told him that, "I beg to inform you that at a meeting of the president and fellows held April 7, 1975, your retirement as Thomas Morgan Rotch Professor of Pediatrics was recorded to take effect August 31, 1975."[23] At the same time, he was duly appointed Thomas Morgan Rotch Professor of Pediatrics Emeritus. In a less formal vein, President Derek Bok wrote to him,

> I do want to add my personal thanks for your thirty-seven years of service [to Harvard]. You have over the years given so generously and so often to the programs, the goals and the students of the medical school . . . of your own wisdom, knowledge and resources that it is impossible adequately to express our appreciation—your warmth, understanding and willingness to listen and help are qualities which have made you *the* deeply and respected and beloved teacher of younger doctors . . . I think those who follow your example . . . will themselves be your greatest tribute.[24]

Clement Smith, in an editorial, probably summed up best the feelings so many at Children's had for Janeway, commenting that those who have known Dr. Janeway best and longest felt, as he did, that his greatest contributions to American pediatrics were not the usual ones. But "Far more important," he observed, "have been the intangible things learned from him and surely (even if unconsciously) transmitted through the country by numerous past members of his staff and residents. For three decades these intangibles have been acquired by them not by precept but by example, the example of a rare mixture of intelligence, of integrity, of insight and humility, of reserve and generosity."[25]

Although Charles A. Janeway began his formal retirement from his professorship at Harvard and from his position as Chief of Pediatrics at the Children's on September 1, 1975, he continued to remain active. He saw patients at the hospital in the rheumatology clinic, traveled, supervised the Cameroons project (which is discussed in Chapter 10), and responded to continuing requests for help, advice, and support. He was always available, it seemed, to anyone who needed his advice and the benefit of his expertise.

Janeway continued to reap honors and awards and was in demand as a guest professor and speaker. On May 12, 1976, less than a year after he retired, the trustees and alumni of the Children's Hospital honored him with an all-day scientific program that climaxed with a banquet at the Ritz Carleton Hotel. In 1978, Ralph Feigin, the new chair of pediatrics at Baylor, asked Charles to be the first Dr. Russell J. Blattner lecturer.[26] On April 26, he received the John Howland Award of the American Pediatric Society, the highest award of the society and of American pediatrics. Also in 1978, Steven Mueller, president of Johns Hopkins University, invited Janeway to participate in the installment of new members of The Johns Hopkins Society of Scholars, of which CAJ was a member.[27]

The last of his "big" lectures (in the sense that it was published and was given at his alma mater, Johns Hopkins, and summarized his career and philosophy) was the Thayer lecture, named after the professor of medicine who was a close associate of Osler and who, after Theodore Janeway's death, succeeded him as Physician in Chief at Hopkins. In this lecture, Janeway summed up his broad view of medicine, perhaps sensing that it was to be his last publication. He advocated that "learning medicine is a lifelong task, in which one's prime method of learning is observation, at the bedside and in the clinic, laying the foundation in experience for the examination, and evaluation of the condition of patients—their diseases and their responses." Toward the end he wrote, "the responsibility devolving from investigative work is to make sure that valuable new knowledge is not only applied to better diagnosis and treatment of the individual patient, but wherever possible to prevention . . . by its institutionalization as part of a public health program.[28]

Despite the many honors and accolades that came to him, many of Dr. Janeway's final years were plagued by illness and pain. In the late

1970s he was diagnosed with Waldenstrom's macroglobulinemia, a disorder of unknown etiology in which the B lymphocytes or plasma cells produce excessive amounts of IgM, a high-molecular weight macroglobulin that produces hyperviscosity of the blood and crowds out the normal bone marrow cells, producing anemia, fatigue, weakness, bleeding, and susceptibility to infections. In CAJ's files is a report from Dr. William Maloney, hematologist at the Peter Bent Brigham Hospital, dated March 30, 1976 and stating, " Dr. Charles A. Janeway was first seen on August 25, 1975, complaining of weight loss (10 lbs.) and a gradually falling hematocrit." The bone marrow "contained lymphocytes with a plasma cell like cytoplasm. His IgM was 3400 mg%." A diagnosis of Waldenstrom's macroglobulinemia was made and Janeway was started on Leukeran. His condition at first improved. By 1979, the medical report states, he had required intermittent corticosteroids, was not on cytotoxic drugs, and was receiving transfusions. A follow-up letter, dated April 27, 1979, described his treatment with "cytotoxic drugs." There is also a three-page summary of his medical record, undated, but in the same folder as the two other letters.[29] Dr. Fred Rosen tells of CAJ submitting a sample of his blood in 1974 for electrophoresis, at which time Rosen found an elevated IgM component; it is likely, therefore, that Janeway knew the diagnosis before 1975.[30] After the diagnosis was made he received many transfusions and underwent plasmaphersis to remove the excess macroglobulins. After these procedures he would regain some strength. In his folder of letters from 1977–1978 there is a record—in uncharacteristically poor handwriting—of his procedures, symptoms, weight, blood counts, and medications, with dates in June (probably 1980).

These records are themselves indicative of the man: CAJ maintained his discipline, recording his own illness as he had always done with his patients. He also collected literature on the illness. For example, in his files is a clipping of a letter from a practitioner to the editor of the *Lancet*, entitled "Survival in Waldenstrom's Macroglobulinemia." The author states that, from his experience with seventeen patients, those with diffuse bone marrow involvement (in contrast to the nodular form of the disease) have a shorter survival.[31] Janeway did not note his disease type, but his survival was relatively short, suggesting that he had the diffuse form. The same folder also contains a *New York Times* article on this disease.[32] Rosen, however, recalling a day in 1975 shortly after Dr. Janeway had learned of his diagnosis, informed us that "He read about the disease and announced that he would live for seven years. This he almost did."[33]

Dr. Thomas Cone told us that he drove Janeway home from the Children's during the last two years of his life, "leaving about 4:00 p.m. so that he could be home in Weston about 5:00. En route Janeway would relate stories of his early life as a boy in New York City." Cone recalled that Janeway would reminisce about Dr. Edwards Park, who, after CAJ's father died from pneumonia in 1917, became a father figure during Janeway's growing years. Cone says he learned then that Park had shared an office with Janeway's grandfather for three years and had worked with Theodore Janeway on a number of studies, including the measurement of blood pressure in man. CAJ would recall that his father was the first to describe essential hypertension and to make clinical use of the mercury sphygmomanometer. Cone noted, sadly, that Dr. Janeway's memory faded toward the end of those two years of car rides.[34]

During this time, CAJ received a letter from his long-time colleague, Louis K. Diamond, who was then semi-retired in California. Diamond wrote that he hoped CAJ would "write three biographies (for Park, Edwin Cohn, and his own)."[35] Diamond opined that the biography of Park would have great appeal to the Hopkins group, and added the name of an editor at the Boston publisher Little, Brown & Co., who, he thought, would be happy to publish it. Diamond went on to recall Park's modesty: he recalled a time when Park had referred a patient with possible leukemia to him (Diamond) but the call was taken by a resident who told Diamond that "an LMD [local medical doctor] from somewhere in Canada" wished to send a child, but the resident questioned his diagnosis. When Diamond phoned back and learned that the caller was Dr. Park (who was on vacation in Canada), he apologized for the delay. Diamond recalled that Park was not resentful, as "anyone in his position" might have been."[36] Charles Janeway most probably read that note with empathy and understanding, for he was like Park in many ways; Park was the role model for him, professionally and personally. The book, however, never was written: it appears that CAJ was not up to the task at that late time in his life.

Janeway's seventieth birthday was formally celebrated in England. Among those who attended the festivities were noted British pediatricians. A glimpse of CAJ's catholic interests is revealed in a letter associated with this party from Professor Tizard, a highly respected English pediatrician who was then chief of Pediatrics at Hammersmith Hospital. He wrote Dr. Janeway after the party, "I am glad that you are enjoying Pliny's letters." We were not aware previously that CAJ enjoyed reading classical writings.[37]

As Janeway's life was drawing to a close, he wrote several letters to his close colleagues expressing what he had found difficult to say in person. For instance, to Dr. Berenberg he wrote, "I should have written this letter long ago, but since it is perfectly clear that I am now in some kind of terminal phase of this illness . . . I am taking this opportunity to write to tell you how deeply I appreciate the loyalty and fine service you have given this department over the years. It is the kind of dependable collaboration that one can lean on and be helped by. You have been a particularly loyal contributor from the first day I took over here . . . most of all, however, it is the personal aspects of this association of long standing which have meant so much both to the department and in my own life.[38] This is typical of Janeway's feelings, so difficult for him to express directly, but when expressed, beautifully delineated and much cherished.

In CAJ's final years he took great pride in his children's accomplishments. Anne had achieved her goal of working in India with a mentor; Carlie had gained prominence as one of the leading immunologists of his day and was a full professor at Yale School of Medicine; Elizabeth was the mother of two children, wife of an academic pediatrician, and a skilled photographer; the youngest, Barbara, had received her degree in nursing from Yale the same year that Janeway celebrated the fiftieth anniversary of his graduation from the same university.

For those of us who studied under Dr. Janeway, learned from him, and admired him, his final years were sad, yet encouraging. On the occasion of a dinner party at his home in April 1980, I (RJH) was surprised to see how feeble CAJ was and how "out of it" he seemed for most of the evening. He did not respond to several requests for advice about a new job that I was then undertaking (the presidency of the William T. Grant Foundation). Yet, at the end of the evening, Dr. Janeway put his arm around my shoulder and said, "Bob, bet on young people." This statement, so simple yet so profound, was one that Janeway had exemplified all his life, both in his clinical work with children and as a teacher of young professionals all over the world. It became my (RJH's) guiding principle at the Grant Foundation and in all of my international activities thereafter. That was how it was to be taught by CAJ. Bedrock wisdom would be expressed in simple terms, and it would stick.

Dr. Janeway died May 28 1981 at his home in Weston. His family and close colleagues—Drs. Fred Rosen, Fred Lovejoy, and David Nathan—were present. His last days were difficult for all. His breathing was so labored that he required oxygen. He faded gradually and took his last breath at 7 p.m. on that late May day. CAJ's eldest daughter, Anne, recorded her father's terminal thoughts a few days earlier. Janeway said,

> Here I am as always. My mind more alive and vivid than ever before; my sensitivities keener, my affections stronger. I seem for the first time to see the world in clear perspective; I love people more deeply and more comprehensively; I seem to be just beginning to learn my business and see my work in its proper relationship to science as a whole; I see myself to have entered into a period of stronger feeling and understanding. And yet here I am, essentially unchanged except for a more concentrated me—held in a damaged body which will extinguish me with it when it dies. If it were a horse I was riding that went down or broke its neck, or a ship on which I was traveling that sprung a leak I would leave the old vehicle behind. As it is, my mind and my spirit, my thoughts and my love, all that I really am, is inseparably tied up with the failing capacities of these outworn organs.

"Yet," he continued, apostrophizing in a serio-comic mood,

> poor viscera, I can hardly blame you. You have done your best and have served me better than could be expected of organs so abused. When I think of the things that have flowed over and through you, innumerable varieties of fermented hops, malt and the grapes of all so many countries and climates—no, no my organs I cannot feel that you have let me down. It is quite the other way around. Only now it seems so silly that you must take me with you when I am just beginning to get dry behind the ears.[39]

Many are said to have remarkably clear perceptions on their deathbeds. It was so typical of Charles Janeway that he should be so analytical and yet express his love of family and the whole world, and at the same time do so with a dash of humor.

As for afterlife and similar aspects of religious doctrine, Betty told us that her husband believed in some sort of superior being but was not an active participant in formal religions. Indeed, as was noted earlier, for many years the Janeways, together with their next-door neighbors, the Cummingses, held a Sunday service in their home. (Betty later was active in the Unitarian church.) We believe that is where Charles Janeway's beliefs lay: in a superior being that created the universe but not one expressed in a sectarian church nor one to whom one prayed for intervention or micromanagement of human affairs. His tolerance for all the world's religions and beliefs, his worldwide travels and friends from all cultures and religions, probably made him skeptical of narrow sectarian forms. Dr. Cone, in his interview, said that CAJ had become disillusioned with the Weston Episcopal Church because there were no black faces there (very few blacks lived in Weston at that time). It is interesting to speculate on what he thought, coming from such a long line of distinguished religious leaders, but his more immediate lineage of physicians was probably more influential on his beliefs. His religion was a love for all peoples and an advocacy for the children of the world. He was, as many of his obituaries described him, "the foremost pediatrician to the world's children." That would seem to be a satisfactory and sufficient religion unto itself.

Condolences poured in to Janeway's family from all over the world. The Japan Pediatric Society sent "our deepest sympathy in tribute to the lifetime work of Dr. Charles A. Janeway." Prof. Noburo Kobayaki of Japan, a former president of the International Pediatric Association, wrote, "I wish to express great sadness at this moment. The loss to the international pediatric community is immeasurable. Beyond his pioneering work in child health, Professor Janeway was a citizen of the world—interested in the problems of children in developed and developing countries."[40] Janeway's former students, numbered in the thousands, sent similar letters. Dr. A. Izzet Berkel, at the time Professor of Pediatrics at Hacettepe University in Ankara, Turkey (a new university founded by Professor Ihsan Dogramaci), a close colleague of Janeway in the International Pediatric Association, wrote, "His exceptional personality and humanism are among his characteristics to remember."[41] Professor John Davis, of Cambridge, England, who spent a year at

Children's, wrote, "becoming his disciple marked a turning point in my life, as in that of many friends . . . not only because in expecting the best in everyone, he usually got it . . . but because of his genuine kindness and concern at a personal level which was reflected for me in the hospitality as a family to an obscure and lonely visitor from abroad."[42] Betty received over 400 condolence letters from colleagues in the United States and abroad. William W. Wolbach, Chairman of the Board of the Children's Hospital, characterized "Charlie" as "the epitome of what Children's was, is, and should always be;" as "Scientist, teacher, world-wide ambassador, pioneer, and beloved friend to generations of colleagues and students, Charlie WAS Children's to much of the world. We, who knew him, vividly remember him and will always miss him."[43]

A page-long obituary in the *Boston Globe* reviewed Janeway's accomplishments and told its readers that "he trained a whole generation of leaders in medical child care, not only in this country, but in underdeveloped countries," and that Janeway was "a pioneer in the modern science of immunology" and was among the first to recognize that some children die of infection because their systems fail to produce antibodies. The article reviewed Janeway's wartime experiences with plasma proteins, noting that he was a consultant to the Secretary of War as a member of the commission on neurotropic virus diseases. The article added an appealing personal note, "Although rather small and frail of build, Dr. Janeway was a good-looking man with close-cropped silvery hair, a wide grin and crinkly eyes that had a characteristic squint when he smiled." It also quoted a colleague, who said, "His word was as good as anything in the world. He never did a dishonest thing in his life. He was a rare individual. A decent, compassionate man of total integrity. A model for all to look up to."[44]

The Harvard Memorial Minute, which was read at a faculty meeting on December 15, 1982 and later published in the *Harvard Gazette*, summarized the view of a committee of Charles Janeway's Harvard colleagues and peers.[45] Speaking about Dr. Janeway at a Janeway award ceremony in the early 1980s, the author (FHL) spoke of the chief as follows:

He was a marvelous teacher. He taught us by word; intelligent, wise, experienced, and he taught us by example, purposeful example. By word, who shall forget the beautifully organized consideration of a case at Monday Student Rounds; or the quiet, probing, thoughtful questions and final summations that seemed to pull it all together so well at Thursday's Chief Rounds; or the voluminous fund of information on almost any subject balanced by the perspective of the wisest practitioner as seen at Senior Rounds; or on Wednesday afternoon Ward Rounds . . . And he taught by example: when we understood a disease poorly and when we would do much, he would advise caution and suggest we do little. When we became slack and our efforts faltered, we found his notes in the charts longer than ours. When we wondered whether we worked too hard, we would see him hard at work in his office on Saturdays and Sundays. When we would sleep through a conference we would remember nothing; when he slept through, he would awake and summarize all. When we were too sure, he showed us his great humility . . . and when our purpose in medicine would occasionally falter, he would show us his true concern for his patients. We will miss him.[46]

On Thursday, June 18, 1981, a celebration of Charles A. Janeway's life was held at the Memorial Church in Harvard Yard. Several hundred people attended. After hymns had been sung and prayers read, Dr. Fred Rosen spoke in elegant terms of this extraordinary man. How could one raised as he was, "basking in . . . Protestant prosperity" . . . have turned out to be "a democrat, the healer of the unwashed, the supporter of the irascible and the dispossessed, the man of peace?" Rosen asked, admitting that, while he could not answer that question, "there dwelt in him in perfect harmony the two most irreconcilable forces of the Western mind, for he had at once a stern Calvinist asceticism and a deep rational humanism. And in him they found in each other comfort, plausibility and peace." As for Janeway's "Calvinist asceticism," Rosen added that Dr. Janeway

> was so full of purpose and conviction that anger and depression were dispelled from his person, even in the most trying times; that he eschewed comfort and luxury . . . While he was not unmindful of that paper product of the U.S. Mint, he just found it less important than the work we were doing in the privileged vineyard of healing . . . he brought great moral authority to all his endeavors . . . [and] dealt with everyone as though they too were mature adults. And this

gave him a certain quality of remoteness and distance—his clean, incisive, and objective reasoning—that lifted everyone around him out of the gutter of gossip and pettiness to more noble standards of human behavior.[47]

Clement Smith, long-time director of the newborn service at Boston Lying-In Hospital and one of Janeway's longest-time colleagues at the Children's, wrote of him in a private communication,

> Charlie Janeway was a remarkable man, but one with an odd elusiveness and self containment. Polly [Bunting-Smith, Smith's wife, and a former president of Radcliffe College] knew him and Betty, his wife, more than 10 years before I did, for she was Betty's roommate at Vassar, in the class of 1931. Yet neither Polly nor I, both of us feeling we knew Charlie as well as anyone, think we shared any real intimacy with him. Yet, insofar as one may love such a man, we loved him. And few persons [who] gave us the sense of strength and stability we got from him are left to us.[48]

Smith, in an editorial he had previously contributed to the February 1977 issue of *Pediatrics,* probably summed up best the feelings so many at Children's had for Charles Janeway, commenting that those who have known him best and longest felt, as he did, that his greatest contributions to American pediatrics were not the usual ones. But "Far more important," he observed, "have been the intangible things learned from him and surely (even if unconsciously) transmitted through the country by numerous past members of his staff and residents. For three decades, these intangibles have been acquired by them not by precept but by example, the example of a rare mixture of intelligence, of integrity, of insight and humility, of reserve and generosity."[49]

Betty Janeway reported that the idea of scattering CAJ's ashes in the Adirondacks came as she and her children Anne and Barbie were walking Betty's dog, April, up Concord Road after the family service, at which the twenty-third Psalm had been read. Betty wrote that suddenly it came to her: "I know. The still water . . . He leadeth me." Stillwater Reservoir was the place in the Adirondacks where she and her husband had spent many happy summers. Betty went on, "I knew he had wanted to be cremated, but we both felt that what lived on would be in people's hearts and minds and ways of living. This is clear from the more than 400 letters, in people's remarks and eyes and in my heart. As I told everyone in the family that we wanted to scatter his ashes in the Stillwater, the plan began to take shape. Even so, the actual carrying out of the mission seemed a miracle."

The miracle took place not long after, when the moon was full and the upper lake was nearly abandoned. At 3:00 a.m., she and several of the immediate family canoed out on the lake amid pouring torrents, with thunder in the distance. Betty wrote, "There were some tears and a lot of hugging as we took turns scattering handfuls of my darling's ashes on the water and on the green in the secluded places," and added,

> We talked about Charlie and how long ago, 51 years [ago], he'd taken me there because he loved it, and Katie, who remembered it least, glowed with pleasure as we reminisced for her. Then Marty said a prayer about the beauty of the place, Francesca read Josephine Goldmark's poem, "Maminess Juvat," and others spoke quietly and movingly about Charlie. We said the 23rd Psalm. Marty read the 121st and said another beautiful prayer about Charlie as a man of peace who had spent so much of his life trying to make the world better. We sang "Dona Nobis" and "Simple Gifts." Then Barbie played on her recorder and, as we heard the simple flute-like notes in the clearing air, [Mount] Marcy came out of the clouds to join the rest of us.
>
> Now, in Tunbridge, a place he dearly loved, I've left a bit of him here, in Lee's resurrected flower bed and the pond. But it's the spirit that counts, and the things people wrote in the guest book, and what lives of him in all of us.[50]

That rare mixture that made Charles Alderson Janeway the premier pediatrician of the twentieth century explains why he lives in the hearts and minds of all who knew him, and why he was deservedly looked upon as pediatrician to the world's children.

6 THE JANEWAY FAMILY AND FAMILY LIFE

CHARLES JANEWAY's family was very important to him. In spite of an extremely busy schedule, he always made room for family events. To us it appeared that his home life was the foundation upon which he built everything; indeed, as we came to know Dr. Janeway in the years we worked with him and learned from him, it seemed that our relationship with him was but an extension of his home life. We think his concern for the children of the world was another such extension. Family began with Janeway's love for his wife, Elizabeth, known during his life as Betty. She was his constant source of strength. His children were his legacy.

While Janeway was interning at the Boston City Hospital in 1934–1936, he and Betty lived with Betty's mother, Mary Bradley, at the Bradley family home on Beacon Hill. Their first child, Anne, was born on February 15, 1936, while they were living there. She was followed by Elizabeth, born August 5, 1938; Charles A., Jr., born February 5, 1943; and Barbara, born July 2, 1947. Charles took special pride in his children and their accomplishments. While he made time for them as best he could, Anne did tell us that she was quite ambivalent toward medicine, partly because it was so demanding and took her father away a great deal. She allowed, however, that Janeway gave himself over completely to the family every Sunday. Betty was instrumental in arranging for Charles to be at home on weekends.

Anne was graduated from Smith College, and early in her career was a teacher for the Peace Corps at the Center in Experimental Living. Her ambivalence toward Western medicine has continued; her major activity in the last several years has been to spend nearly half of each year in India with a teacher-guru, studying Indian complementary medicine. Anne said that her father was a very private person even with his children. He did not talk about medicine at home. He expected much from his children, Anne reported, and that an element of keeping a stiff upper lip ran very deep in her family. Her father expected them not to complain and was tougher on them when they were ill than he was on his own patients. He was parsimonious with the use of antibiotics and told the family that "one of my roles is being certain that physicians don't overuse drugs." Anne felt that Betty was the disciplinarian in the family, and that her father's greatest attribute was his fairness, as she put it. Even as Anne described her father as somewhat aloof, she also thought he had a very common touch. She told of a visiting French professor of pediatrics who "was shocked that Dr. Janeway would allow his residents to see him swimming in a bathing suit!"

Elizabeth (familiarly known as Lee), like Anne, was graduated from the Windsor School in Brookline, Massachusetts. She later was graduated from Radcliffe College, became a skilled photographer, married a pediatrician, Dr. Ronald Gold, and has lived in Toronto for many years. She is the mother of two children, one of whom is also a pediatrician. Charles and Betty's third child, Charles Alderson Janeway, Jr. (called Carlie by the family), followed his father's footsteps, deviating only in his university and medical school: he attended both at Harvard rather than Yale. After preparatory school at Exeter (which, he told us, he did not want to attend since he was happy at the Weston public school), he achieved advance placement as a sophomore at Harvard. He did return to the family university, Yale, where he became a world authority on immunity and was a distinguished professor of pathology. Carlie died in 2003. It is ironic that Dr. Janeway's scientific contributions and his death from Waldenstrom's hypergammaglobulinemia, and Carlie's death from a brain tumor, were both related to the B lymphocyte.

Barbara Bradley Janeway (Barbie) is a nurse practitioner; graduating from Yale School of Nursing. She is married to Donald Wilder and has two sons. Unlike Anne but like her other siblings, she felt little or no ambivalence about Janeway's medical career. She recalled one illustrative story for us. In the summer of 1955, during the last great poliomy-elitis epidemic in Boston, her father said that she and her friends could go to the town pool because no one else would be there. This was at a time when people were so frightened of polio that they stayed away from all pools and crowds. His reasoning was characteristic: while he always emphasized hand washing and meticulous infection precautions in the hospital, it made good sense to him that the town pool would be safe since, if no one else used the pool, there was little or no risk. Janeway did not usually let emotions drive his decisions, although, in retrospect this may not have been such a wise decision since any one of her friends could have had asymptomatic polio and be infectious. Memory may have altered the circumstances, or Janeway may have known that the odds of getting polio at the pool were low enough to take the risk.

Charles and Betty lived most of their married life in Weston, Massachusetts. After briefly living in an old house on the south side of Weston, they built an unpretentious modern home on a little more than six acres on Concord Road. They bought the land in 1948 for $4,250. The neighborhood then was in wooded, suburban land but is being overbuilt now, which the Janeways would have bemoaned. They lobbied hard to keep Concord Road narrow, twisty, and bumpy in order to keep traffic slow. The architect of their house was Janeway's roommate during his first year at Milton Academy, as well as his classmate at Yale, John Whitcomb. The Janeways' next-door neighbors, the Cummingses, with whom they shared ownership of a driveway, were always the closest of friends. They shared a well with the Cummingses and Howes. Together the three families owned about sixty acres in a common trust.

In Janeway's files is a letter from Charles Cummings, written upon the latter's retirement to New Hampshire.

> In scores of ways you have been the central spirit in the events concerning our little community, and we all feel it. Whether it was a tree operation, a big fire, a tag football game, building the tennis court, planning policy for parcel D, selecting an MD for some ailment, cheering a sick child, building a stall, reroofing a shed, operating on impacted crops (the families owned chickens), celebrating Christmas Eve with song and eggnog and carols to our neighbors—and lots

more—you have always been the wise and tender guide and helper.
And we have all felt it.[1]

This accolade from a neighbor and friend captures the feeling felt by almost everyone who worked with Charles Janeway. The feeling extended to the younger Cummingses, too. At the memorial service held
after Janeway's death in 1981, the son of Charles Cummings, Charles
Kimball (Kim) Cummings III, reminisced about life on Concord Road:
"There was a whole line of people with advanced academic degrees
down Concord Road, but we neighborhood children reserved the title
'Doctor' for Dr. Janeway. We didn't need him for simple things . . . but
when we felt downright lousy and nobody could figure out why, that
was a case for Dr. Janeway. One of my clearest memories was of him
coming to my bedside on Christmas Day."[2] The Janeways and the
Cummingses were the closest of neighbors. On Sundays, the Janeways
held joint religious services with the Cummingses, who were Quakers.
They would sing a hymn, read a passage from the Bible or other
sources, or sit in silence as at a Quaker meeting. Each family would
lead the service for two to three weeks.

Anne Janeway mentioned an incident that elucidated her father's
views on religion. She told us about a letter she wrote to her father
concerning her views on religion, and noting her own conflict between
science and religion. His answer was a long time in coming; CAJ wrote
it on his way to the Cameroons (probably in the latter 1970s). Anne recalled her father writing that he "had waited so that he would have
enough time to respond appropriately." She told us that this letter was
one of the most meaningful that she had received from him. Sometimes, in letters such as this to his children, he expressed his deeper
views: "Let me tell a little of my experience since I share your feelings
that we do have a destiny, and whether we make it or not, if everybody
that passes contributes something to the brotherhood of humanity, we
are at least in tune with man's inner and deeper urges and with whatever the principle is that every part of humanity has called God in
some guise or other."[3]

Charles Janeway reported in the 1950 Yale Twenty Yearbook that
their modern but modest home

was on six acres carved out of a large place purchased jointly with friends, which gives us lots of room to work in but which can be subdivided and sold as our efforts to improve the schools and raise taxes for better education in Weston [the sale of some of this land financed the college education of his children] . . . Our main interests, aside from trying to learn something about forest management, fruit and vegetable growing and chickens, are skiing and the outdoors in general.[4]

He embellished the remark, adding, "We built a house in the country part of Weston in 1949 and, perhaps foolishly, are adding the study to it we couldn't afford then, and probably can't now. A community tennis court gives us a chance to enjoy our favorite sport, and in the winter we indulge in the other, skiing in New Hampshire."[5]

When the children were growing up, Betty insisted that they do things as a family. Tennis was a major competitive activity, and family camping, fishing, and skiing were frequent. Charles worked Saturdays at the hospital, making "Chief's Rounds" at 11 a.m. and doing paperwork the rest of the day, but Sundays were family days. Charles and Betty rarely went out on Sunday while the children were home, keeping the day instead for the family. At times Janeway would take work with him on skiing trips and work in the car while Betty drove, but once at their destination, he devoted himself fully to the children and the activities. He did not work at home in the evening but arose very early in the mornings to do paper work. He needed little sleep, although all who knew him realized that he frequently fell asleep in meetings. He liked to read; often he and Betty read to each other aloud. They both enjoyed the Boston Symphony Orchestra; Betty was a long-time Friday afternoon subscriber. Charles liked the theater, and he and Betty joined the Theater Guild. In activities related more directly to his profession, Janeway was active in the Boylston Society at the Harvard Medical School.

Life on Concord Road was not confined to family and neighbors. Most house officers at Children's recalled being invited to the Janeway home for Sundays of tennis and food, which was always well received by young house officers, and yes, work. Most remember bringing in hay and doing other strenuous chores on those Sundays. Usually the pleasure of being with the chief and his family, especially for the single men (and most were single in the early years), was reward enough. But a few remember working most of the day and then suddenly having Dr. Janeway appear to say that the last train to Boston was leaving in a few minutes, and rushing them off to the Weston station, sans dinner. We suspect that such occasions happened because Janeway suddenly realized that there was some other engagement that evening. We also suspect that such events occurred rarely, but were remembered vividly because the Janeways were always such good hosts.

The Janeways were one of about twenty couples who held a monthly group meeting to discuss Town of Weston matters. The group met at various homes and was called the Cracker Barrel. Meals were simple sandwiches, consistent with the conservative New England attitude. The politics was distinctly on the liberal side. Charles and Betty also entertained foreign guests frequently, as their home address book attests; it contain the names, with compliments to the hosts, of most of the great pediatricians of the world of that time, as well as many other guests.

John Kennell, who has had a distinguished career as pediatrician at Case Western Reserve University, recalled his early days at the Children's. Kennell started in 1946, the year Janeway assumed the role of Physician-in-Chief and chair of the department.

> I have a wonderful overall memory of Charlie as extremely kind and thoughtful. I remember he telephoned me while I was busy working, and invited me to have Thanksgiving dinner with his family . . . This was before they moved into their new home. I was the only single intern on the pediatric service [a result of returning servicemen; later, most were unmarried, though today there is a return to the majority of residents being married]. Betty's children were small [Barbie was an infant] and were obviously occupying a great deal of her time and energy so I was particularly impressed by the Janeways' generosity and thoughtfulness.[6]

When Kennell returned to The Children's after military service, by then married to Dr. Gross's former chief operating nurse, Peggy, he noted that they had the good fortune to be invited frequently for the famous "work Sundays" at Concord Road in Weston. Peggy and I enjoyed the outside work, the Janeway children, the Janeway singing, stories and family evenings together. Therefore we were surprised that some of our fellow residents did not take so kindly to the Sunday work. I remember one period when we would spend all of Sunday collecting manure at another farm then transporting it and spreading it around the trees.[7]

Dr. Janeway's personal library was a window to his interests. Most of the books were about medicine, but his preoccupation with managing the property was evident in several brochures on *Pruning Apple Trees* and *Pesticide Safety Guides: For People Who Love Trees*. A more scientific book was *Ecological Energetics*, published in 1969, a sophisticated analysis of the interrelation of energy, food, and human population growth as well as agriculture. The interrelation of different sciences was one of his remarkable interests and carried over to his professional work. In view of his vigorous outdoor life, it was not surprising to also find the *Report of the President's Council on Youth and Physical Fitness*, 1961, in his library.

Annisquam, a small village about an hour north of Boston on Cape Ann, where Betty's father and uncle had build a summer home in 1902, was, like St. Hubert's, a place of refuge, relaxation, and recreation for Dr. Janeway. After Betty's mother's death, the home at Annisquam was jointly owned by Betty and her sister, Mary. Charles and Betty shared many good times in Annisquam. In the early 1950s, Janeway was a Governor of the Annisquam Yacht Club. Dr. Georges Peter, who would become a leading infectious disease expert and pediatrician at Brown University, spent summers there also, as did one of the authors (FHL). Peter noted that people in Annisquam had little idea of the national and international respect that Janeway commanded, "for in his private life Dr. Janeway was a very modest, unassuming person who was well liked and respected as a friend, but he didn't talk much about his professional role." Peter also recalled that by chance he once was Janeway's doubles partner in a local tennis tournament, and that "Dr. Janeway was a very crafty, intelligent, and serious tennis player. He didn't have strong ground strokes, but he had great court sense and obviously loved the game."[8]

The house at Annisquam, sometimes called the Bradley house, was Betty's great love and became Charles's love as well over the years. It was an ideal location for anyone who worked in Boston because of the one-hour commute. It allowed Janeway to go to work on Saturday in the morning but get to Annisquam for afternoon and evening activities. It became the home of all of the Janeway clan; they came to Annisquam nearly every summer. They were very much a part of the community and were exceedingly active in all of the activities. Betty was an excellent tennis player and played often with Charles on the tennis courts immediately below the house. They made an excellent mixed doubles team. Charles and Betty also were active on the water; they owned a 16-foot sailboat, which the children used when they learned to sail.

Because Charles and Betty were in Annisquam all summer, they were involved in many social and recreational activities. Betty, along with my (FHL's) father and Richard Mechem, a teacher at St. Paul's School, established a Junior Program that taught sailing, tennis, and swimming at the Annisquam Yacht Club. Betty also served as a trustee of the Old Wharf Lot Association, which had tennis courts, a beach, a dock for rowboats, and a location for mooring sailboats. Charles participated in the ritual of weekend swimming on the small beach below their house with friends. He sailed with Betty and the children and participated in activities at the Annisquam Yacht Club. He and Betty entertained often, bringing friends, especially physicians from throughout the globe, to Annisquam. As well they would, for Annisquam was, and is, an ideal place to relax, enjoy swimming and the good weather, and to have time for thoughtful conversation. The water was exceedingly cold. We suspect that Charles and Betty took pride in their New England roots (even if Janeway's were transplanted from New York) and their ability to tolerate the cold water, which sometimes was somewhat threatening to their visitors.

Dr. Janeway influenced a number of people from the Children's to come and spend a month or so in Annisquam. At one time or another Alexander Nadas, the David Daniel Teeles, and Edward Neuhouser spent summers in Annisquam. In addition, Janeway held periodic retreats for the department at this house, and during my (FHL's) four-year tenure as chief resident he regularly brought the house staff to

Annisquam for tennis, swimming, and a cookout. Anne, Lee, Carlie, and Barbie all grew up in Annisquam and were very active in the summer activities. Anne was a particularly good fish boat sailor, winning the championship in her boat, *Grayling*. Lee was an excellent tennis player and won many of the junior and ultimately senior tournaments both in women's and mixed doubles. Carlie played tennis and sailed regularly, as did Barbie. In addition to friends whom they invited regularly, Betty's sister and her husband, the Meyers, who lived in Baltimore, came regularly with their family to share the house. Mary Meyer, too, was a wonderful tennis player, and the two families jointly lived in the house in a most satisfactory and congenial way. At summer's end Charles and Betty would go to St. Hubert's in the Adirondacks, Janeway's summer home and the home of his family. This part of their summer was important to the family because they would depart for a week in late August, prior to returning to Weston.

For those of us who trained with Dr. Janeway, the opportunity to share a part of his life away from the hospital was tantamount to an education all its own. But for one of the authors (FHL) and for Dr. Georges Peter, the experience was magnified because we, in a sense, grew up with Dr. Janeway, at least in the summers. In the early years, we boys knew that Dr. Janeway was a doctor in Boston, and perhaps even an important doctor in Boston. Sailing, tennis, and summer activities, however, were far more important to us. We played tennis often with members of the Janeway family in tennis tournaments and competed regularly in sailing as well. Their house was a particularly wonderful place on rainy summer days.

As we grew older, we came to realize Dr. Janeway's importance as a pediatrician. The many visiting physicians from foreign countries impressed us. We often joined the Janeways before dinner; there, we noted that the conversations were serious and more focused on important worldly activities that went beyond the narrow confines of Annisquam. We also came to realize the importance of Janeway's work. He would often be gone on Saturday and (rarely) Sunday mornings, working in Boston, then returning to join the activities during the afternoons. I (FHL) periodically would join the Janeways for small cocktail gatherings, where the discussions would be thoughtful and stimulating. Both Peter and I knew that Dr. Janeway could be preoccupied with his work. On occasion he would walk by us, seemingly not recognizing or addressing us, his thoughts deeply centered undoubtedly on issues and challenges at the hospital. Later in life, Charles and Betty built a small studio next to the Bradley house. They often would stay in the studio, especially when there were large gatherings of other family members. This afforded Janeway the protected time and quiet to work, study, and reflect.

Annisquam was a very important place for the entire Janeway clan. In addition to providing the setting for Charles and Betty's wedding in the garden next to the house, their granddaughter, Katie, was married on the lawn of the Annisquam house. Charles and Betty came every summer until Janeway's death, and the remaining family continued to come every summer thereafter. Near to the time of Betty's death the house was deeded over to one of Mary's children, although Betty had use of part of the house each year until she died. The wonderful old house, like its contemporaries at Annisquam, saw many changes in the families, but the house stayed the same. The large Janeway/Meyer house received paint on a periodic basis and repair of leaks and damage from the harsh winters, but essentially it changed little. Betty continued to come to Annisquam every summer with the children and grandchildren until her death. The importance of Annisquam for her and the family was clearly very evident at her memorial service in New Hampshire at the end of her life. Annisquam was a remarkable part of the life of both.

In the 1970s, Charles and Betty bought a farm in Tunbridge, Vermont. They meant it to be a retirement home. The property consists of a simple farmhouse with a small pond. They thought of it as a place of their own; the Janeway family place in the Adirondacks and the Annisquam summer home both belonged to multiple members of the family, but the Tunbridge place was to be theirs. Tunbridge was a special place for Betty after Charles died. Whenever the Haggertys would visit her at the retirement community of Kendall at Dartmouth, where she lived after selling the home in Weston, she delighted in being driven to Tunbridge for lunch, cross-country skiing, or bird watching. It was home.

In Dr. Janeway's files are diaries of family vacations. Detailed day-by-day accounts of every family member's doings show a vigorous family. One family vacation was spent in the eastern U.S. and Canada; they visited the Janeway family place at St. Hubert's in the Adirondacks before commencing a trip around eastern Canada. They spent few days in hotels but many nights were spent camping, a demonstration of the family's ability to "rough it," which helps explain their adaptability to the rigors of some of their later trips abroad. Charles spent many a day fishing; all family members swam in rivers wherever they were. Eastern Canada was Dr. Edwards Park's country, and fishing the Margaree River and in pools with Park pleased Janeway immensely. They caught several good-sized trout, all recorded as to length and weight. Evenings were often spent as a family, reading such works as *Winnie-the-Pooh, The Secret Life of Walter Mitty,* and other lighter literature. One night in Nova Scotia, several of the Janeways went to a local square dance, "a gay, crowded affair—wonderful music—An almost fight . . . all tried to dance and everyone home happy." On the way home to Weston via Dr. James Gamble's place at Sorrento, Maine, the family diary shows the usual problems of children on a long ride. "This seems to be the breaking point, 'I want toys,' 'I feel sick,' etc." At the Gamble home the diary notes, "First hot bath in 15 days." Dr. Janeway's summary of the trip, "it's probably the best of all vacations for all of us—the vagabond life is good but we've been fed nearly everywhere." They had stayed with friends or had meals with them, a characteristic of most of the Janeway trips, at almost every stop.[9] The picture was of a vigorous, outdoors-loving, gregarious family, visiting friends, making new ones, doing things together with gusto.

A second family vacation, equally well recorded, was spent in Wyoming. Although the Janeway family were based at a ranch, they went off as a family, hiking into the mountains for several days at a time. The sheer joy that Charles expressed in his diary of Carlie's skills as a cook on the range, and the excellent fishing they all had, showed this to be, as he said, the best vacation of all. The vigor of the family was remarkable: bathing in cold mountain lakes, catching many of their meals by fishing, hiking to high mountains, expressing joy at the vistas from the tops, and sleeping in tents or in the open.[10]

Skiing was a vital activity. In Janeway's files is one labeled "Skiing," with maps to places in Aspen, Austria, and Switzerland, letters arranging visits to such places, and the inevitable list of expenses, carefully noted.[11] Frequently these skiing trips were tacked on to a medical meeting, as was the trip to Switzerland in March 1967 after a meeting of the International Children's Center in Paris. Throughout our research we have marveled at Dr. Janeway's ability to be hosted wherever he and Betty went. A letter in the skiing folder, from the wife of Dr. Raymond Martin Du Pan, of Geneva, explains why Du Pan's wife wrote, "how kind Professor Janeway . . . was to him last spring during his journey to the U.S.A. and how much he was looking forward to seeing you in our country next winter. My husband ordered me . . . to stop all plans for your sake."[12] (She was asking for the dates of the Janeways' visit.) Hospitality given, hospitality received.

The record and numerous anecdotes reveal that Betty was a major influence on CAJ. Theirs was a true partnership. Dr. William Berenberg wrote,

> There is no doubt that Betty was a driving force behind his own aspirations and it was clear that he was occasionally irked by some of her efforts to prevent him from hiding his own light under a bushel. On the other hand he was extremely proud of her career [as a social worker] and did make frequent references to her accomplishments with pride. I believe her strong commitment to children, and to pediatric social work had something to do with his eventual choice of pediatrics as a career.[13]

While she was raising their children, Betty volunteered in a variety of arenas, local and international, as well as working part-time as a social worker at Massachusetts General Hospital. When Janeway went abroad she broadened her horizons and saw new approaches to maternal and child health. She was an active recruiter for UNICEF and lectured on her experiences abroad with this group to encourage support. She was an active member of the Social Action Committee of the Unitarian Church of Weston.

When she was fifty-seven years old, Betty returned to the paid work force as a medical social worker at the Boston Lying-in Hospital, working with pregnant teenage girls. Her efforts were concentrated on getting supports in place to enable these women and their children to make an effective transition from the hospital to their homes. She tried to get the medical establishment to recognize the links between the social issues and the health and well-being of these mothers and their children. She continued in this job until her late sixties. Betty tells of an amusing incident when Katherine (Katie), Carlie's daughter, was a third-year medical student in the neonatal intensive care unit (NICU) at the Boston Lying-in Hospital. A nurse remembered Betty with great fondness as the social worker in that hospital and asked Katie, "Wasn't her [Betty's] husband a doctor?" Betty took great pleasure in telling this, for it was one of the few times that she was remembered for her own sake rather than as Dr. Janeway's wife.

In November 1999 the Family Service Association of Boston dedicated The Elizabeth Bradley Janeway Center for Maternal and Child Health, honoring Betty for her work with pregnant women there in the 1960s. This organization, founded in 1838, received $500,000 from the Meyer Family through their Island Trust of the New York Community Trust to renovate the second floor of an old brewery in Roxbury at the corner of Bromley and Heath streets. The dedicatory plaque states that it is dedicated to Betty, "for her work in social work with high risk mothers." For once Betty got recognition on her own.

Betty and Charles suffered from chronic illnesses. Charles had back trouble in the early 1950s and had a spinal disc removed in 1953, but had relatively little further trouble with his back. In the middle 1970s, however, Janeway developed Waldenstrom's macroglobulinemia. (In the late 1970's Janeway met Dr. Waldenstrom at a meeting of the blood research group. Dr. Waldenstrom reviewed Janeway's records and felt that the disease should proceed at a moderate pace.) In 1943, when Dr. Janeway was studying gamma globulin fractions with Dr. Cohn, he repeatedly injected himself first with the fractions. This was a custom of ethical investigators at that time, before institutional review committees became a fixture in research; in fact, Dr. William Berenberg gave Janeway the first dose of gamma globulin ever administered to a human being. On that occasion in 1943 he had a severe reaction, with high fever and shock, and was admitted to the Peter Bent Brigham Hospital. Dr. Fred Rosen states that the gamma globulin was contaminated with staphylococcal endotoxin.[14] In Janeway's own record of his medical history he records it as staphylococcal endotoxin reaction, and the Peter Bent Brigham Hospital record of the visit records it as a result of staphylcoccal toxin contaminating the gamma globulin. Dr. Berenberg notes that there were other episodes of serum sickness after he received batches of gamma globulin,[15] and several of his colleagues have speculated that his later illness with hypergammaglobulinemia could have been the result of this early stimulus of his immune system. It is ironic that the man who did so much to unravel the disorders of the gamma globulin system succumbed to a disorder of that system.

Betty had a number of illnesses throughout her life, including migraine headaches and lower back and coccygeal pain, but the most difficult illness was with her neck, a problem that began in the early 1970s. She developed a severe spastic torticollis that no therapy could help until she finally underwent an excision of her trapezious muscle on the affected side. This left her with a neck that tilted to the right unless it was supported by a neck collar or held up by her hand, accounting for a familiar pose during the last years of her life. Neither Betty nor CAJ complained to outsiders about their physical problems. Both had a stoical attitude to adversity. They tried not to let these afflictions interfere with their zest for life. Betty went cross-country skiing with the Haggertys until she was well into her eighties.

In 1991 Betty moved to Kendall at Hanover, New Hampshire, maintaining a two-bedroom apartment there. She changed her first name to Lizza because, she said, there were too many Bettys at Kendall! She remained an avid birdwatcher and, when the Haggertys would take her to her beloved Vermont farm in Tunbridge, she relished sighting birds. She started a large asparagus garden at Kendall and, true to her New England upbringing, sold the extras to the other residents. She also took creative writing classes at Dartmouth and participated in many activities there. When we (RJH and Muriel) visited her she introduced us to many of the residents, whom she knew by their first names. She remained vigorous, although slowed by her neck problem, until a year or two before her death, when she suffered a stroke. Her mind remained clear. We last saw her in the spring of 2000. Anne, her eldest daughter, was living with her, otherwise she would have needed to go to the nursing home at Kendall. Betty spent that last summer at Annisquam, in what Anne described as a tranquil and peaceful time. She died October 20, 2000.

A memorable memorial service was held later at Kendall, with several hundred people in attendance. Many people who live to be nearly ninety years old have lost most of their contemporaries and failed to make new friends. Betty never failed to make new friends. She was engaged in the events of the day, decrying the Republican agenda, especially their opposition to abortion, for she had seen at first hand the misery that overpopulation caused for the third world and among pregnant teenagers in Boston. Little wonder that so many people came to pay their respects. At the memorial service Anne presented a brief life of Betty. In it she quoted her mother's statement in 1959 to her Vassar classmates: "My friends range in age from five to ninety-five. The five-year-old helps me feed the hens and collect the eggs while the eleven-year-old brother rides horseback with my youngest daughter. The ninety-five year-old discusses books she has read recently on archeology in the Middle East and on how to stop Atomic Bomb tests. Our friends encircle the globe." Betty Janeway almost made the ninety-five year mark herself with her faculties intact. Anne's final paragraph summarized her life: "Eliza has four children, seven grandchildren, and one great grandchild, numerous nieces, nephews and a wide circle of friends, new and old, as well as young and old. She has traveled extensively, read widely, been an avid birder, a great cook, and a generous and caring member of society, characteristics she tries to pass on to her children and their children."

Toward the end of Charles Janeway's life, several friends wrote to him, commiserating on his illness but rejoicing that he had the companionship of a loving wife. One said, "I hope your good wife appreciates how much she has been a large factor in your career. Love and peace at home I know make a man capable of living up to his potential."[16] Another, commenting on Janeway's Howland address, remarked, "I liked, in particular, the way you gave Betty credit, for she has indeed been a major influence on us all."[17] It is interesting that in 1985 Betty was elected to the Board of the Center for Blood Research, the successor of the Protein Laboratory in which Dr. Janeway had done his early research over forty years earlier.

Charles A. Janeway had a deep commitment to all of his family, both those of origin and his descendants. In spite of a punishingly busy career, he kept in touch with the family and helped them with the many problems, medical and otherwise, that occur in every family. It is no accident that in his final years he was appointed to a committee of the Institute of Medicine to report on family medicine and primary care, and wrote several papers on the future of Family Medicine. It was not his professional career but his personal rearing and dedication that led him to see the importance of the family to medical care.

7 IMPROVING THE LOT OF MANKIND: EARLY INTERNATIONAL ACTIVITIES

CHARLES AND BETTY JANEWAY were internationalists. They believed passionately in the United Nations, in the need to solve international disputes peacefully, and in the duty of the developed world to assist the developing one to grow and prosper as the best way to avoid war. We speculated earlier as to how this passion might have had its beginning. Janeway worked with an international Christian group while at Yale and made many visits to Germany as a college student. His family had traveled abroad frequently. In time, he began to see himself as a citizen of the world as well as of the United States. It is not clear how Betty came to join him in this outlook, but when she did, the emotion was equal for both. It continued in their children, manifested especially in Anne's work in India, a special place in the hearts and minds of the Janeways.

Even in family activities in Weston suggest intense involvement in international affairs. The Janeways' son, Carlie, said that when the family had breakfast together, his mother and father would divide the newspaper and comment on international affairs with the children, rather than discuss sports or local activities.[1] Their view was distinctly a liberal, international one. Betty listened to the television commentator Louis Lyons on the Boston PBS radio station and would comment on the news of the world that he had reported. Their liberal Democratic leaning during the McCarthy affair led Betty to be concerned that her husband might lose his job, since he was so outspokenly opposed to McCarthy. In retrospect, this probably was highly unlikely. In writing this chapter, which first looks into Janeway's involvement in the International Pediatric Association and afterwards at his activities abroad during two sabbatical leaves, one in 1956 and the other bridging the years 1965 and 1966, to help advance pediatrics and child care in the third world and in developing countries, we have been fortunate to have available extensive documentation in the form of detailed diaries Janeway maintained or summary typed letters he and Betty sent to family and friends throughout their travels.

On most of his trips, Dr. Janeway kept notes in pocket-sized notebooks that describe what he did, the patients he saw, the lectures he gave, and statistics and history of the countries he visited. He also described whom he met, and recorded his frank opinions of people on each of his trips. It is a pity that such details do not exist for his work at Children's Hospital. That is true for many of us, however; we are inclined to report on the trips and exotic places to which we go and neglect to record details of our everyday activities at home. The quality of the Janeways' written reports of their sabbaticals and the insights into their beliefs and character support our detailed excerpting from these notes; they provide clues to the Janeways' keen powers of observation, their superior writing skills, and their basic values and international commitment.

In a tribute to Dr. Janeway given in 1977, Dr. Steven Joseph, then director of international programs at the Harvard School of Public Health, used the phrase, "Pediatrician of the World," to describe him. He noted Janeway's many contributions as a teacher, researcher, and wise clinician on his many trips abroad, and how these were remembered by pediatricians throughout the world.[2] During the 1950s and through the 1970s, Charles A. Janeway was the most famous named pediatrician everywhere in the world because of his well known commitment to the health of the world's children. In his thirtieth anniversary book of the Yale Class of 1930,[3] Janeway mentioned his involvement with India during his 1956 sabbatical and also wrote, "I received another lesson in the problems of world health as a member of the United States delegation to the 11th World Health Assembly in Minneapolis in 1958," an experience that further strengthened his involvement in international activities. The initial part of this chapter will focus on the origin and early expression of these interests, and on Janeway's membership in, and work on behalf of, the International Pediatric Association.

Relatively early in his career, Janeway was asked to become active in international activities because of his eminence as a pediatric scientist and because he was from Harvard. Although he gave many lectures on his scientific work and reviewed many research programs of faculty around the world, observers such as Dr. Ihsan Dogramaci of Turkey felt that Janeway's major contributions to pediatrics was not scientific but humanistic: "he inspired in residents, and especially in fellows from abroad, a sense of dedication to children and a sensitivity to the needs of children all over the world."[4] In a biographical note for a Yale update,[5] Janeway observed that the Children's was attracting students from all over the world. Accordingly, when he took his first sabbatical leave in 1956, he and Betty traveled through the Middle East, India, Ceylon, and Indonesia in order to study the pediatric and educational problems of their medical schools first hand. They spent nearly two months in Madras, where he served as visiting lecturer in pediatrics at the Government General Hospital, which had been founded during Elihu Yale's tenure as the first British governor at Madras.

As a result of the vivid experiences and many friendships formed on that trip, Charles and Betty became deeply interested in helping those countries in their efforts to raise the living standards of their people. This feeling of friendship and helpfulness brought many visitors from many lands to their home, and even more students to the hospital. He also told his classmates of becoming involved in the affairs of the Iran Foundation, that operated a group of philanthropic institutions founded by a wealthy Iranian family, the Nemazees, for the advancement of health and education in Iran, of which in 1958 he had become president. He mentioned at the end that he would be glad to hear from any interested volunteers who wanted to give blood, sweat and tears, and even a few dollars for some satisfaction. Early on, CAJ derived many satisfactions from his own blood, sweat and tears. By 1956, he was solidly hooked on his commitment to international affairs. In 1979, he wrote in the introduction to a Children's Hospital publication that the children who benefit from the activity of the hospital lived around the corner and around the world and that the impact of the hospital's teaching and research programs was felt nationally and internationally. "Ours is an international, not a national, profession."[6]

Not everyone was overjoyed with Janeway's commitment to international pediatrics. Alexander Nadas, for example, was troubled by Janeway's long absences and urged him to cut his outside commitments drastically and spend more time at the Children's when he returned from his 1965–66 sabbatical. During that same year, 1966, Janeway's mentor and father figure, Ned Park, wrote to him to say, "I am more interested in your progression in medical science than I am in your mission in various parts of the world, although I am sure that the latter results in a good deal of good."[7] Park's comments at this time mirrored an extensive comment he had made a decade earlier about Janeway's involvement in giving talks and doing administration in the United States, at a time when Janeway was being considered as chair of pediatrics at Hopkins, which, Park opined, would allow him to remain a scientist, as opposed to his position at Harvard, which involved a great deal of administration and continuing education. "But I have feared that you were spending too much time traveling around the country, giving papers and talks that did not represent the fundamental contributions to knowledge of which you are capable."[8]

The comments of Nadas and Parks are interesting rebukes from two of Janeway's closest friends and mentors. Both were concerned about his over involvement in administrative and educational activities in the United States and his commitment to international child health, which, inevitably, consumed a large amount of his time and energy. These pieces of "unsolicited advice," coming as they did from persons he respected deeply, must have caused Janeway some anguish and reflection. That he continued, nevertheless, to devote much time and energy to international health is evidence of his deep commitment to the health of the world's children. As noted in the previous chapter, upon his return from his sabbatical, Dr. Janeway did recruit and promote more faculty at the Children's, thus addressing one of the concerns of Nadas. He continued to do so in subsequent years, but he did not reduce his commitment to the world. In our opinion, his course demonstrated that he felt so deeply about international health that he believed he could disregard advice from two of his most trusted friends.

In 1967 or 1968, Dean Rusk, then Secretary of State, asked Dr. Janeway if he would be interested in going to Vietnam with a group of eight physicians to determine the effect that napalm and its consequent defoliation had on children's health. CAJ replied that he would indeed be interested, but felt obliged to let Rusk know that he was opposed to the war. When replying months later, Rusk wrote that the government had not allocated enough money to send all eight; funds were available to send only seven pediatricians. Janeway was the lone omission. It seems clear that the United States government did not want an anti-war pediatrician on that mission, even one so fair-minded, so scientifically rigorous, and who represented a prestigious institution.

From his early days, Dr. Janeway believed in international collaboration of the sort ultimately exemplified in the United Nations. In a letter to his mother just before America's entry into World War II, he wrote,

> The War news is terrible . . . it is a complete vindication for the people who believe in a federal union of the democracies. The little nations will certainly have to learn that the only way they can keep their freedom is to become part of a large whole but not an organization like the League of Nations, which is international, but allows every individual country freedom of choice to conduct its foreign policy as it pleases. No one can contend that the people of Delaware would be as well off it they were a small independent country, surrounded by large nations such as Pennsylvania and New York. I only hope the Allies will have the wisdom to put through some such scheme when this mess is finally over.[9]

Janeway's faith in what was then only a vision of the United Nations would be a source of unhappiness to him today, at a time when the United States has disregarded the U.N. and most of its members have been willing to give up autonomy.

The International Pediatric Association

The International Pediatric Association (IPA), an organization of national pediatric societies, was a source of great satisfaction and engagement for Dr. Janeway. The Association was founded in 1912 by European pediatric societies. In 1947, its traditional triennial meetings had lapsed for over a decade owing to World War II and the disturbances leading to and following it. In that year, Janeway and L. Emmet Holt, Jr., chair of pediatrics at New York University, organized the first post-World War II meeting of the society in New York. The event was held from July 14 to 17, 1947. Several young European pediatricians were invited and their expenses were paid so as to enable them to become more familiar with scientific developments in American pediatrics. These pediatricians were selected for their potential and future leadership in a rebuilt Europe, and many fulfilled that promise. This meeting was the first example of Dr. Janeway's explicit involvement in international pediatrics. It came only a year after his appointment to the pediatric chair at Harvard and was to be a continuing commitment until his death, a span of over thirty years.

In his history of the IPA, Professor Guido Fanconi expressed gratitude to American pediatricians who, with several philanthropic foundations, contributed $200,000 to make the meeting possible. He was impressed with an American innovation at the meetings, exhibits by investigators (these are called poster sessions today): "Visitors to the exhibition who stopped at a booth had an opportunity to discuss the subject informally and personally with the investigator." This was in contrast to the traditional European plenary session lecture, which did not offer discussion. Fanconi also marveled at the advances in scientific discovery by the Americans. "For us Europeans, the plasma fractionation technique [thanks mainly to E.J. Cohn and partly Janeway] was also a revelation."[10] So began Janeway's deep involvement with this international group of pediatricians.

Janeway became a member of the IPA Executive Board in 1956, at its meeting in Copenhagen. He chaired the Executive Committee from 1962 to 1968, and stayed on the Executive Council until 1978. At the 1956 meeting in Copenhagen, he was critical of the congress:

> Biggest ever, 3,500 registrants. Little new in papers . . . a mixture of (a) grammar school pediatric education . . . (b) a few original scientific papers, c) occasional outstanding reviews of big subjects like Achar (India) on kwashiorkor or DeSilva (Ceylon) on ascariasis or Walgren on tuberculosis . . . International complications require

acceptance of every paper, so a few [from Germany and USA] abominable ones got on the program. Congress now too big to permit taking in all of papers or exhibits you want to see or hear.[11]

Dr. Janeway also wrote, "On the positive side, it brings together people from many countries you seldom see . . . it was good and impressive to find physicians from behind the iron curtain talking, acting and being received like human beings, social life was wonderful. Best event was informal party for organizing committee, a small group of friends, 150 . . . in Copenhagen's finest club . . . after dinner danced till 2 a.m., when we left, party was going strong."[12]

Janeway, attending his first session of the Executive Committee as a delegate from the United States, summarized his impressions of the meeting: "Meeting almost a farce. Professors in Europe [Fanconi in this case] don't understand democratic system of parliamentary rules." He noted that Asian and other colonial countries' representatives were affected by their sense of inferiority based on their colonial experience, while, "The European group, which has dominated these congresses, has not really aligned selves with new world, in which Latin America, Asia must be heard in some relation to their importance in present day world . . . Best things for me were the insights into world, meeting those from Communist countries, seeing Asiatic physicians like Achar and DeSilva, talking with Gomez and Cravioto from Mexico to get a feel of what very fine people they are."[13]

As Dr. Janeway gained greater influence in the IPA, one of his major contributions was to increase the presence of members from Latin America and Asia. Like many revolutions, the process is still not complete. The IPA has still to learn to see its strength in its wonderful people from all over the world and not emphasize one or two areas. Janeway was invited to go to East Germany and, although there was not time on that 1956 trip, he added, "I must go there and to other Russian orbit areas and to Finland. One gets the idea the Iron Curtain is breaking and we may be missing the boat."[14] It was to take another two decades before CAJ's suspicion came to pass.

Dr. Janeway's next documented involvement with the International Pediatric Association took place in Zürich, Switzerland. For four days, starting on Monday April 10, 1961, he met with other members of its Executive Committee, while Betty went to ski with friends in the Alps. He listed each member of the committee and indicated their strengths and weaknesses. "Meetings were good. Debated purpose of IPA, answered Fanconi's questionnaire and wrote a new constitution . . . Major conclusions: a) International Congresses must be every three years. It is one chance for those behind the Iron Curtain to get out and talk freely . . . b) quality of papers main consideration." His second point was that regional meetings were important. "Child health emphasized. Watkins and I wrote definition [of Child Health]. Obviously it meant nothing to many Europeans." CAJ was continually concerned that European pediatrics was still dealing primarily with a small group of children with rare diseases rather than focusing attention on the health of the whole population of children with prevention the main focus. As a fourth point, he noted that the structure of the IPA depended on money available, but dues could not be raised. Some societies could make contributions, but industrial and foundation contributions were needed. At the meeting, the Executive Committee was renamed "Advisory Board," which, Janeway thought, it really was. They also made provisions for regular meetings and agenda to obviate occasional problems. He noted in his diary, "Good meeting. Very harmonious."[15] Elsewhere in his diary, CAJ made note of "great" lunches and of dinners of the Executive Committee participants, at which each hosted a small group dinner in rotation, allowing more intimate conversation. He considered this a very satisfactory advance over the Copenhagen meetings in 1956 and as being very helpful in the organization of the IPA.

Janeway participated in the September 1962 IPA Congress in Lisbon, one of the regular triennial major gatherings of the organization. His diary of that event includes twelve pages of detailed notes on the main plenary lectures and round table sessions, but no description of the Advisory Board's activity. At the Tokyo International Congress in 1965, Janeway chaired the Advisory Board and faced some delicate issues that required his diplomatic skills, including the orderly transition of the long-time and internationally famous but somewhat dictatorial Secretary General of the IPA, Professor Guido Fanconi, who was seventy-four, in favor of a younger person. (To his credit, Fanconi, it seems, initiated the transfer.[16]) Numerous letters exist in CAJ's files to and from members of the Advisory Board concerning the suitability of several different candidates. In addition to the problem of selecting a suitable successor was the difficult and sensitive matter of effecting the transition without hurting Fanconi's feelings, which, much to Janeway's relief, occurred easily, with Professor Thomas Stapleton elected as Executive Secretary. Initially, a problem had erupted over the appointment when, at the last moment, three names were proposed for the position, requiring Janeway to resort to some politicking that he did not relish. After the three names had been proposed, Janeway diplomatically adjourned the meeting.

Afterwards, Professor Bo Vahlquist proposed Stapleton, an Englishman who originally was at St. Mary's Hospital in London, but at the time was Professor of Child Health at Sidney, Australia, thus adding an Asian flavor to the IPA. Janeway then suggested an additional candidate, causing Vahlquist to respond that "if there is any chance that you yourself might consider the post in spite of the penalty of U.S. leadership," he would be very happy.[17] As the process continued, the reasons for the selection of Stapleton became clearer. He was a young man who might carry on for a number of years; and he was much traveled and had a first-hand knowledge of pediatrics and the health problems of children in many parts of the world. It is easy to understand, then, why Dr. Janeway breathed a sigh of relief when he recorded in his diary, "Best of all, Fanconi retired in a blaze of glory and I think happy . . . and made Honorary Secretary for life."[18] But his diary mentioned some narrow squeaks, such as trying to get a "real African" on the Advisory Board and dealing with the inflammatory Israel-Arab question. While Janeway continued to be worried about the quality of the presentations at the Congresses, he was pleased about the quality of the sessions at Tokyo.

The "Israel question" was a vexing one, then as now. At this time, Israeli pediatricians sought to attend meetings of the Middle East Pediatric Society but were not permitted entrance. Later, Israel joined the European Pediatric Society as an alternative. In a letter to Fanconi about the problem of Israel participating in the Middle East Pediatric Society meetings at Athens, CAJ wrote that he was distressed about the difficulties of the Middle East and that he wanted to keep that kind of political thing out of the IPA. He added in a postscript that the "IPA should take punitive action against any group which cannot arrange to admit Israel, or any other nation, regardless of its political beliefs, to any congress," and went on to say, "Of course, I think it would be quite interesting if the Pediatric Society of Communist China were admitted to the IPA and the next congress were to be held in the United States." Would the U.S. State Department permit Chinese Communists to come to our country, he wondered? "This would be a real test case which would be fun to fight, but I'm not sure at all how it would come out."[19] Dr. Stapleton subsequently wrote to Janeway, saying, "I think that I have been able to organize myself another Chinese visa . . . This might give me a chance to find out if the Chinese would join."[20] The sticking point was the relationship to Taiwan, which ultimately was solved by the admittance of both. Janeway was getting an education on the political aspects of international pediatrics. While much has been made in this book about his liberalism, he was, at this time, very critical of the People's Republic of China and North Korea as being totalitarian and aggressive. Like many, his views of communism were mixed. He saw neither an "evil empire" nor a "worker's paradise." His was a nuanced and thoughtful view of complex issues that were difficult to solve.

Another of Dr. Janeway's constant worries was the IPA's financial problems, which have continued to plague the organization to this day. He wrote to Bo Vahlquist about forming a fund-raising committee. In reply, Vahlquist suggested "the very able and successful Dogramaci . . . or one of the 'professional fund raisers' at a U.S. medical school" as the right man for the purpose.[21] This was the first mention of Ihsan Dogramaci of Turkey, who was to become such an important force in IPA in subsequent years. It is interesting that Fanconi reported that dues had been received from all but four of the member societies (sixty-two in all at the time) and those four had assured him that they would pay.[22] This stands in marked contrast with the IPA's situation today, when it is difficult to get even two-thirds of the 143 member societies to pay dues. Among other financial issues, there were discussions of the importance of corporate exhibitors as a source of income. Fanconi had reported that contributions had been made since the year 1962 to support IPA by three Swiss pharmaceutical firms, which, it appears, he had solicited. Although Janeway did not accept such contributions from pharmaceutical companies for his own department, he did not object to the IPA practice.

IPA's relationship with Nestlé has been difficult. In his history, Fanconi lauds Nestlé for its financial support of the organization's work; and, indeed, Nestlé has continued its support to this day. The issue lies with breast feeding; most pediatricians strongly favor breast feeding of infants when possible, but they also want a safe—as close to human as practicable—milk substitute when not possible, or when the mother does not want to breast feed. However, the marketing practices of Nestlé, which manufactures a milk substitute, had been to discourage breast feeding, especially in developing countries, leading to boycotts of Nestlé; thus, accepting the company's support has been a continuing source of rancor and controversy within the association.

In his opening remarks at the 1968 International Congress in Mexico City, Dr. Janeway observed that "we must not forget that every child who becomes ill and requires hospitalization represents a failure in pediatrics." He assigned such failure to ignorance on the part of the child's family, or to the lack of an adequate system of health care, or to poor clinical judgment on the part of the doctor or other health care worker, or to the failure of medical research to determine the cause, and thus provide the means of prevention or rational therapy for a particular disease.[23] His concluding remarks at that Congress are considered by many to be the crowning statement of his vision concerning international child health:

> As physicians concerned with the health of children—who make up over one-third of the world's population—we are drawn together by common interests, which bring us closer to one another than we are to many of our countrymen. Ours is an international, not a national, profession. Disease does not recognize political boundaries. A sick or hungry child is equally pathetic, whether his skin be black, yellow or white; the happy smile of a healthy child has universal appeal to all mankind. We are a privileged profession, whose daily work deals with the recurring freshness of opportunity which life presents in every newborn infant, whose task it is to heal rather than to kill, and whose major goal is to prevent disease so it will not need to be cured . . . The Children of the world are Our children . . . By the nature of our Association, linking us together in friendship as physicians, who

share our pediatric experiences with one another "for the benefit of children everywhere in the world," we are demonstrating that scientific knowledge can be applied constructively to solve the health problems on this small planet, where it has become essential that men and women learn to live together in peace or perish.[24]

In his day-to-day work, Charles Janeway tried to advance the aims of the International Pediatric Association, which was founded to foster the collaboration of pediatricians throughout the world.

It was at the Mexico City Congress in 1968 that Janeway completed his term as chairman of the IPA Executive Committee, perhaps recognizing the criticism (from some at home) of his extensive involvement in international affairs; nonetheless, he led the process of reorganization of the IPA at that meeting, and the process would have far-reaching impact. He believed that there was a need for a strong president to replace the chair of the Advisory Committee; he thought that the Executive Director and president should each serve more than a three-year term, in anticipation of the succeeding Congress and to help prepare for it. The person he had in mind for president was Ihsan Dogramaci, whom he knew would be a strong leader. He called Dogramaci from Mexico City and convinced him to take the presidency. Dogramaci was at the time in Ankara, unable to attend the 1968 Congress, although he had been elected to his initial term on the Advisory Board in 1966 and had been a member of the Ad Hoc Advisory Committee that met in 1961 to discuss IPA's future. Dogramaci told us that he was reluctant to take on the responsibility that Janeway pressed on him, as he was fully engaged in building a university from a medical school he had begun in Ankara. However, CAJ was persuasive and Dogramaci accepted the office.[25]

Three years later Dogramaci saw the need for a long-term, powerful Executive Director (chief administrative officer) rather than the then existing office of secretary. To the dismay of Thomas Stapleton, then secretary, he was successful in getting himself appointed Executive Director, a position he held for three decades and in which role he contributed enormously to many successful IPA activities. Dr. Janeway's contribution was to convince Dr. Dogramaci to become actively involved. The rest of the IPA story requires another publication, for it occurred after Janeway's time as chairman.

The 1956 Sabbatical

Dr. Janeway's first sabbatical occurred in 1956, after ten years at the helm of the medical department of the Children's. He utilized this opportunity to make a seven-month tour of Europe and the Middle East, in the company of his wife, to teach pediatrics and assess the health of children in those areas. The 1956 sabbatical was Charles and Betty's first trip abroad since college days; and they decided to have the children accompany them on the first part of it as a family experience; hence, the family spent the months of July and August travelling about Europe, taking in the sights and enjoying its culture and pleasures. At most stops, in addition to sightseeing, Janeway gave lectures and made rounds in children's hospitals, thereby exposing himself to leading pediatricians in Europe and learning about pediatrics in the countries he visited. One of his goals was to attend the IPA meeting in Copenhagen, referred to previously.

After the Janeway children returned home in late August to resume their schooling, Charles and Betty traveled east to Madras, India, where Charles served as visiting professor at the Madras Medical College for two months (see chapter 8), observing the conditions and medical treatment of children in an underdeveloped area of the world and taking short side trips to Ceylon and Indonesia for the same purpose. The 1956 sabbatical was supported by a Rockefeller Foundation grant.[26] In his final report, Janeway gave a characteristically careful accounting to the penny. In his initial letter following the submission of his report, CAJ noted that having his wife accompany him, which allowed her to make contacts with Indians while he was at work, made that part of the experience far broader than would have been possible had he made the journey alone.[27]

The sabbatical started in Europe, with the entire family embarking from Montreal on June 10 on the MS *Seven Seas*, a dumpy but comfortable German transport, where they found much "Gemütlichkeit" during the long, slow voyage to Southampton. After landing, they immediately took a third-class coach to London, where they passed the next three days partaking of the sights and wonders of England for the first time, before leaving for Newcastle to catch a ship that would take them on to Norway.[28] Janeway communicated to his diary, "The 7 hour boat ride . . . one of the most beautiful trips I've ever taken, threading our way between islands all the way to Haugesund and Bergen."[29] In Bergen, he visited the new children's hospital, built after the war, and was much impressed with its "nice able staff, alert and good . . . nurses do technical work . . . Friendly warm atmosphere."[30] He found Norway lovely, simple, and decorative. He was impressed with Norwegian medical education that included a mandatory one-year internship and four months as an assistant to a practicing doctor who was also a public health officer. The Janeway family fell in love with Norway. "Norway cannot be described," he wrote in his diary, "it has to be lived and absorbed . . . it's the one country to which I'd like to return for a real vacation of simple outdoor life."[31] This trip was not to be a leisurely one, however, for the next day it was on to Oslo, where Janeway visited the new children's hospital.

On the following day they drove on to Copenhagen and the pediatric congress, at which Janeway was introduced to Professor Plum and Carl Friderichsen of Waterhouse Friderichsen Syndrome fame. The fact that he was attending a medical meeting did not alter Dr. Janeway's parsimonious ways; the family stayed in an old boarding house on the outskirts of the city rather than at the congress hotel. While in Copenhagen, CAJ gave a lecture to medical students on special problems of infectious diseases in early childhood. At the lecture he noticed, "students dressed worse than ours. A few in polo shirts, a few existentialist beards." Dr. Janeway was fastidious about neatness in hospital. At the close of the meetings, the family traveled on to southern Denmark, where, on one of the small fishing islands, he noticed the cleanliness and pride in boats and little boys working with their fathers on them. "No juvenile delinquency when you go to work and try to copy your father at 8 or ten years old," he told his diary. They stayed in Seogoardin in, as one would expect the frugal Janeway to note, "a wonderful and cheap country inn . . . and Danish maids in blue uniforms and white caps whom I'd give my eye teeth to kidnap for nurses aides at CMC."[32]

In Germany, on the way to their next point of arrival, they picked up a hitchhiker who was a student. They took him to Hamburg, where, within a "half a mile from harbor," they noticed "everything had been reduced to rubble . . . rebuilding is beginning among some empty shells . . . one of which had geraniums in boxes in its skeleton window ledger, a strange flicker of life in a dead wasteland." They spent their first night in Germany in Hildesheim, which CAJ remembered from 1929 as one of the loveliest medieval German towns. When he asked where the old town was, the answer was "alles kaput!"[33] On the trip south they came within a mile of the Iron Curtain, where passage down the roads was forbidden by signs indicating the boundary of the Russian zone. They were afraid they would get on the wrong side inadvertently and have trouble getting out. When they reached Heidelberg they found, seated at a table in a beer Stube, drinking beer, Edward G. Janeway, Jr., Private, U.S. Army, Janeway's nephew, the son of his brother Edward. The young Janeway was a reporter for the army newspaper. The Janeways had dinner with him.

Then it was on to Switzerland, with main stops at Basel, Zürich, Bern, and Geneva. At Basel, they stayed at the home of Hans Habich, who had worked in CAJ's laboratory in Boston. The family skied for a week in the Alps, where they opted to stay in a very small village that "kept us from the Americans." Dr. Janeway attended a symposium on "Digestion in Infancy," where he met more European pediatricians and observed the wide gulf that existed between Anglo-Saxon and German pediatrics. His comment: "the latter . . . concerned with problems we ceased worrying about 15 or 20 years ago" (such as the "ideal" baby food). He also noted that, at informal meetings, there was little discussion at the end, interrupting a speaker was unthinkable, and research was still thought of as an individual undertaking rather than a broad approach to a basic problem by collaboration between groups with different techniques, as in America.

In Zürich, Janeway spent four days attending an IPA Executive Board meeting and visited Professor F. Rossi, Fanconi's assistant. In Bern, he visited the Swiss Red Cross and made an inspection of its unified blood program. Afterwards, the family passed a week's vacation in the Swiss Alps, during which they took a train trip to Zermat and spent three days in the tiny village of Evoline, which captivated him: "Scenery today was magnificent . . . best of all the view of Dent Blanche up valley in golden afternoon light and tonight in moonlight. Will miss Evoline. It is beautiful, unspoiled and remote, though like St. Huberts [the Janeways' place in the Adirondacks] in the late 1800s, a group of devotees who like to walk."[34]

They entered "La belle France" on August 18, stopping at small towns for the night on their way north to Paris. After wandering their way to the Loire valley, they stayed for a few days with Professor Debré, the leading teacher of pediatrics in Paris, in his eighteenth-century summer home, a large country chateau where the Janeways had a wing to themselves and were served breakfast in bed. Their stay was enlivened by visits by Professor Royer and Mme. Masse, Debré's assistants, who would become Janeway's colleagues in the IPA. When the idyll with the Debrés ended, the Janeways journeyed on to Paris. Then, after a brief stay,[35] the children all departed for the United States and Charles and Betty prepared to proceed to the East, with the first stop in Ankara, Turkey, where they inspected Dr. Dogramaci's new institute. Here they saw under construction a ten-story medical science building for the university and an addition to the modern hospital that would contain several hundred beds. Charles and Betty were impressed with the energy of Ihsan Dogramaci, who had in three years moved from a rented two-room ambulatory clinic to build a children's hospital along the lines of that in Boston. It had a full-time staff and a research institute, serving as a model for Turkey.

Janeway was quite taken with Dogramaci. "All in all, an extraordinary performance," he concluded, his assessment being based primarily on "(1) enough wealth or business sense to permit him to devote full time (rare) to his work, (2) complete dedication and conviction regarding his goal, (3) personal charm and political skill." Janeway met with a group of faculty and was also impressed with their earnest desire to learn how to accomplish better education of health personnel. "Except for the delay to translate into Turkish . . . we might have been in HMS [Harvard Medical School's] faculty room." One day he visited a rural health center and was impressed by the marriage of curative medicine with public health, including home visiting. Dr. Janeway worried that the Turks would have less success recruiting doctors for more remote health centers, but Dogramaci, ever the optimist, said that with rising incomes in rural areas, free housing and opportunities for fellowships, after spending a few years in rural areas, they had no problems with recruitment.[36]

The Middle Eastern part of the sabbatical continued with a journey to Beirut (September 13–18), where Janeway lectured on plasma protein physiology and was much impressed with the high caliber of the American University staff. Dr. Zellweger, professor of pediatrics, took Charles and Betty to Byblos to view the remains of its 7,000-year history and afterwards to Baalbek, a city on the caravan route, where they saw huge Roman buildings, including the largest temple the Romans built anywhere, "a feat of engineering and slave driving;" and they also inspected the American University Farm, which served as a research station for both agricultural as well as public health research programs. Nevertheless, CAJ was worried even then that in the process of adapting to Western medicine the Lebanese were adopting what was ugly in America: large cars, ugly tourist buildings, and unrestrained growth.

Janeway's education in international assistance was developing rapidly. He was beginning to see that scientific teaching and research might not be enough and that there were things to learn from these older cultures, even in medicine. Betty was also getting an education. The letters she wrote for family and friends describe their visits with officials of the United Nations Relief and Works Agency (UNRWA) for Palestinian refugees in the Near East and visits to refugee camps in more detail than CAJ's diary entries. And on this trip as well as later ones she was often taken by UNICEF officials to social programs while her husband was visiting medical facilities. On later trips she was a certified UNICEF consultant and became, upon her return to the United States, a spokesperson for UNICEF.[37]

Charles and Betty's whirlwind trip continued with a drive to Damascus, Syria, where they saw, among the ancient sites, one of the three oldest mosques in the world. They went to Tehran the next day, and then on to Shiraz, Iran, for a week-long stay to inspect the Nemazee Hospital that had recently been opened (see chapter 9); they afterwards made a trip to Karachi, in the new country of Pakistan, before heading on to Madras, where Janeway served as visiting professor of pediatrics for the next two months (to be discussed in chapter 8).

In December, following their visits to Iran and India, the Janeways proceeded homeward, stopping in Rome, Florence, Davos (where they went skiing), and Vienna before returning to France. In Florence, Janeway was taken by Pat Young, an American pediatrician who had organized a research project comparing children in Florence with a similar number in Boston to determine genetic vs. environmental factors in child health, on a visit to a clinic that did not impress him: "Drug companies finance much in departments of medicine . . . a pernicious influence as they expect results."[38] In one hospital he met a pediatrician who was "insecure particularly over hormones he gave to a large number of adolescents," which Janeway attributed to another example, if he needed one, of the bad influence of pharmaceutical companies as a support of academic departments. However, the Ospidale delle Innocenti, built in 1440 by Brunelleschi and featuring wonderful Della Robbia sculptures, won his heart. Here he found expectant unmarried mothers, along with many others nursing their newborn babies. There were new cribs, murals with bright colors, and blue ceilings, imparting a cheery effect.

On New Year's Eve, a train brought the Janeways north from Davos, where they had been skiing. Dr. Stapleton, who was in Vienna, inveigled Janeway to detour and visit a Hungarian refugee camp while Betty went to France. These camps were the result of the recent Soviet invasion of Hungary, and the subsequent stream of refugees into Austria. Janeway was impressed with the work being done at the camp by the Canadian Immigration Service, which was processing some of the 150,000 refugees who had crossed the border for resettlement. In the camp where Stapleton worked, Dr. Janeway came face-to-face with the dismal life of the refugees, who lived in buildings without windows and had no furniture save cots. CAJ was deeply troubled. The disposition of such people, many of them children and adolescents, needed to be decided fast, before they deteriorated. He was most emotionally involved when he talked to families. "Met one wonderful family—mechanic, wife and two kids. He came out 3 weeks ago because, as active volunteer from workers group, feared for his life. Then went back last night, brought out wife and children, 16 kilometers on foot carrying kids. Fine, honest, simple group. Would be an asset anywhere."[39]

After the harrowing experience at the Austrian refugee camps, Janeway was relieved to join Betty in Amsterdam, from which they traveled to London, where they remained for three weeks while CAJ visited Dr. Reginald Lightwood, the chief of pediatrics at St. Mary's Medical School and Paddington Green Children's Hospital, who had been a visiting professor at Boston in 1953 and had delivered the first Blackfan Lectureship that year. During his visit, Dr. Janeway was shown most of the pediatric hospital units in London—the Institute of Child Health, the research part of the better known Great Ormond Street Children's Hospital, and some internal medicine units of other teaching hospitals. He taught students at St. Mary's Medical School, gave lectures to London pediatricians, and was wined and dined almost every evening. Lee, their second daughter, came over to join her parents on this phase of their sabbatical trip. CAJ was impressed with the St. Mary's Home Care program, which cared for children with serious chronic diseases at home, and which had served as the original model for the Family Health Care Program at the Children's in Boston. "Primary objective to demonstrate better services, but wonderful teaching material," was Janeway's brief comment.[40]

Dr. Janeway seems to have been impressed with the work of the research units. He described the research being done with Dr. Rowley, a Reader in Bacteriology at St. Mary's, who enhanced nonspecific resistance in mice by injecting them with killed enteric bacilli, and he gave lectures on resistance to infection at the Great Ormond Street Hospital. He was pleased to meet several of the former exchange residents to the Children's who had been part of the St. Mary's exchange program, and to find them doing well. He had a talk with Dr. Kenneth Cross, a distinguished investigator on newborn physiology, who was being considered for an administrative job but told Janeway he did not wish to leave research.[41] This discussion with Cross occurred only a year or so after consideration of Janeway for the chair at Hopkins and the admonition from Dr. Park that he too should return to the laboratory and devote himself to research. In our opinion, the very fact that CAJ wrote of this conversation with Cross in such detail in his personal diary suggests that at times he was sorry to have left the laboratory. Nonetheless, because he selected outstanding personnel to work in his laboratories, he accomplished the multiple tasks of being an academician-researcher, clinician-administrator better, and for a longer period, than anyone else in academic medicine in the latter half of the twentieth century. At the end of his London trip, Janeway knew all the heads of pediatric departments and research institutes in London on a first-name basis. Many subsequently became visiting professors at Children's in Boston.

Overall, Charles Janeway's 1956 sabbatical made a much wider impact and impression on him than did the teaching of medicine in Britain alone, for it widened his view of medicine in the bigger world and helped him to determine the place of pediatrics in it. If any published work can be considered Janeway's masterpiece, it would be his 1957 philosophic paper, "Pediatricians for Peace;" and it was no accident that its formulation followed on the heels of that 1956 trip, encompassing a great many ideas that he had been developing while abroad and which became an important part of his thinking for the rest of his life. In this paper, Janeway reviewed the progress made in child health in the western world and called attention to new areas of concern, such as adolescence, mental health, and chronic diseases in children, although he noted that in the developing countries the old traditional disease problems were still dominant. He then spoke about the education of pediatricians who came from developing countries for training in the west.[42]

As a result of what he had seen and learned on his sabbatical, Dr. Janeway was concerned that pediatricians coming from developing countries for training in the West would not experience what they most needed to learn at many of the West's best institutions, for their needs at home were public health measures, family planning and preventive medicine, as well as the new curative techniques they were coming to the West to learn. He recommended that there be an exchange of learning on both sides of the world, feeling that such an experience would be beneficial. He then spelled out his vision of a pediatric peace corps program analogous to the then "Atoms for Peace" plan, "which had brought about cooperation between physical and biological scientists all over the world for the general good." Janeway made these remarks three years before President Kennedy initiated his own Peace Corps program. He suggested that pediatricians from the West should spend some time in developing countries (as he had done) and he made it very clear that the program must be associated with the World Health Organization or under UNICEF administration, not any one nation's. His view of pediatrics along a world-wide scheme of things continued to widen and grow, owing to his involvement in the IPA and as a result of additional trips that he would make abroad; for the Janeways added several footnotes to the foregoing account by way of additional European visits from 1957 until 1964.

The first of these took place in April of 1961, approximately five years after the foregoing sabbatical, the main purpose of the trip being to allow CAJ to attend an IPA Executive Committee meeting in Switzerland. However, that business was prefaced with a vacation (with some pediatric matters interposed) in England, Norway, Finland, and Denmark, as well as Switzerland itself, and he and Betty also visited France. At each stop the Janeways stayed with friends, usually pediatric friends, often with pediatricians who had spent some time in Boston. They were treated as royal visitors and, true to Janeway's frugal nature, without the need to pay for hotel accomodations. As usual, Janeway kept a detailed diary of events, doings and thoughts.[43] In London, the first scheduled stop, they lunched with Bernard Schlesinger, a leading British pediatrician, and they spent some time with Reginald Lightwood at his farm. Lightwood had spent time in Iran, which by now had become one of Janeway's main interests, and was enthusiastic about the progress that was being made there and the work that Boston-trained Mohsen Ziai was doing. The Children's exchange program with St. Mary's claimed some of Janeway's attention as he met with Abraham Bergman, then the exchange resident, and arranged for his flat to be used by the following year's resident from the Children's. He also met with a "very nice Scot," an obstetrician he was interested in recruiting for the Nemazee Hospital in Shiraz. His diary devotes an entire page to that interview and the problems of the hospital's financial support. But there are details of much recreation also—shopping, the theater, and sightseeing—in between.

Then Charles and Betty went off to Norway for what was largely a skiing vacation. Their next stop was Finland, where they spent considerable time with Professor Niilo Hallman and his wife, who were now among their closest European friends. In addition to enjoying the pleasures of the Hallmans' summer cottage and hospitality, Dr. Janeway gave a lecture to the Finnish Pediatric Association, was interviewed on local radio about preventive medicine and the problems of adolescence, and was shown cases of congenital nephrosis, a disease first described by Hallman. Except for a brief visit to Copenhagen, the remainder of the trip was devoted to skiing in Switzerland. His diary does contain, however, a long, detailed, almost wide-eyed description of his experiences in Finland, notably his first sauna. Never one to be content with socio-cultural aspects, he commented that the sauna experience raises corticosteroids four-fold for two to three days!

In early December 1961, while on his third trip to Iran on behalf of the Shiraz Medical Center, Dr. Janeway stopped briefly in Athens, where one of his hosts was Dr. Doxiades, a strong proponent of social pediatrics. One of his programs was devoted to illegitimate children. In contrast to other places, where such children were warehoused, Doxiades had developed a program in Athens to assign three such babies to each nurse for an extended period, "As a real foster mother pavilion with babies," Janeway recorded. "Ultimately adopted, but real problem with handicapped and retarded. Quite a paradise."[44] He also made a trip to Ankara, where he was again impressed with the continued progress made by Ihsan Dogramaci. He wrote in his diary about the contrasts with Iran, to which he was now travelling. His diary has a wistful tone, a feeling of what might be accomplished in Iran with leadership there such as Dogramaci's. In Turkey, the cultural history of no landed aristocracy and the location of Dogramaci's hospital in the capital city, where relations with the national government could be more easily maintained, were factors missing from the Iran project that made all the difference. He commented, "Of course, major factor is money, but money comes from the things they do."[45]

In August and September of 1962, Charles and Betty undertook another journey to Europe. Like so many of his trips, their reason this time was another of the International Pediatric Congresses, at the time being held in Lisbon. Prior to the meeting, Charles and Betty and their daughter, Barbie, spent nearly four weeks touring northern Norway (August 8 to September 2). They went by land and sea, north of the Arctic Circle, over difficult terrain requiring a Land Rover automobile, taking long walks along the way and sailing in small ships into fiords. On these treks they were gregarious; in his diary Janeway recorded in detail the wonderful people they met and dined with, and old friends visited, as well as the height of mountains climbed (1847 meters) and the cost per day per person of the trip ($4.50).[46]

In the spring of 1964 (May 4 to June 8), the Janeways traveled to Germany and then to Czechoslovakia and other lands then under Soviet hegemony. In Germany, they found Würzburg a "delight," despite the fact that, as Janeway noted, it had been destroyed in a British air raid in

March 1945, although the city had no strategic targets at all.[47] Janeway made rounds in the local hospital with Professor Stroder, who had been assigned by the Nazis to direct the children's hospital in Krakow, Poland. Stroder made friends with many there, and was even hunted by the Gestapo. He cared for the Polish people so well that the postwar Polish Peoples' Republic honored him with the Gold Badge of the Order of Merit. Janeway commented that "he is the best type of liberal German, a strong humanist who should be backed and helped."[48]

In Prague—by now Janeway had attained his earlier stated wish to come into contact with pediatricians actually behind the Iron Curtain—he gave a lecture to about 100 persons, but noted that it was slow going because each paragraph had to be translated. His diary commented: "Questions after were exhaustive and intelligent."[49] He described in detail the hospital, laboratories, medical education and patient care, "Medical care and service obviously good."[50] Their stay in Prague was short, and their subsequent visit to Warsaw even shorter, only a quick day's tour. The next stop was Krakow, where CAJ received an honorary degree in the Philharmonic Hall. Most of the recipients of honorary degrees at this time were Russian or Polish physicians, but a few were awarded to Americans, including Paul Dudley White and Henry K. Beecher of the Harvard faculty, and Linus Pauling in addition to Janeway.[51]

Following their stay in Poland, Charles and Betty motored with a Hungarian couple through Czechoslovakia into Hungary. Their first stop was in Pec, where Janeway delivered a lecture on protein metabolism. They were exposed to differing views of the then communist country. Their first hosts lived on top of the hill overlooking the city; they still had a large home and vineyards, but they told Janeway that they could not afford to keep it up under the communist regime. Later, at a resort lake, they saw many laboring families on vacation, "who certainly would never have had anything like this week's tour under any other regime. This is positive, as well as books, records, music and plays cheap . . . Only question is, 'how big is the price'."[52] They next went on to Budapest. During the hospital tour, CAJ was concerned to learn that 2,500 abortions were performed in the obstetric department for every 500 deliveries, and the prematurity rate was high owing to the multiple abortions. Among teens, suicide and accident rates were high. A highlight of their Budapest stay was their visit to the home of Alexander Nadas's aunt, who, Janeway was distressed to learn, was with her family among the dispossessed; they had formerly owned their own home but now had only a flat. And Nadas's uncle, a radiologist, had to work from early morning to mid evening just to make ends meet. The Janeways got an earful on the downside of the Russian occupation. Nonetheless, CAJ got a contrary impression of the occupation from his good friend, Dr. Kerple-Fronious, who told that one could freely buy books in English if one knew how to read them and could listen to the Voice of America and the BBC on the radio.[53] At the end of his visit he jotted into his diary, "Alex must go [i.e., visit]. They love him and need him."[54]

On May 20, Charles and Betty were in Berlin and saw the Wall, which was then still new. Janeway found it sad. Here, too, was the stark reality of a Communist country. One suspects that what he would have liked was some combination of socialism and capitalism, for he wrote, as they left for Scandinavia, "Now for Scandinavia where social reform has been made without the Communist price."[55] Copenhagen, their next stop, was another world. "What a contrast," he wrote. "Gone shabby dress, drabness, dirt and the feeling you must look around and see who's there before you talk freely."[56]

After going on to Sweden and staying two days in Göteborg, where Janeway attended hospital rounds and lectured on plasma proteins, they traveled on May 22 to Norway for a three-day vacation visit with friends in Lillehammer, after which they went to Oslo. Then, with Professors Wallgren and Zetterstam, they drove to Uppsala, where, on May 29, CAJ received the Rosen von Rosenstein medal, the most prestigious award a pediatrician could receive. His friend, Bo Vahlquist, who represented the Swedish Pediatric Society on the occasion, was probably responsible for seeing that Janeway received this honor, as he did also with Guido Fanconi and Emmanuel Pepper of New York. This award must have meant much to him, for, in a folder amongst Janeway's papers, labelled "CAJ Honors," is the program from that event, the menu for the formal dinner (to which Betty was also invited), and a brochure about the Castle of Skokloster, which he and Betty must have visited. The Rosen von Rosenstein medal was, in CAJ's mind, a very prestigious award; he was justly proud of it, albeit his diary recorded his embarrassment at not wearing a dark suit during the daytime ceremony: "Everyone dressed up. I felt shabby in tweed jacket and grey flannels." Nevertheless, he gave his lecture on "Problems of Immune Deficiency," and noted that it was, "good, I think." By now Janeway was an inveterate traveller and had seen his share of sophisticated ceremonies, but he was impressed with the formal ceremony in the evening, for he described the seating, dinner menu, speeches, dancing, and decorations, "High point was singing with candles by students from a window above looking down on hall." Subsequently, the Janeways flew to Zürich for an IPA Executive Committee meeting in Fanconi's home.[57]

On the plane trip home, Janeway summarized his impressions. In the Eastern countries, he reflected, a certain amount of economic leveling had been achieved, "but it's leveling down whereas in West Europe it's going up for everyone." He noted further, "The free play of human initiative [in the West] taking advantage of human nature instead of trying to remake it gives a vigor and richness to life . . . which the East somehow lacks . . . If we can avoid war I don't see how we can fail to stay ahead of Communist Europe, but we mustn't underestimate the dedication, the idealism, and the willingness to sacrifice that gives the movement its power."[58] Charles Janeway's views had changed since his college days, when he flirted with communism and utopian ideals.

The 1965–66 Sabbatical:
Travels to Southeast Asia and the Far East

The Janeways devoted a little more than half of the year 1965 and the first two months of 1966 to foreign travel, again to gain a better understanding of the nature of pediatrics and life in two new (to them) countries, Australia and New Zealand. From late March until early June of 1965, he and Betty toured Australia, New Zealand, and also the Philippines; then, after a hiatus of about four months spent at home, the couple made a five-month journey through Korea, Japan, and a number of other Far Eastern countries under the sponsorship of the Alan Gregg Fellowship in Medical Education of the China Medical Board of the Rockefeller Foundation, returning by way of India and Egypt.

There is no evidence in Dr. Janeway's papers to indicate that the first of these two trips was taken as part of a planned sabbatical or had a connection to a sponsored program other than a formal, report-like summary of that trip.[59] However, the later trip in 1965 and into 1966 was undertaken as part of a sabbatical. Ten years had passed since the previous earned leave of absence, and Janeway was due for another period of change and relief from the burdens he had been obliged to shoulder as chairman of the medical department at the Children's Hospital.

On the first of these extended tours Charles and Betty left Boston on March 25, 1965; they returned on June 4. The first stop was in Australia, where they visited the cities of Perth, Canberra, Melbourne, and Sydney over the period of a month. They then spent another month almost entirely in Auckland, New Zealand, and on the way home stayed a week in the Philippines. The previously mentioned undocumented report or summary of their activities during this time began with the comment, "Opportunities were afforded to make observations in the fields of pediatrics, virology, public health practice, the organization of medical education [and] the role of universities in tertiary education, including technical and the general developmental pattern of these two 'new' countries."[60] It would appear, upon reflection, that the two journeys may have been part of a sabbatical taken in two parts, the first funded by the Rockefeller Foundation and the second by its China Medical Board.

In Perth, Janeway gave three lectures and attended three seminars. He noted that there were no university hospitals in Australia that had all clinical services under the full control of a professor; instead, individual clinical pediatricians each had a ward they administered. He was exceedingly impressed with the potential for this area to become a training site for Asian students, and he was intrigued with the possibilities of using marsupials for studying the ontogeny of the development of the immune system.[61] Canberra was the site of the meeting of the Australian Pediatric Society, at which he was one of the visiting professors. He found the papers to be of high order, and that there was a striking degree of cooperation between pediatricians, pediatric radiologists and pathologists, and pediatric surgeons."[62] He was most impressed with the high caliber of the Virus Research Institute in Australia and its concern about the ingress of animal viruses from New Guinea, which could be devastating on health and the nation's economy.[63]

At Melbourne Children's Hospital Dr. Janeway was, as an experiment, given a ward during his stay. He lectured on enterovirus infections, viral vaccines, emergencies in infectious diseases, and acute respiratory obstruction, all different from his usual immunology lectures.[64] Visits to the Fairfield Hospital and the Commonwealth Serum Laboratory, as well as to MacFarlan Burnett's laboratory, and making daily ward rounds, occupied fully his time in Melbourne. Thereafter he went to Sydney, where he spent most of his time in the Royal Alexandria Children's Hospital; here he gave the same lectures and seminars. He was impressed with the vigor and flexibility of Australia and its spirit of "thinking big."[65]

In Auckland, he was impressed that New Zealand's tranquil social security program had a bearing on medicine with a lesser degree of vigor for growth and change than in Australia. He was surprised to find severe rheumatic fever in young Maori children, much as he had seen in India. He was given a ward for a month at the Princess Mary Hospital for Children. He was surprised at the limited amount of money being spent on health promotion, scientific research, and medical education, owing to the good state of health of the population and the environment. New Zealand, he commented, considers itself "as a European outpost; its sense of belonging to Asia is not as deep as in Australia."[66] The British tradition of maintaining pediatrics as a branch of adult medicine was even more apparent in the former colonies than in Britain. On the way home, Charles and Betty spent May 29 to June 4 in the Philippines, where Janeway gave the Luis Guerrero Lecture. The rector of the University of Santos Tomas impressed him for having reduced the size of the entering medical school class from 1,500 to 300. He hoped that the "move to a full-time system will . . . Stimulate all the other Philippine medical colleges toward achieving a higher standard."[67]

The Janeways' later five-month trip to the Far East came about because CAJ was a consultant to a number of medical schools in the region, schools that the China Medical Board now deemed to be in its area of responsibility. (Before the fall of the Republic of China in 1949, this organization had supported the Peking Union Medical College; following the revolution that produced the People's Republic of China, it moved its interest to other areas of the Far East and supported medical education reform in several countries of the region.) Their trip started with South Korea, which had become a primary United States concern following the cessation of hostilities with North Korea in 1954.

Charles and Betty's journey across the Pacific took them first to Hawaii, then to Tokyo, and finally to Seoul, where they were met by a "huge crowd, wildly waving from the roof."[68] Drs. Se Mo Suh and Kwang Wook Ko, both former residents at the Children's, and their families, made up the reception committee. One of their first functions was to visit Yousei University Medical Center, a Christian university where the medical science building had been provided by the China Medical Board. They toured the pediatric wards, apparently to Dr. Janeway's disapproval, owing as much to the presence of religious pictures and the chaplain passing out tracts as to its improper design, "no scrub sinks, no place for parents."[69] At Seoul National University, which they visited on the following day, he was equally unimpressed. The former president had been ousted recently by student demonstration, and a new president, who was alleged to have an armed bodyguard, impressed him as "A man frightened by his new job he didn't ask for, looking for help"[70] Furthermore, its forty-year-old Japanese barnlike building was poorly maintained, "but good work going on."[71] Days passed as CAJ taught and lectured. He compared his experiences in Korea with those in Iran. Korea, he wrote, "seems remarkably stable. The main difference from Iran—this is a country recently liberated from traditionalism but not feudalism. The farmer owns his own land and there is a middle class."[72] He saw problems, however: "1.2 million cases of tuberculosis out of 25 million . . . coolies pulling huge loads . . . and riding bicycles piled 8 feet high with loads . . . more soldiers, both R.O.K. and U.S. than I've seen anywhere."[73] He was later taken to a private clinic that had a few beds for obstetrics as well as pediatrics. The physicians were well trained and were full-time faculty, but could not afford to educate their children on full-time salaries. His comment: "I am not convinced that the full-time system is good for clinical departments of the medical schools of these countries any more than it was when medical education first started in U.S.," no doubt recalling the stress his father faced as the first full-time professor of medicine at Hopkins.[74]

The Janeways got the red carpet treatment on this trip, as they often did while travelling. When they visited the National Museum, they were given a tour by its director. They attended an evening reception hosted by the president of South Korea. Mainly, however, their diaries and letters suggest that medical matters were uppermost in their minds. Visits to other hospitals, lectures and rounds, discussion of diseases endemic to the area always elicited a long description in Janeway's notebook, especially the epidemic hemorrhagic fever that seemed unknown to him before. One comment jumps out of his diary, when speaking of one rounds: "No hand washing till end!"[75] On another day he visited a family planning clinic, where he was impressed with the "Testing variety of methods of reaching people beyond mass media."[76] Dr. Janeway settled into a fairly routine period of work that sometimes kept him busy from 7:45 a.m. to 7:00 p.m., although one weekend (October 14–17) he and Betty took a train trip through the mountains to the east-coast city of Kangun, where they were hosted by a rich winery owner whose daughter had been very ill with dysentery; Kwang Wook Ko had saved her life and Janeway, as that physician's mentor, was being repaid.

Back at work in Seoul, Janeway discussed curriculum with the faculty, trying to help them add electives to the course of study. His days were also filled with rounds of lectures as well as discussions with faculty. Each patient seen was described in detail, but CAJ was discouraged by the difficulty of getting students and interns to provide exact details of a case history.[77] In summarizing his impressions, Janeway commented that "Korea needs to cut numbers in higher education and get quality; it needs to loosen lock-step education to develop initiative and thought; and most of all it needs to develop a vocational practical education, glorifying working with our hands."[78]

Not all dinners that Charles and Betty attended were hosted by Koreans. The Janeways were guests of the American Ambassador one evening. They were among a large, impressive guest list at the eighty-year-old building, said to be the oldest U.S. Embassy in the world. Here again they seemed to find friends wherever they went. Betty saw a woman who had formerly been a Smith College and Winchester School roommate of one of her good friends; she afterwards took the Janeways to lunch at the Officer's Wives Club to hear the Ambassador speak. Betty liked the Ambassador, Winthrop Brown—Yale '29—the cousin of the wife of a pediatrician in Cambridge, Massachusetts. The Janeways shopped for antiques, attended other social events, and spent an entire day at the sports stadium, seeing soccer and rugby games with Betty sitting in an armchair at mid-field next to President Pak. On another evening they were taken to a night club where there were "more and more naked girls in every act . . . what gets me is all the missionaries have been here. They all go 'Ya Hoo'." CAJ was not impressed by formal religion, especially if it seemed insincere.[79]

At a final lecture that Janeway delivered to the Korean Pediatric Society, Janeway was made an honorary member. He commented that "I've . . . lectured more in three weeks than in a year at Harvard."[80] Dr. Janeway's mission from the China Medical Board seems to have led him to meet with several groups that were doing community development work, including the U.S. Agency for International Development officer who wanted to connect Korean researchers with those in the United States via xerographic copies of the Americans' published articles, rather than have Koreans travel to the United States. CAJ felt the plan "has much merit."[81] Dr. Kwang Wook Ko wrote a poignant letter of thanks to Janeway for giving him the opportunity to train in Boston and show that he, as a poor boy who grew up in a tiny village where there was no electric light, had become a professor and director of the children's hospital (he later became president of the university). This must have warmed Janeway's heart and gave him more enthusiasm for offering training in Boston to those who would later provide such leadership in their own countries. Janeway's relation with the China Medical Board was demonstrated when Semo Su wanted to get a flame photometer but had been turned down by the board. CAJ wrote in his notes, "Urge CMB to help."[82]

One day Janeway was taken to a contagious-disease ward of a hospital and was disturbed by "no hand washing till end of all rounds, charts all over beds, screens on windows in typhoid room but open to let air and light in. Only isolation is geographical."[83] On a visit to a rural health center he was disappointed by the lack of patients and was told that only about 10% of the population used the center. He suggested that they use home visiting nurses, as was the practice in Turkey.

A visit to a Protestant mission hospital in Taegu impressed him as the, "best I've seen yet," but he was worried by the evangelizing. "Christianity does mean something but wish there wasn't so much evangelizing. And wish they seemed more [in tune] with Korean culture—i.e., they built a Gothic cathedral that sticks out like a sore thumb."[84] At a Maryknoll Sisters hospital, where a Duke-trained pediatrician was doing a good job, he was impressed with the outreach, home nurse visiting. He commented, "Less self conscious in some way than Protestant missionaries. Their chapel made to make Koreans feel at home—mats on floor."[85] In summarizing his trip to Korea to that time, Janeway noted that Korean medical education was good in the best schools, but that clinical material and training were too limited while lectures were overemphasized. He noted that hospitals were fair, with the mission hospital the best; however, the government had no real disease-prevention program and that private practice in cities resulted in intense competition for paying patients. He thought that government support was needed for private institutions; that missionaries would have to give ground on evangelism; and that pregnancy was the most serious public health problem in Korea.[86]

From November 3 through 5 Janeway organized a large medical congress in Seoul to share with Koreans some modern medical advances. The speakers were to go on to the IPA Congress in Tokyo and included several American pediatricians as well as some from Europe. It attracted 400 attendees. Janeway had organized the meeting to demonstrate the relationship of basic patho-physiology to clinical disease with an emphasis on prevention. The participants left the pre-congress meeting on November 5 for Tokyo and the International Congress (described earlier). After the IPA Congress, Charles and Betty toured Japan from November 12 to 21, returning to Korea on November 21. Coming back was like coming home, with Se Mo and Kwang Wook meeting them. Janeway went back to teaching in Korea and was still concerned with the didactic lecture system.

On a train trip to the country, Janeway was so concerned about the "coughing, spitting and drunken" passengers that when he returned to

the hotel he "washed and gargled and prayed for health."[87] His exposure to social pediatrics continued with visits to large orphanages and
to an anti-tuberculosis project. He and Betty visited rural health centers and South Korean medical schools, obtaining an even more extensive view of Korean medicine and culture. He was besieged by young
doctors who wanted to come to the United States. It is clear that
Charles and Betty developed a real affection for the Korean people they
met. Before departing, they threw a party, featuring a hired folk dance
troup, for over 100 guests. When they left Korea on December 5,
Janeway noted in his diary, "To airport—large crowd, about 20 to see
us off, 3 bunches of flowers each. Could have cried as we turned for
last look at wildly waving group on airport tarmac. Good people.
Hope they can make it."[88]

Charles and Betty were in Japan from December 5 to 11, staying at
International House, which was "built by private donations, mainly
Japanese, plus Rockefeller family funds."[89] At Tokyo University he discussed curriculum and gave one of his stock lectures on the development of immunology. The contrast with Korea in the type of patients
seen was clear; few had infectious diseases and many had allergies.
"Research the big thing—source of funds commercial—small government budget . . . Tokyo University would not think of appointing new
professor except from Tokyo University graduates. Autopsy percentage—about 70–80% in pediatrics—less in rest of hospital."[90] On a day
of great significance for Americans, Janeway wrote in his diary, "Pearl
Harbor Day—no mention in Japanese papers."

In Tokyo, Janeway also visited St. Luke's Hospital, with its cross on
top. "What a difference," he noted, "Spotlessly clean, good medical
care obvious . . . One would have no hesitation being a patient here,"
the ultimate accolade.[91] While he toured the hospital, Betty was shown
its social service department. His impressions from what he had seen
up to then: "Tokyo University—emphasis all on research, not patient
care . . . Japanese Professor too powerful, he holds fate of all in his
hands. Has low salary, so has to work for Pharmaceutical Companies
(dangerous). And student who gets degrees from him give him presents (equally dangerous)." After their visit, Charles and Betty received
lavish hospitality and presents. At Keio University, they were given a
wonderful Japanese dinner—"hate to think of expense"—and again

presents. "Very nice," Janeway recorded, "but I wish they wouldn't outdo themselves so in giving presents."[92] During their Japanese tour the Janeways visited Hiroshima, which elicited emotions common to most Americans, "very impressive and guilt producing."[93] In addition to tourist activities, CAJ attended a medical conference in Kyoto, where he reported on immunological disorders. And so ended their visit to Japan.

The Janeways spent the week of December 11–18 in what Americans then referred to as Formosa, now known as Taiwan. Sightseeing, ceremonial dinners, presentations of medical education in Taiwan, as well as health programs in the country, were all duly noted by Dr. Janeway in his diary, as also were causes of death in children and other statistics. They were happy to see at a maternal and child health center that UNICEF had provided bicycles for the midwives to conduct family planning services and deliveries in the home. The first part of their visit concentrated primarily on public health, on visits to supplemental milk programs, pure water supply systems, farms, and to a new university in the country. In Taipei, Janeway paid more of the usual visits to laboratories and medical schools. There was an obvious presence of American physicians: Dr. David Barr, former chair of medicine at Cornell; Dr Russell Alexander, an epidemiologist from Seattle; Dr. Ward Bullock, formerly of Yale, and others. Bullock and Alexander were doing work that interested Janeway a great deal, for his diary records much detail about their research; however, he noticed that there was not much involvement of Taiwanese physicians in the research. There was an obvious presence of U.S. AID as well. A dynamic Taiwanese physician, identified only as Dr. Hsu, told Janeway of his success in getting Madame Chang Kai-shek to approve a $30,000,000 program to supply 600,000 IUDs in five years with a goal of getting population increases below 2.0%. CAJ commented that he is "Like Martha Eliot, very smart politician to win support and to carry out program at grass roots level."[94]

At the National Taiwanese University medical school Janeway was briefed on the curriculum, which was similar to that in the United States. He commented that while the school had a Japanese tradition, it had "gone American fast" in recent years.[95] He was impressed by the new buildings and laboratories, provided in part by the China Medical

Board as well as by the military presence that was all about. Dr. Barr took him to the National Defense Medical Center, an institution much like the Walter Reed Army Medical Center in Washington. CAJ noted, "This is PUMC [Peking Union Medical School], has had CMB plus ICA and China Lobby support, but clearly superior to anything seen elsewhere."[96] The Veterans Hospital was even more impressive. Again, the presence of an American, William Jordan, a visiting professor, helped CAJ suppress his natural qualms about the military. They had made a superior medical school, in stark contrast to a new school, Taipei Medical College, which had been started by successful practitioners "to provide scientific doctors to replace quacks." After seeing that school, CAJ wrote, "I would be scared of product now, Brave attempt but [needs] vision and courage."[97] He also recorded that there were then six medical schools in Taiwan and that he had visited them all. The pace was maddingly fast, and while he kept detailed notes on each place, he seems not to have reached any general conclusions about the state of Taiwanese medical education.

The Janeways spent only three days (December 18–21) at their next stop, the Philippines. He was immediately impressed with its difference from other Asian countries: "The country—culture very reminiscent of Mexico, Spanish culture including disregard of high birth rate, paternalism, happy-go-lucky, poor-rich contrast, with friendly nice Asian people."[98] He gave his usual lectures, made ward rounds, was made an honorary member of the Philippine Pediatric Society, toured hospitals, and saw many UNICEF projects separately. He was impressed with the Children's Hospital Center and with Dr. Fe Del Mundo, whom he described as an indomitable, dedicated woman, and how the hospital stood in stark contrast to the University of Philippines General Hospital, which he described as "really disgraceful." He was impressed with the wide range of pathology he saw in the Philippines. He saw a hopeful note at Catholic University, however, which had a family planning clinic. Betty was even more concerned with the population problem, for, after the meeting, she met "a charming young American Jesuit," and related, "I openly discussed family planning with him!"

The Janeways spent a little more than a week (December 22–31) in Hong Kong, staying at the apartment of a pediatrician friend, Dr.

Eleina Field. They visited the usual child health services of the Department of Social Welfare, including a settlement house, nursery school, a health clinic and "too neat" housing estates. Christmas was spent in part visiting hospitals, where each service had a party. On another day, Charles and Betty were taken to several different housing projects, from squatters' shacks to the new, huge high-rise apartments. They were impressed that 40,000 people, 8,000 families, were housed in one high rise, with the "marvelous city hall—restaurants, and theater, concert hall, big courtyard, art museum and crowded."[99] On the evening of December 28, Dr. Janeway gave a lecture on staphylococcal infections; another evening, he visited the basic science facility. To Janeway, Hong Kong was a marvelous laboratory in which to study urbanization, crowding and the Chinese capacity to adapt.[100] It was clear that Janeway was thinking much more about the role of social factors in health than he had before. Betty's notes show that they spent a good deal of time discussing the future of Hong Kong when it reverted to China.

The Janeway's visit to Cambodia was also short (December 31, 1965 to January 2, 1966). Part of it was devoted to attaining a long-sought goal: "We took advantage of New Year's weekend to visit the ancient ruins of Angkor."[101] In their flight over southern Vietnam, they viewed hilly jungles that had no vegetation and commented on the defoliation that had been caused, presumably, by American troops. They spent only one and a half days at Angkor, "not enough time to do justice to the place."[102]

The Janeways spent January 2–10 in Bangkok, Thailand. An old friend, Dr. Thavi Tantiwangse, who was at Children's Hospital Medical Center from 1955 to 1958, paved the way. In Bangkok, Dr. Janeway got more involved with the medical schools and hospitals. At Siriraj Medical School and hospital, the oldest, brought up to modern standards a generation before through the aid of the Rockefeller Foundation, they found a large volume of patients, 350 beds, 120 bassinets, 200 outpatient visits per day and much pathology, including a good deal of inherited diseases such as thalassemia and glucose-6-phosphate dehydrogenase deficiency. It was a wonderful place to study infectious (acute hemorrhagic) fever, hereditary and respiratory diseases, and a new and growing problem—many abandoned children.[103] On January 4, Dr.

Janeway had dinner with a group of old CHMC fellows and residents. On January 6, he and Betty flew north to the new medical school supported by U.S. AID, the University of Illinois, and the Rockefeller Foundation, at Chiengmai. "Don't ever think that the tropics lack diseases of the north," was Janeway's comment. "Strep throat, glomerulonephritis, nephrosis and rheumatic fever with both carditis and joint symptoms are common . . . there are unique diseases besides."[104] Janeway was concerned with the population increase that likely was related to some of these diseases, but noted that the Thais "are now waking up and starting family planning."[105] He visited all departments and met with the dean, who mentioned his problems with the faculty, which CAJ duly noted, "Work at play, play at work. They will work ears off for celebrations or parties but not at regular work." He commented, "Many things like Shiraz, but seem more gentle, less driving, easier to work with but harder to enthuse than Iranians."[106] In addition to the time spent in India (January 15–30, 1966, see chapter 8), during this long trip Dr. Janeway spent time in Iran (February 1–6, see chapter 9), Egypt (February 6–10), Switzerland for a skiing vacation, France (February 12–20), and Britain (February 24–March 1). "We're on the home stretch," Betty wrote in her letter home, "having skipped Afghanistan reluctantly because of transportation difficulties, we're full of impressions of India, Iran and the UAR [United Arab Republic; Egypt]."[107]

In Cairo, their next stop, they could see the pyramids from their bedroom window at their host's home. The host, Dr. Namet Haskem, had trained in hematology at the Children's. Betty commented on the strains evident in the country: mail was opened and censored; Dr. Haskem did not slow down as they drove past President Nasser's home for fear her license place number would be recorded; newspapers were full of anti-Americanism because of United States support of Israel. Nevertheless, "the revolution here has been a real one . . . it is planned socialism, but definitely not communist," she noted.[108] Janeway believed that although the Egyptian government was committed to socialism, it was trying to draw the best from the East and West, and that Egypt had a tremendous drive to be leader of the Arab world, suppressing criticism and subversion from both the right and left and intrigues in the affairs of other Arab countries."[109]

Janeway's Cairo diary recorded the usual visits to the dean of the Cairo University Medical School for talks on medical education, and to the Children's Hospital, where he gave a lecture. He and Betty were also shown a model community center that UNICEF had established in Cairo, which Janeway described as containing "mothers' clubs, fathers' clubs, and a family planning unit, social work as well as health care. An impressive program of training and research."[110] He was also impressed with "the pure water from deep wells . . . and latrine installations . . . given free. These have cut ascariasis from 47% to 7%, hookworm only slightly"[111] Dr. Haskem took them to various hospitals and laboratories. She had a National Institutes of Health Grant arranged by L. Emmet Holt, Jr. About this CAJ commented that the money was well spent, as Dr. Haskem was doing "a beautiful job and has a good group," although a rival group was trying to undermine her efforts.[112] At another hospital he gave a lecture on staphylococcal infections and was embarrassed by the flowery introduction given him. His final diary entry in his visit to Cairo was upbeat. After a visit to a UNICEF training and demonstration clinic he wrote: "a first class institution . . . with a model community center" that included a family planning center.[113] Family planning had become, by this time, CAJ's highest priority in the developing world.

The Janeways returned home by way of Switzerland, Paris, and London. In the first, they met Lee and her husband and their grandson, and Carlie and his wife, and skied and skied and skied! In Paris, they dined with the Masses and Debrés. They had been away four and a half months, living out of suitcases. When they departed for home on the first of March, Janeway wrote in his diary, "Off for home—now die refreshed."

One offshoot of his Asian trip was a paper Dr. Janeway wrote upon his return and presented at the dedication of the Wyler Children's Hospital at the University of Chicago in August 1966. In that paper, entitled "Asia: Home to Half the World's Children," he wrote that Asia "is too vast an area to portray adequately in a brief address, but I hope I can bring you some sense of feeling of common humanity, which is the smile of every healthy child and in the apathy and misery of every sick one, as well as some appreciation of the tremendous problems and the great suffering going on throughout this part of the world to give

children an opportunity for a healthier life."[114] It was a source of satisfaction to him that most of the Asian students who had come to the
United States and then returned to their own countries were making
important contributions to medical teaching, giving superior care to
patients, and sometimes carrying out clinical investigation. He did not
subscribe to—and refuted—the allegation that it was a waste of time
to train international students because most would stay in the United
States. He was most impressed with what two international agencies,
UNICEF and WHO, were doing by providing expert personnel from
all over the world: "The minuscule sums they are investing in the
health of the coming generation, when compared to the fearful cost of
war and our military assistance programs, are doing more good to root
out the causes of instability in the developing countries than you can
imagine." And, voicing his opposition to the then current events, he
stated that "it is tragic evidence of our failure to solve the world's basic
problems that the U.S. Government spends as much in two days on the
war in Vietnam as UNICEF and WHO spend in a year all over the
world."[115]

8 THE ENCHANTMENT OF INDIA

INDIA OCCUPIED a special place in the hearts and minds of the Janeways. It was there that they chose to spend a substantial part of their 1956 sabbatical, and to which they returned in 1966 and again in 1977. In view of their international outlook, they were curious to find what they, from a developed country, might do to help a different culture and a developing democracy. They always felt the need to share their good fortune with those less fortunate. In a letter to Dr. John Weir, Associate Director of the Rockefeller Foundation, Charles Janeway revealed some of the reasons for visiting this vast subcontinent at that time:

> In selecting India, I have done so, not so much for the academic advantages which it might offer as its importance in regard to relations with United States. My objectives in wanting to go to the Far East are several. First, I want see at first hand the pediatric problems in an underdeveloped area. Second, I wish to get a sense of the level of medical education in these countries since we are getting many students from these areas. It is important that we learn how to train them best for what they will return to. Third, and as a very important by-product . . . I will have the opportunity to act as an ambassador at large . . . for our country. It is in this later regard that I have thought particularly of India because India is the largest and most important free country in the Far East and is one little understood by Americans and yet is crucial as a bastion of democracy.[1]

Dr. Janeway and his family were wonderful ambassadors at large; the family, notably their daughter, Anne, were forever attached to India after their first visit. Madras was probably chosen as their focal point because Professor S.T. Achar, the first head of a department of pediatrics in India, had spent some time in Boston. CAJ admired him and wanted to help him establish his department.

Since the trip was sponsored by the Rockefeller Foundation, which helped arrange the Pakistan and India portion of the trip, Mr. M.C. Balfour, based in New Delhi, India, and director of the Medical Education and Public Health division of the Foundation, wrote to suggest an itinerary and arranged a dinner party on the Janeways' arrival in Delhi. In CAJ's files is a long letter from Balfour outlining people and places he should visit in India. Balfour noted, "I am pleased to know that Mrs. Janeway will accompany you. For a mother with four children she has certainly been active. There are several schools of social work in India, notably in Delhi and Bombay . . . Surely there will be many opportunities for her to observe and advise."[2] Betty did not go along only for the social and touristic aspects. She visited hospitals with CAJ and in addition visited social work programs, day care centers, agricultural developments, and schools. She gave CAJ added insights to the countries and the non-medical institutions. Theirs was a partnership in all ways.

The Janeways left Iran on September 30, 1956 for Karachi, the capital of the newly independent Pakistan. Their arrival occurred shortly after Muslim refugees had come from India after Pakistan was partitioned from India but before Bangladesh had separated from Pakistan. Charles and Betty found Karachi to be a "raw" city: modern homes were surrounded by refugee camps of tents and cardboard.[3] Pakistan was intended by the Rockefeller Foundation as the family's first stop on the Indian subcontinent mainly as a way of orienting them to this vast area. Dr. Janeway met with U.S. AID groups and visited the Microbiological Institute in Karachi, where he got his first view of the differences between the previous British organization of medical research; that is, institutes that did little teaching and little patient care compared to the integrated form in U.S. medical schools.

Dr. Kingsland, a former Boston physician now with the international aid groups in Pakistan, pressed his view on Dr. Janeway that "they should have put their emphasis on teaching in medical school departments in realistic situations rather than by training teachers in unrealistic situations [i.e., research institutes] with no roots."[4] Kingsland felt that "the only way is for some American institution to take over one medical school for a good period of time, so Americans can revolutionize system and work side by side with Pakistanis and really indoctrinate them."[5] While this was in a broad sense CAJ's vision for Iran and India, it is unlikely that he would have used the word "indoctrinate;" he would have preferred "educate." But Kingsland's view that "This is a real U.S. obligation"[6] coincided with Janeway's view as well.

After a visit to the Director General of the Health Service, Janeway noted that he was an "honest, dedicated public servant, whose only flaw is a devotion to British system of 'qualifications'."[7] There is a bit of "inside" humor in his description of the minister's office: CAJ recorded that the minister "was slumped behind desk with papers piled a foot high covering whole desk (made me feel better),"[8] an allusion to his own desk at Boston, where papers also were piled high. Janeway was impressed with the job being done by American engineers to develop a safe water supply. "These down to earth guys with technical know how are our best ambassadors. They're not afraid of anyone, blunt, they know their stuff and there's none of the high level nonsense of the striped pants big shots."[9]

Kingsland had told Janeway that Pakistan was receiving $100,000,000 a year from the United States, while India, with a population several times larger, was receiving only $60,000,000. CAJ's note about that was "Ideological?" One of the International Cooperation Administration (ICA) officials said that his biggest problem was "visiting congressmen."[10] Janeway was concerned about the failure to meet basic needs owing to "political fiddling"[11] caused by conflict within the political parties, some wanting a pure Muslim country, while others desired a truly democratic one. He felt very sympathetic toward the efforts of a "country trying to lift itself by its own bootstraps"[12] without the oil revenues that Iran could use to help pay for modernization.

Balfour had advised him that he need not spend much time in Pakistan. (Balfour, as the Foundation representative for India, may have been prejudiced.) Dr. Janeway had his own contacts there, but he did spend only a few days. It was apparent that he was not happy with the theocracy. The split with East Pakistan, later called Bangladesh, was festering. CAJ's comment about the feud was "Their arguments sound hollow to me and totally irrelevant in a country which is disorganized

and trying to get on its feet. It is a theocratic state which seems anach-
ronistic."[13] It was "democratic" India that he was anxious to visit.

Charles and Betty arrived in New Delhi on October 4. The start was
not auspicious; they were not met at the airport, they did not know
what hotel they were going to, and no one was able to cash travelers'
checks. They eventually contacted Balfour and settled into life at the
Cecil (hotel), where they were impressed with "an old British tradition
we're not likely to live . . . again . . . a bearer brings us tea at 7 and after
drinking it in bed, we take a plunge in the pool. If we play tennis we
have three ball boys and a marker who lends us his racket or makes a
fourth at doubles."[14] They attended orientation courses the first three
days of their visit and met a number of Americans: members of the
press, professors on sabbatical, fellows on Fulbright scholarships, and
Hugh Leavell, Professor of Public Health at the Harvard School of
Public Health, who was working on a community health program in
Indian villages. Janeway spent each day at the Rockefeller Foundation
offices but spent much of his diary on the, to him, "incredible street
scenes; crowds, people sleeping on the streets, sacred cows interrupting traffic, lepers being pushed in wooden home made carts and
men carrying huge loads on their heads."[15] Balfour had arranged
for "official" calls to a hierarchy of ministers, the ICA U.S. mission,
UNICEF, and WHO; the Rockefeller Foundation arranged the many
visits and provided introductions to government officials and medical
school faculty. Janeway was amazed at the number of outside agencies
working with the Indian ministries and, while there were attempts to
coordinate their efforts, it was clear that there was overlap and lack of
coordination.

Janeway possessed that awareness of the cultural subtleties he encountered on all his international visits, even this first prolonged one in
1956. He was also learning. He met with the Minister of Health, as
well as Point IV and WHO officials. The Rockefeller Foundation, interested in improving medical education, and the Ford Foundation, interested in health education as part of its community development program, were educating CAJ. The ministry of health had asked him to
give four lectures, so every afternoon, from 4 p.m. on, was spent in a
lecture hall at Lady Hardinge Medical College before a large crowd. He
also visited several outpatient clinics, where over 400 patients a day

were seen by one full-time staff, two registrars and four house physicians, and toured the new Children's Hospital, "where the Russians have sent a full time team who are running the show."[16] He was generally pleased with the Russian-run children's hospital, but was disappointed that it excluded mothers. He was also bewildered by "Much physiotherapy hocus pocus—oodles of fancy Russian electrical equipment . . . After my visit what I'd bring to India would be a first rate lab technician who could set up micromethods + lab procedures close to patients and doctors who need training."[17]

Fourteen pages of Janeway's diary list references about India and detailed tables of health and population statistics. He was a collector of facts as the basis for his conclusions. The Janeways did not spend all their time collecting facts, however. They relished the opportunity to see the countryside and the great tourist spots as well. A day's trip to Agra to see the Taj Mahal and its surroundings led them to exclaim, "bigger and more beautiful than we'd expected."[18]

Back at work, Dr. Janeway continued to get briefings from the big agencies. He saw first hand the lack of coordination between the multiple agencies, both Indian and foreign. While the Indians had a coordinating council (to try linking the Ministry of Health with WHO, the Rockefeller and Ford Foundations, and ICA), there was still much duplication. CAJ's lecture one afternoon to the Lady Hardinge Medical College focused on a survey of American pediatrics. The following day he went to the Irwin Hospital, where he was amused by a sign on the wall: "822 beds . . . Occupancy 917!"[19] Professor Dr. Pran N. Taneja, chief of pediatrics, was a "young, attractive, able man. Slated for service at the All India Institute, he has DPH and FRCP accreditations but no research experience."[20]

Dr. Janeway certainly felt that research was needed and was impressed with the opportunities for research that were unexplored in India, but with only two senior physicians at Irwin Hospital, it seemed unrealistic to think that there would be much time for research. (Taneja was later to come to Boston for some exposure to research, spending six months with Dr. Samuel Katz in the Enders laboratory, where he worked on measles, a great problem among the children of India.)[21] Then, as now, it was difficult for an American physician to appreciate the sheer volume of patients' needs in India without seeing it firsthand. Janeway saw an example of the huge patient load in the out-patient department at Taneja's hospital, "incredible jam of people re-quiring cops to control . . . in pediatric clinic mothers shrieking to get in."[22] He found the wards simple but pleasant, having been built by UNICEF, but he was unhappy, as he always was when there was inade-quate hand-washing facilities, "only one scrub sink in a side room for 20 beds!"[23] Later that day, in another hospital, CAJ noted that it "had more scrub sinks . . . than most but no rigid individual isolation."[24]

At another hospital he visited, Janeway's belief in research was confirmed by the presence of a young physiologist who had, under a Rockefeller Foundation grant, spent a year at Yale and then received a grant to study central nervous system control of vegetative and regula-tory function in various animals. He had discovered two centers in the hypothalamus that controlled anorexia and another that regulated ap-petite. He too was slated to go to the All India Institute for Medical Science. It was evident that the "best and brightest" young Indian phy-sicians were being drawn away from smaller hospitals to this central, showcase institute. CAJ visited the Institute and his diary contains sev-eral pages of statistics about it. He was impressed with the young, good, bright, staff but noted, "lots of teaching as everywhere but less time for research."[25] But soon, Charles and Betty had to continue their journey.

The next stop was Lucknow, where the schedule was much the same: visits to the hospitals, five lectures given by Janeway, and sight-seeing plus nightly dinner parties. Janeway commented that "Pediatrics here about where we [the United States] were in 1910."[26] He had added a lecture based upon the Survey of American Pediatricians to his usual lectures on infectious diseases and immunology. This outline of the state of American pediatrics in the 1950s was of great interest to Indi-ans. Most of Dr. Janeway's work was at the Gandhi Memorial Hospital, about which, Betty commented, "The new 80 bed Children's Unit is quite a contrast to C.H. [the Children's Hospital in Delhi] . . . wards of 6–10 beds are light and airy."[27] They were impressed by all the mothers or deputy-grandmothers, or sisters, staying in the hospital with their children, "in spite of dreary hospital construction. Mothers sleep there, so climb in bed with child. Children more relaxed than at Russian hospital." Dr. Janeway thought highly of a young pharmacologist who "got badly treated in Boston. I could scream, as he's best man I met."[28]

At Lucknow, as was usual at the conclusion of the tour of each city he visited, Janeway outlined several major impressions, made a list of existing problems, and suggested solutions. These were sent to the Rockefeller Foundation, but it is not clear what, if anything, happened as a result. One can sense his frustration at the close of each of these four or five day visits to the major medical schools in India. They all had the same intractable problems of lack of money, too many students, and overwhelming numbers of patients. But, ever the optimist, Dr. Janeway kept meeting with dozens of people at each stop and sharing his perceptions of what needed to be done to improve medical care and medical education in a developing country such as India. Becoming discouraged or admitting failure were not part of his psyche. He continued to push for more research training but was most impressed with the effort in some places to develop urban and rural health centers that emphasized prevention. This would become especially clear to him in a program he visited on his next stop, Calcutta. Here, as in Lucknow, he felt that Western physicians "must train people to encompass curative and preventive services and do it with less equipment and help than was possible in the West.[29] He was also exposed to those who felt that medicine was not the highest priority for a developing country, was beginning to question whether Western medicine was the right answer for a developing country such as India. In later diary entries he wrote repeatedly that community development, population control and preventive services should be the priorities.

Dr. Janeway recognized that progress would come from strengthening agricultural services as well as medical services. He and Betty wanted to see village life; they were taken to one that had an Extension Training School, with models of latrines, showers, and pure water as well as medical facilities such as clinics. The dean of the medical school, however, warned them that most villages were not like this one, that most were totally unimproved. They were impressed with the model, a multi-purpose work: starting at the bottom, getting the cooperation of the people and selling the program.

Before visiting Calcutta, they spent two days (October 15 and 16) in Benares, the holy city on the Ganges. In Benares, they thought their hotel, Clarke's, was "the pleasantest we've stayed in . . . until they discovered that a rat got in and chewed pieces out of both shoulders of Charlie's best suit!"[30] They viewed the holy days, during which thousands bathed in the flooded river. In Calcutta, CAJ gave four lectures at various institutes and medical schools, and the morning of the second day he and Betty visited a rural health center that they found "more fascinating than the Lucknow villages . . . which Dr. Chaudhuri—a charming man with a very attractive doctor wife—has dreamed, planned and built on his own."[31]

After a weekend of leisure, Charles and Betty were off again to Singur, a rural health clinic twenty-three miles away, "eighteen of them hair raising, 30–40 miles per hour down narrow concrete roads with people, animals, bicycles on both sides . . . Somehow nobody got killed. Why I don't know."[32] He was impressed with this health center as a service but was "Not sure students stay long enough or get hands dirty enough."[33] He liked the model of a community center integrated with economic development, nutrition, agricultural modernization, education, especially of the mothers, and health services. The research carried on in this center pleased him. His lectures at every place exemplified modern science but also were a means to an end, leading to better health through integrated services. Research, education, and services were of equal importance to him, but he believed, and tried to emphasize, that they should be pursued together rather than be separated in different institutions.

On October 23 they reached Madras, their main destination. The Janeways were to spend almost two months there (until December 13) while CAJ worked as visiting professor. During the trip they made a two-day side trip to Vellore and visited Ceylon (November 10–17) and Indonesia (November 18–26). Why did Dr. Janeway pick Madras for a prolonged stay? His diary provides no clue, but it appears that Professor Achar probably was the lure: he had recently been appointed the first professor of pediatrics in India; all previous pediatricians were appointed in departments of internal medicine because, as will be noted later, internal medicine resisted the separation of pediatrics from medicine. In addition, Janeway wanted to immerse himself in one hospital long enough to understand its problems. Achar, Chief of Pediatrics there, was well known for his work with pediatric cirrhosis of the liver, and this fact also may have attracted CAJ as an opportunity to see and study a disease with which he was not familiar, perhaps in hope of finding an immunological cause.

Janeway was appointed to the staff of the Madras Medical College and kept a regular schedule of alternate daily teaching with Prof. Achar. Betty observed the institution keenly. "On our first visit I counted 10 little girls in a row on the floor, . . . but with 50 children's beds there is never room enough."[34] One of the other students, Dr. N. Sundaravalli, who later spent some time at the Children's in Boston, reported that in his teaching Dr. Janeway stressed a good detailed history and a thorough clinical examination. "Many of us did not make otoscopic exams as a routine and we learnt its importance after his visit." Sundaravalli also related that Janeway came to know the clinical trials in children with childhood cirrhosis and conducted trial treatments with steroids and gamma globulin. Because gamma globulin was expensive, the trials were limited to a very few children. As soon as he returned home, however, Janeway sent enough gamma globulin to last for two years.[35]

As a footnote to this story, Dr. Sundaravalli reported that when she later went to Boston for study and research, she was surprised to see Dr. Janeway himself waiting to receive her at the airport. She added, "An international authority in pediatrics was so simple and carried my luggage himself."[36] Few chairs, then or now, go out of their way for such visiting fellows. A medical social worker and a nurse from Dr. Achar's institute also described how Janeway included them in all rounds and "imbibed in us the team spirit." His humanity shone through: "Everyone knows Dr. Janeway's clinical acumen and academic brilliance, but few know the love and affection friends from India received from him, which was unique."[37] Janeway published one paper during this stay, a privately printed outline of his educational philosophy. Produced on the occasion of the Eighth Annual Conference of the Indian Association of Pathologists and the Committee Meetings of the Indian Council of Medical Research, this was one of his first forays outside the world of infectious diseases, immunology, and plasma proteins. In it he outlined his belief that research must be a part of medical education.[38]

Janeway described the Madras general hospital in his usual detailed way. He observed that the Indian offices were "all the same—bleak, bare, piles of records. Files etc. of terrible quality, frayed paper tied together with string. Big overhead fan which cools you but blows papers around . . . Achar avoided isolation of a Children's Hospital, instead remained in Madras General Hospital."[39] Janeway was especially concerned with the lack of good lighting in the wards, "3 dim hanging bulbs—impossible to see anything." Achar and his colleagues had a six-bed study unit where many liver biopsies were performed in connection with their well-known work with cirrhosis. Janeway was interested in why so much cirrhosis occurred in India, feeling that it was caused by hepatitis but was intrigued by the clinical observations. "Funny thing—familial incidence in 20–30%. One man, two wives—1st all sibs well; 2nd, 4 boys, all got cirrhosis. More in middle class. Not seen in very poorest classes."[40] He was always anxious to see therapy given and pondered in his notes, "Could do two things; 1: Use lots of cortisone to prevent fibrosis; 2: give gamma globulin to supply antibody and quiet down necrosis."[41]

The wards of the hospital were filled with preventable diseases: malnutrition, diarrhea, infectious diseases. He observed, wryly, "I don't feel they put enough emphasis on prevention . . . How, Mr. know it all? All you have to do is change the pattern of life that's gone on for 3,000 years!"[42] After outlining the steps he would advocate, Janeway recorded his recommendations to improve the situation: "I think weak link is health education + concerted will to defer hospital and curative medicine improvements until health needs really filled. They've got to get tough on latter and have cultural and social anthropologists at All India Institute of Hygiene working with expert advertising men to work out effective approach to the masses."[43] Ordinary life for the Janeways in Madras was different. Betty wrote, probably with tongue in cheek, that Madras was a prohibition state and that, while they had come with a bottle of scotch, they were running low, so "Charlie applied for a permit stating that he was an addict and needed 8 units of liquor a month."

World affairs were on Dr. Janeway's mind, even here. His diary entry for November 3 reads, "Hard to think of anything but war."[44] The Egyptians had seized the Suez Canal and English-French forces had bombed Egyptian airfields while Israeli troops had invaded the Sinai peninsula. CAJ reports, "Little sympathy [*i.e.*, in India] for British-French position, less awareness of Arab-Egyptian intransigence—hope to God way found to stop it." In fact, the United States and the Soviet Union joined in pressuring the English and the French, and a cease fire was arranged on November 6. At about the same time, the Soviets invaded Hungary. Janeway observed, "At first it seemed as though India and most of Asia would see only the mote in England's eye and not the beam in Russia's eye, but both Nehru . . . and the papers have linked them as parallel instances of aggression."[45] Betty was even more angry at Britain, fulminating about "Eden's policy incredibly stupid example of relying on military force and overlooking the minds of men . . . just when Russia was unmasking the nature of her imperialism [by invading Hungary] . . . the whole case for democracy and morality . . . of the West has been spoiled."[46] The Janeways were for peaceful resolution of these national tensions. In the United States they hoped that, now that Eisenhower had been re-elected, the U.S. could find a way to admit China to the United Nations, although they felt it was "too bad to waste a good man like Stevenson . . . we really should have a coalition government."[47]

On November 13 the Janeways departed on their excursion to Ceylon. The visit lasted only five days. There, Janeway was most impressed with Dr. deSilva, the professor of pediatrics in Columbo, "a good candidate for the Blackfan Lecturer . . . A real feel for preventive health work. Probably most able man in this part of world."[48] CAJ's diary during that visit is filled with page after page of statistics about Ceylon: health, diseases, hospital beds, history, and economics. The children's hospital in Colombo, built in 1951, was the "most attractive I've seen in the East. School much more up and coming than most places I've been except Lucknow . . . what a contrast to Indian provincial offices . . . many things about Ceylon people seem more western and more on the ball. But basic socio-economic and health problems the same." (Most impressive to him was a "scrub sink available and used.")[49]

The Janeways' Indonesian visit (November 18–26) was organized as part of a University of California program. The University had a contract using U.S. Point IV funds, matched by Indonesian funds, to help set up laboratories and train physicians. The Janeways were housed in a compound in a modern suburb, which, CAJ remarked, "could be

U.S."[50] Janeway had a habit of using the first pages of his diary in any new country to write a detailed history of the country. He did so on his Indonesian trip as well. He was impressed that the Indonesians had only achieved full control of their nation in 1950—six years before. He thought they were "Still in [their] early formative period."[51] He noted that the university was "due to get autonomy from government. Very necessary to get chance to organize properly . . . Medical school has Dutch tradition—all lectures and theory, little practical work."[52] The California project was established to reorganize the curriculum. The Children's Hospital CAJ visited was "a real pleasure—light, airy, clean wards, cubicles all glass, needed for enteric disease."[53] His continuing education in public health was implemented by a visit to a health center run by a graduate of the Harvard School of Public Health and organized for a defined population of 200,000, "What impressed me," he recorded, "was what a good job was being done in clinics by midwives, records good, babies really being looked at and fine job in very simple houses." He contrasted the situation with India: "here buildings were put last. The professor of public health emphasized that [the] secret of public health is working with people and getting them to help themselves."[54] (We in public health are still trying to get others to understand this view.)

Visits followed to other hospitals, a leprosy research center, a tuberculosis hospital, the veterinary school and the Pasteur Institute of Indonesia, where CAJ was impressed with all the vaccines being made. All these visits filled his short time in the new nation. In his report of a closing interview, Janeway reported that the "Dean said that it might be good to send some of his people to Calcutta, but won't send people to India [as they] learn bad habits; if [they] got to Europe or America [they would] learn good habits."[55] Indonesia was and is a Muslim country, which certainly colored the dean's views against India. Overall, CAJ was impressed with Indonesia, commenting, "all doing good job."[56] The Janeways stopped briefly in Singapore on the way back to Madras. There he discussed the city as a possible place to hold the South East Asia Pediatric Congress in 1958. Janeway learned that the government of Singapore might support it, which would allow people to be officially invited, thus allowing them to come with government support.

After their return to Madras in the last days of November, the

Janeways made a side trip to Vellore on December 7–9. They visited the Christian Medical College, a small missionary hospital medical school where Dr. John Webb, a British pediatrician, was chief. CAJ liked Webb, whom he considered a "Good guy, English, outgoing person with nice wife."[57] The school had some Rockefeller Foundation Funds for research. Janeway "liked the way they tackled vital problems, did neat NH2 acid analysis and careful studies of biological value."[58] Once again its rural health center impressed him. In his diary he drew pictures of the floor layout and commented favorably on the center's Student Family Advisory Plan, whereby students visited families, examined all members, and provided curative and preventive services under supervision.[59] In the teaching hospital CAJ noted the "general feeling of a U.S. or British hospital."[60] However, he was put off by "Scripture quotations all around hospital and evangelist on staff. See why Hindu said 'people seem to care about you here at Vellore.' But gospel business would get me down. Can't get far from it."[61]

An amusing incident occurred in Vellore during the Janeways' stay at the Webbs' home. During the night, the Webbs heard a crash and wondered what had happened. The Janeways' bed had collapsed. The Webbs were anxious that the famous visiting professor and his wife had been hurt, but when Charles and Betty emerged they said that they were willing to spend the night on the floor; all laughed at the implications of what had been happening just before the bed collapsed! Charles and Betty remained life-long friends with the Webbs. After Janeway's death, Webb wrote, "I was initially deferential towards this [professor] but he quickly cut across all that with 'We are contemporaries. Call me Charlie.' He was ready to teach: offered to speak on any topic . . . but he was even more anxious to learn." Webb summarized his many contacts with Janeway,: "I unhesitatingly rate Charlie as one of the finest human beings I have ever had the privilege of knowing. His greatness was peculiarly individual and marked by the way in which he cloaked his eminence and distinction with a disarming, almost self-effacing humility. Therein lay the secret of his gift for friendship through which he contributed so much to pediatrics around the world."[62]

During their final stay in Madras, Dr. Janeway talked about medical education with Professor Achar, who was discouraged by diffident, unmotivated students, persons interested only in the examinations that were given for all the schools in the province. Since pediatrics did not have an examination, students did not take it seriously. Even though Janeway was opposed to examinations as a basis of determining "good" students, he felt it was necessary for Indian pediatrics to have a final examination, similar to medicine and surgery in that country. (In 1994, when RJH visited India for the Indian Pediatric Congress, India still did not require a final examination in pediatrics to graduate from medical school. The International Pediatric Association strongly recommended to the Ministries of Education and Health that such examinations be mandatory; a few years later they were finally required.)

As he did wherever he went, at the end of the Madras visit Janeway outlined needs he thought should be met. In the case of Dr. Achar's bailiwick, he identified six obvious needs: 1. organize chief residents, right hand men who could take the routine running of service off Achar's back; 2.residents to assure continuity of care; 3. laboratories of biochemistry, bacteriology, and clinical pathology attached to the pediatric service; 4. more staff and more beds; 5. enactment of Achar's scheme to spread out by putting pediatricians in 6 health centers, thus relieving pressure on Achar's outpatient department; and 6. residents in training for the degree of MD in pediatrics (the MD was an advanced degree based on a thesis, similar to the British tradition.)[63] Even as Janeway advanced these suggestions, he recognized the difficulties of achieving them. "Biggest problem—terrible load with inadequate staff and space and self-satisfaction of rest of medical college, making change difficult." Nonetheless, Janeway visited the vice-chancellor of the university and pressed Achar's needs.

The importance of Dr. Janeway's visit to the Madras medical school, and especially to Acher's service at this time, was pointed out in a long letter that Dr. P. Chandra sent to one of the authors (RJH) in 1993.[64] Dr. Chandra began by setting Dr. Janeway's visit within the context and important time-frame for India within which it took place. Dr. Janeway's visit, Chandra pointed out, occurred fourteen years after the Quit India movement, which was a tumultuous period and a time of crisis for the Indian people, occurring less than a decade after the attainment of Indian independence in 1947 and the closing of the colonial period. Chandra related that India had to struggle to recover from moral and material impoverishment, and famine and epidemic disease were prevalent. The British influence was obvious in every facet of Indian civilization, including medical care. Medical professionals had to carry over the effects of pre-independence days, as most medical teachers had received postgraduate training in the United Kingdom. They were concerned with maintaining academic excellence in order to obtain the approval of the General Medical Council of Great Britain, ignoring prime needs of national relevance.

Further, independent pediatric care was non-existent at the time. For centuries pediatrics had been tied to the apron strings of mother medicine (*i.e.*, internal medicine) and lacked emphasis on preventive pediatrics. The creation of the chair in pediatrics (in 1947, the first in India) by Madras University was an historic milestone in child health development in India, Dr. Chandra noted. Dr. Achar was appointed to the chair, becoming the first Professor of Pediatrics in India. Pediatric training for undergraduates was unknown in India previously, and Dr. Janeway's visit was well timed to strengthen Achar's efforts. "During Dr. Janeway's visit," Chandra wrote,

> I was a final year student undergoing one month pediatric training. We were excited and curious when we were told a visiting professor from the United States will be taking classes for us. Dr. Janeway's tall figure [an interesting comment, as Janeway was only 5' 9" tall], long white coat and smiling face left a long and lasting impression. He took about four classes for us with clinical demonstration. When my turn came to present a case I was nervous with no previous exposure to pediatrics and totally ignorant of diseases of children. I chose a case of patent ductus arteriosis as it was the fashion to present rare problems. It must have been a very bad presentation with no assessment of growth and development. His following statement is still ringing in my ears. "If a child is growing well the child is well. If a child is not growing, then there is something wrong."

Dr. Chandra related that the other topic Dr. Janeway presented was on immunization; that in very simple language the visiting professor explained immunology, active immunity and the role of immunization in bringing down child mortality and morbidity,

> He was so kind and homely [*i.e.*, homey]. We students, all below 24 years, wanted to know whether legal action was taken with mothers who failed to immunize their children [in the United States]. He nodded his head strongly and said, "the USA is a free country and no

punishment is given. It is by health education through various chan-
nels [that] parents are motivated to accept immunizations volun-
tarily." Many students wanted to know about opportunities in the
USA to specialize in pediatrics. He said, "First learn and specialize in
pediatrics in your own country and later think about visiting advanced centers in the USA." That sound advice impressed me and I
got trained in India and did not seek higher training abroad. He was
committed to spread the importance of child care to all professionals. He addressed members of the clinical society of Madras Medical
College on preventive pediatrics. We witnessed the resistance of senior professors of internal medicine for an independent department
of pediatrics. One of the senior and popular physicians said, "You
shouldn't be talking about preventive pediatrics but on the prevention of pediatrics!"

At the final party in Madras, Dr. Janeway noted that he was "Glad
Achar brought sisters [i.e., nurses], social workers, secretary, and house
staff . . . very good thing." He went on to note his "Major impressions
of Achar: has vision + integrity . . . very good ideas of what needs to
be done—poor organizer. More a thinker. Leave Madras with affection
for place, people like Achar and for its fascinating pageant of people."[65]
Janeway probably realized his profound debt to Achar in 1956, but he
certainly did so more than a decade later, when he wrote a paper in
Achar's honor.[66] CAJ said that, "as a younger man who learned a great
deal from opportunities to observe professor Achar at work in Madras,
I have been the beneficiary of his willingness to share not only his successful experiences but his problems." He paid tribute to Achar's careful planning of the first pediatric department in Madras, where he established a teaching clinic, a clinical laboratory, peripheral clinics in
different areas of the city, where preventive pediatrics was practiced,
and for writing an Indian version of Dr. Spock's book for parents. He
believed that Achar was ten years ahead of the United States in such
comprehensive preventive and curative programs. Further, Achar conducted research on prevalent liver diseases and, together with a colleague, was one of the first to apply liver biopsies to study cirrhosis in
children.

Betty was very active during the entire Madras visit. She went
to leprosaria and child care centers, as well as spending three days
(November 11–13) touring Madura and South India as a sightseer and,

at the end of November, visiting Hyderabad. Before leaving Madras, the Janeways tried to return some of the hospitality they had received by giving a dinner at the Oceanic Hotel for Dr. Achar, his assistants and their wives.[67] At the end of the Madras visit Janeway wrote, "Madras is picturesque, with its naked fishermen, cows brought in the door to provide milk, coolie carts pushed by four straining, sweating men in pink loin cloth, and colorful women carrying loads on their heads . . . On my last night there I walked the six miles home from the hospital. There is something to remember every step of the way." He and Betty felt a real nostalgia at leaving Madras.[68]

On their way to fulfill the last phase of their trip, in London, they visited Bombay (December 13–18), which they found different than Madras: larger, more masses of people, poverty with opulence side by side and, "more Westernized," in dress, speech and manner than Madras."[69] During their five-day stay, Janeway delivered lectures on nephrotic syndrome and the physiology of plasma proteins, attended fancy dinners, and made tours of hospitals. Charles and Betty took weekend trips to tourist sites. Betty wrote, "Charlie's program was staggering. From hospital to hospital. Speech to speech. Dinner to dinner. I follow when I could keep up, shopped, saw a bit of Bombay, and collapsed when I couldn't."[70] There can be no doubt that Charles and Betty Janeway were changed by this experience in India. The nation never was far from their thoughts during the rest of their lives. The bonding with the subcontinent became even stronger when their daughter, Anne, began her life-long work there.

Dr. Janeway's seventeen-page, single spaced, final report to the Rockefeller Foundation of his experience in India covered medical care, rural health, and more. It could well be the outline for a book on medical education reform in the developing world. We trust the Rockefeller Foundation used it in its support of medical education in the developing world. In it, he noted that he had visited nine of the forty medical schools in India and could not speak about all, but from what he had seen in these he listed five major shortcomings of Indian Medical education:

A. Too large a gulf between medical science and clinical teaching, B. Too much emphasis on the examination system, C. too much dominated by government [the civil service mentality], D. teachers are overwhelmed . . . by medical service, E. Pediatrics and preventive medicine are neglected, F. Despite shortage of personnel, those available are not being used as they might be.[71]

He went on to elaborate on each of these points, deploring the over-emphasis on anatomy rather than biochemical science, the creation of separate research institutes independent of medical schools, the separation of medical schools from their parent universities, and the lack of positions for many who were adequately trained. He recognized that recommendations were more difficult than pointing out weaknesses but proceeded to do so. India needed, he said, "A real full time system, freeing medical education from governmental control, revision of the curriculum, more emphasis on microbiology and biochemistry in the basic sciences and more pediatrics, preventive medicine and psychiatry in the clinical departments, reducing the importance of examinations and the establishment of a real resident system in teaching hospitals." He also recommended that a department of social medicine be estab-lished and nurtured at the All India Institute of Hygiene and Public Health.

India remained a focal point of their international mind and heart for the rest of Charles and Betty's lives. Their letter home after leaving is representative of their feelings.

> When we first left India we were too tired and too near it for any pro-found thoughts—too sad at parting and leaving it behind us, too happy at getting nearer home. Now, with a little perspective, we can only say that we're glad we went. Our eyes are wider, our horizons broader, it was worth the separation and loneliness and we'll never be the same again. Its civilization [was] at its zenith when our West-ern one was going into its early medieval darkness; it too has its long decline, its period of demoralization under early foreign rule and the awakening that came later with Tagore and Gandhi. Today it is a gi-ant rousing itself, proud of its great past, determined to have a bright future, humble about the magnitude of its tasks . . . This is a great nation, destined to play a great part in history.[72]

A decade after this first sabbatical, when Janeway took another sab-batical, primarily in Korea and the Far East, he included a second visit to India. Janeway's motive for doing this was his curiosity to know what a decade had wrought since he had last seen India, and particularly Madras. Before reaching Madras, Charles and Betty spent a short time in Calcutta (January 11–14, 1966). They were dismayed at what had not taken place, "Hard to see much change—hordes of people, poverty. Buildings looking blackened and decrepit and sand bags all around important buildings."[73] They stayed at the home of Dr. James Hughes, a former resident at the Children's, who was doing research on respiratory infections at the Institute of Child Health. Janeway was impressed with Hughes's work, which was being accomplished under very difficult circumstances, "with no expert help has organized excellent study of lower respiratory tract diseases in infants. Take hat off to Jim. He feels institute dead except for M [a man's first name initial; apparently CAJ did not want to identify his name]."[74]

One day, CAJ and Betty arose at 4 a.m. to fly to Jamshedpur, a factory town where Telco (Tata Engineering and Home Company) had built a new manufacturing plant employing 58,000 people and where the plant had built a new town with good housing for its employees. The Janeways felt that the accommodations were luxurious by Hong Kong standards (where people were stacked up in high-rise apartments). It seems likely that their host wanted to show an example of what private industry could do to make a livable city.[75] He and Betty returned by train to Calcutta where, the next day, they visited the Johns Hopkins Medical Research Institute. One wonders how it was for CAJ to be at this place that bore the name of his alma mater? "Incredibly dreary place, he noted, "But saw horrible case of rabies and 6 or 8 cases of smallpox. Rash much more extensive than I thought, even on trunk."[76]

Wherever they went, Charles and Betty were interested in family planning. At the All India Institute of Hygiene they discussed family planning with the director. Janeway reported, "a lot of emphasis here as elsewhere in India of sterilization of men . . . They had come to the conclusion that men made the decision and could not hope to succeed unless they talked to men."[77] The Institute of Pathology and Bacteriology and the All India Institute of Hygiene completed the visits in Calcutta. On the way to the airport, Hughes talked to Janeway about his career. Typical of CAJ's interest in all his trainees, he listed in his diary three options for Hughes and ended by noting the one he believed best. He also noted that he had written to the mentor with whom he thought Hughes should go to work upon returning to the United States.

The Janeways also visited Madras (January 15–21), Bombay (January 22–24), and New Delhi (January 24–30). CAJ's diary covering the Madras part of the trip opens, "By noon [January 15] circle in over Madras—like coming home . . . Met by Achar and Webbs."[78] After lunch they were driven to Vellore by the Webbs and stayed in the Webbs' home, "in Anne's room.[79] Their daughter, Anne, had by this time committed her life to work in India. Anne stayed with the Webbs while she was learning about Indian medicine and philosophy, and taught in a local school. She was not there when the Janeways arrived for this visit but the room where she had stayed was then given to the Janeways. CAJ was proud of his daughter, as was Betty, "visited her school, divided into three houses named Nightingale, Victoria and Janeway."[80]

Dr. Janeway was very impressed with the new medical school buildings and the setting aside of 150 of 900 beds in the university hospital for research, but all times were not spent in medically related visits, for in the afternoon they were driven to a village where there were flying foxes (huge fruit-eating bats with fox-like heads). Janeway noted that "Homes here all sprayed and marked MEP (Malaria Eradication Program),"[81] this at a time when DDT spraying was the magic prevention of malaria. Janeway's social conscience was never far below the surface. He commented, "Untouchables still on edges in poor thatched huts, but children seem more active and playful than before, but still get poor little tikes with reddish hair [sign of kwashiorkor] in poor areas."

The following day, Janeway was back at work in the hospital, marveling at the new construction and reviewing the details of the nutrition researchers. Later he visited a village where there was a nutrition supplementation program and went to research laboratories where enterovirus infections were being studied. He was presented several complex cases at a case conference and gave a lecture on "Development of Immunity," followed by the inevitable evening party. At a visit to a community health center the next day, he expressed his concern that it was "too near the main hospital,"[82] but it allowed students to follow two families, making home visits every two weeks throughout at least two years. He was concerned about his friend, John Webb's, future, however. "Webb doing big job . . . a problem . . . Allison [his wife] and children must all go to England next year [presumably for the children's education] . . . he must stay one more year. They won't find many missionaries with his ability in scientific medicine and dedication. A real leader in a top school."[83]

Charles and Betty arrived in Madras nine years after they last had been there. Betty noted that "The Oceanic has gone down hill . . . while the palm leaf huts of the fishermen have largely been replaced by low cost housing blocks. We walked up the beach with Prof. Achar and waded in the Bay of Bengal . . . feeling quite at home."[84] Janeway liked the progress that had been made. He remarked on the new quarters for the Institute of Pediatrics and the fact that there were more special clinics, but even so, "still 70 patients in 48 beds and mothers and children on floor."[85] He gave one of his usual lectures on the "Development of Immunity" and the next day went to another hospital, Stanley Medical College, where he noticed "Dreary old wards with very sick poor children."[86] He had worked with Professor V. Balagopal Raju at the government general hospital when he had been at that hospital before, and he was amazed at the number of children with cirrhosis, now, a decade later . . . 2 series of 600 cases each,[87] but Raju had been "thrown off work . . . in midst of gamma globulin study and records lost. We should try to work out collaborative study with N.I.H. funds."

From this biological problem CAJ went next to a community health center that provided postnatal care and well child care. He observed, "70 patients seen in 3 hours by nurse, post graduate students and staff . . . Very favorably impressed with services, but no real studies of effectiveness."[88] The new children's hospital, which when completed would have 400 beds, was "planned well and will be good."[89] It was not clear, however, what his good friend Achar's role would be at the hospital; another man was to be the chief, but the personnel seemed to be in "Very good spirit, despite what Achar implies. Hope he can be included but won't interfere."[90] Achar was by this time over the Indian statutory age for retirement and could no longer be the chief, but Janeway was concerned that his skills would be missed. He and Betty visited rural temples, with visits to weavers of saris completing their quick reacquaintance with Madras. The next day, Charles and Betty flew to Bombay, where they remained only three days. Janeway could be forgiven if he forgot which hospitals he visited, for his diary lists three different hospitals in one day as well as his lecture on development of immunity. The procession was dizzying.

Then they were off to see Delhi. Visits to hospitals and medical schools occurred in Delhi, too, but Janeway presented a different lecture, this one on Problems of Medical Education, which he noted was "too hasty and not too good for audience."[91] He lunched at the American Embassy with Ambassador Chester Bowles. During this visit Betty was escorted by an official from UNICEF to a variety of centers. Dr. Janeway was depressed with the bureaucracy in Delhi. He observed that at the All India Institute of Medical Sciences the "maintenance was inexcusably bad."[92] Even so, the director could not fire anyone and the chief of medicine had to see 100 VIP's as part of his contractual obligation, keeping him from doing as much research as he wished. Janeway must have wagged his expressive eyebrows often as he pondered such realities. On the positive side, however, visits to a community health center, where students and registrars worked in preventive as well as curative roles, impressed him greatly.[93]

Perhaps some of his irritation had other causes. CAJ was felled by "acute enteritis, now improving with Kaopectate and paregoric."[94] It is interesting that Dr. Janeway's parsimonious approach to giving medications to patients did not apply to himself, especially since it is now agreed that these symptomatic medicines for diarrhea may make the condition worse, albeit these long-used remedies do reduce the diarrhea and allow some normal functioning at the expense of absorbing toxins from the less-active bowel.

Charles and Betty planned their stay in Delhi to coincide with Republic Day, the Indian equivalent of the Fourth of July in the United States. They were impressed with "Indira Gandhi standing in an open car . . . tanks, bands, bagpipes, planes, school children, dancers, and Charlie so excited by gold bedecked elephants, he forgets to wind the film back before opening the camera."[95] Dr. Janeway summarized the

visit to India thus, "Progress in building social capital is real—new in-
dustries, technical training schools, good roads and extensive
electrification . . . Nevertheless, colorful and squalid village life goes on
as it has for ages . . . It's still too early to tell if they'll make it; population control is urgently needed and the combination of defense spending plus a poor harvest has set them back badly."[96] Betty's concluding
remarks about India were more varied. She remarked, "The trouble
with India is overpopulation . . . A lady doctor says 'we should give up
Kashmir and get to work raising our standard of living' . . . The trouble, an angry young man says, is that the U.S. gave arms to Pakistan,
thinking they'd be used against communism, and instead they were
used against India. Ambassador Bowles says, 'We have 600 Peace Corps
volunteers in India and we could use 5,000.' Indira Gandhi has a challenging job."[97]

Charles and Betty returned to India in 1977 to attend the XV Congress of the International Pediatric Association, which met in New
Delhi on October 23–29 of that year. The entire trip lasted three weeks
(October 15–November 6), and the first part of it was a boat tour side
trip. Perhaps because he was now in the grip of his ultimately fatal disease, Dr. Janeway did not keep a diary on this trip; instead, he and
Betty wrote letters home to their children, the first of which was written from a houseboat, *"Triumph,"* in Srinagar (now in Kashmir), which
was occupied by twenty-seven pediatricians from Canada, Syria, Australia, Hong Kong, and the United States. The sights they saw and the
experiences they underwent were dutifully described to their children
as the trip progressed. At the end of the boat tour they moved to New
Delhi and the IPA meeting.

The Janeways were always short of money, or felt they were. That
Dr. Janeway attended the IPA Congress that year was probably due to
Professor Ihsan Dogramaci's personal generosity. CAJ wrote to several
U.S. agencies asking for support to attend, with negative results, and
then asked Dogramaci, who was Executive Director of IPA at the time,
if IPA could support his travel. Dogramaci wrote that the IPA funds in
Switzerland were very limited but that such funds could be found in
Turkey, from Turkish contributions and donations (our guess, Dogra-
maci's own), and that he would send Dr. Janeway a voucher good for
$2,000 air fare on any carrier. CAJ answered, "Betty and I are both ex-

tremely touched by your letter, offering a prepaid ticket . . . as usual you are a magician in these matters."[98]

At the Congress CAJ was asked, together with Dogramaci and Professor. P.M. Udani, to give opening plenary session lectures. Janeway's topic was "Perspectives in Pediatrics—View from a Developed Country." In his files is a note from the organizing committee, indicating that his lecture would be separately published as a monograph in India. He was also asked by Dr. Taneja to give a lecture on "Current Advances in Immunological Prophylaxis." A brief note in his files outlines the main points he would make in his opening address, and includes an apology for his tardiness owing to his illness, the Waldenstrom's hypergammaglobulinemia that eventually would kill him.

> Plan to discuss responsibilities of academic pediatrics in developed countries: First; cooperative research to identify major child health deficits. Second; education for problem solving with clinical experience in a variety of community settings—hospital, urban and rural. Third; biological, social and economic advantages of health promotion over curative medicine. Fourth; health teams of professional and paraprofessionals. Fifth; need to keep health practice relevant to advancing knowledge and changing environmental conditions through research and continuing education.[99]

Dr. Janeway's participation in the IPA Congress has to be viewed in light of his terminal illness. He was often weary and sometimes confused. Nonetheless, Betty reported, "Dad just gave his paper at the plenary session and I was proud of him. So were others. John Webb and Jon Rhode's words were enough for us all."[100]

On Friday, October 28, Charles and Betty met with the Indian prime minister. As Betty noted, "Dad wanted to tell him about the congress and the high calibre of Indian doctors."[101] She also reported the gist of the meeting with the prime minister, who had just returned from a trip to Russia.

> He said, "We don't lack brains and ability here, the Russian trip was good, we don't want to take sides—all countries of the world must get on together, especially the U.S. and the U.S.S.R. Maybe nuclear weapons will prevent war as they will destroy both sides." What was impressive to me was his calmness, humor, and willingness to toler-

ate gaps in the conversation without agitation . . . He may do a lot of good on the international scene. If he can act as a person of reason from a country without territorial ambitions.

Janeway thought that this International Congress had been excellent. Their friend, Dr. Piloo Bharucha, believed that Janeway's help had been instrumental in getting the congress for India and said, "Ah Charlie, ah Betty . . . you are half Indian."[102] CAJ replied, "we don't feel that way but we feel very much at home surrounded by Webbs, Taneja, and many former students who come up to me in the halls." He went on, "The sessions were devoted to nutrition in general and especially in the developing countries and are full of hope despite the vastness of the problems. Breast feeding with love is one of the themes. Family planning of course comes into everything as well as community participation."[103] (How unhappy Charles and Betty would be at the decline in U.S. participation in international family planning today.)

Betty did note that "Politics in the IPA are as complicated as elsewhere."[104] By this time Dr. Janeway was no longer actively involved with the leadership of IPA but was sought out on its political issues. It was at this time that Professor Dogramaci supplanted Professor Thomas Stapleton as IPA Secretary General. At the end of the congress an event occurred that illustrates Charles and Betty Janeway's integrity. As they were about to leave, "a man appeared with a pile of rupees intended as a refund of our congress fees, but as we'd already received this once on the opening day we gracefully refused the duplication."

The Janeways continued on to Bombay. They stayed with Professor Udani and finally went for a few days in the countryside to Kosbad, where their daughter, Anne, had worked. They were impressed with the progress made in ecologically sound farming. "Nothing is wasted here. All human waste is recycled so that water is used for irrigation; excrement is sterilized and spread on the fields for fertilizer and the gas from the fermentation burns with a clean blue flame which cooks the food.[105] They each planted an Ashoka tree, which bore signs saying, "Tree Planted by Mrs. Betty Janeway, 3rd Nov. 1977." Anne wrote to the director, appraised him of her father's poor health and noted that "my father . . . clearly sees that the problems of child health concern all of humanity."[106] She noted the problem with her father's health and, in a poignant and illuminating description, said, "He is very brave and un-complaining, but he tires easily . . . they would not have to be enter-tained . . . they would be deeply appreciative of the quiet, the peace of Kosbad . . . my parents are basically simple and energetic people . . . who will eat anything. They have adjusted well to new places and people."

Janeway was impressed with the visit to Kosbad, for Betty wrote, "High points—wells—gas plants from manure and night soil—multi-ple cropping—people busy year round. Simple tools, variety of fruits and vegs to meet nutritional needs. Training of tribals to be catalysts. Practical, inexpensive, ecological and appropriate."[107] The Janeways were very much concerned with community development. CAJ was less invested in his traditional medical affairs by this time, and the com-munity-based, self-reliant, making-do attitude with resources available impressed him. In his home files, dating from this time, are reprints on water development, family planning, and ecology. In 1977 these were his priorities for the world.

During this trip, Betty was suffering from the neck spasms that so plagued her later years. She wore a neck support. On their last night in Bombay, the Udanis gave her a scarf to cover the neck collar and a bracelet of brass, copper and steel, designed "to cure my ills."[108] On their way back, Dr. Janeway wrote of the problems of India and ended, "We came away with the conviction that self-help must be the key to development; decent nutrition, quite possible within their limits, and the application of science and relevant education to their problems, provided development proceeds on all fronts and health is given scien-tific and programmatic priority over curative medicine, without losing their deep spiritual ideals that Gandhi translated into effective action."[109]

What an intellectual journey Dr. Janeway had made from the 1930s, when he first began to treat patients with the new antibiotics and later spent so much time on rare disorders of immunology. In 1977 he had come to see that the interrelation of community development, democ-racy, and integrated services is essential to improve the health of popu-lations. He applied his thoughtful, dedicated, intense, remarkable mind and dedicated it to the human race to improve mankind. It is

clear from the notes sent home, written by both Charles and Betty, that
they were equally engaged in international activities. Equally clear is
the fact that their dedication was founded on their basic love for their
family. The final paragraph of the last letter home from this trip ends,
"No letter till our last night in Bombay when, bless her, a wonderful
letter from Lee arrived. She ought to think of writing as a career. Her
words, like her pictures, convey a message of great depth and insight.
As we emerge from the world of the 'other half who die' [they are actually nearer 2/3], refreshed, loving each other and our family, the
prospect of seeing them is wonderful. With love to all of you."[110]

CAJ's terminal disease permeated the 1977 trip like an undercurrent.
He procrastinated about agreeing to several invitations to visit other
centers. Even personal, pleasurable things began to be subverted by his
illness. He and Betty had originally planned to stay at the Tanejas'
home during the congress but, only two weeks before leaving, he
wrote the Secretary-General of the IPA Congress, Professor O.P. Ghai,
that he and Betty "could not make plans in advance because of health
problems," and now wished to stay in the hotel.[111] In this letter he
noted that he had been "showered with invitations of hospitality in
several places," but because he had not been able to make plans, "I
have now refused all but one or two." One of these was to spend two
days after the congress with the Tanejas, and he would agree to spend
a day with Ghai after the congress as well. In spite of his illness, he also
said, "I should be happy to participate in any convenient way in teaching . . . particularly if it is informal, using not slides but a blackboard for
illustrations." The latter stipulation was characteristic; Janeway was a
master of developing the patho-physiological basis of disease about
any patient from a blackboard. The oil painting of him at the Children's (see Illustration 21) is typical of him: standing at a blackboard
with chalk in hand. Thanks to Janeway's superb use of this simple tool,
those in attendance, at Children's or at any IPA Congress, could follow
his thinking as it unfolded.

Because of his illness, the only other professional visit on this trip
was to see Professor Udani in Bombay, as noted above. In a letter to Dr.
Deshmukh, responding to a request to visit a second medical school in
Bombay, Janeway wrote, "I have had to limit those places I visit in India
to . . . either where we have not been before [i.e., Kashmir] or where

there is a very special reason to go there [*i.e.*, to see old friends, as in Udani's case]."[112] The days of CAJ and Betty going wherever they wished, whenever they could, were over.

Except for Charles and Betty's trip to England for CAJ's seventieth birthday, the 1977 trip to India was the last trip abroad. In retrospect, it was a sad yet glorious one. Several of the Indian pediatricians who invited him to come to their institutions said, in effect, "You are the most famous pediatrician in the world and it would be such an honor for you to visit our hospital." Professor Ghai told him, "I have always admired you as the giant among pediatricians but also as one of the finest human beings I have ever come across."[113] Ill and weak as Dr. Janeway probably was, these sentiments must have been gratifying to him. His work for the world's children, which, in effect, ended with the Indian Congress, had not been in vain.

CAJ was failing, but his visibility as the leading pediatrician in international child health would live on, longer in many ways than his contributions to American pediatrics. He had visited more countries, been a more visible symbol of modern scientific pediatrics to the developing world than any other pediatrician of the twentieth century. More importantly, he had combined this with humility, understanding of the diversity of the human race, and a deep commitment to improving the lot of all mankind. He was indeed the pediatrician to the world's children.

9 IRAN AND THE SHIRAZ MEDICAL CENTER

CHARLES JANEWAY'S long and deep commitment to Iran began with his appointment to the Medical Advisory Board of the Iran Foundation in 1955. His interest must have been raised even earlier, for in July 1954 he appointed an Iranian, Dr. Mohsen Ziai, to the resident staff of the Children's Hospital. We who were at the Children's at the time (RJH was then chief resident) were under the impression that Ziai had been recruited to receive further training in order for him to return to a new hospital in Iran, and, indeed, Ziai talked enthusiastically with many of us about his plans to return to the new Nemazee Hospital in Shiraz upon the completion of his training. During his residency years he talked with Dr. Janeway several times about the exciting initiative.[1] But Ziai remembers that Janeway did not know about the Shiraz project when he arrived in Boston and thinks that he (Ziai) and Dr. Claude Forkner, president of the Iran Foundation, then on sabbatical in Boston, were responsible for interesting CAJ in the project in 1954 or 1955.[2] Whatever the origins of Janeway's interest in the Shiraz project, it was a deep personal and intellectual one; he made five trips to Iran over a decade and, as president of the Iran Foundation from 1958 to 1965, devoted an enormous amount of time and energy to that work. Although he must have felt a good deal of frustration as well as a sense of accomplishment, for he encountered many setbacks and problems along the way, his optimism and sense of duty never flagged. He always put his best efforts into this high-risk enterprise.

The Iranian project was a succession of peaks and valleys. From the heady early days of the building of the Nemazee Hospital, when he enlisted an American staff and recruited and trained its replacement Iranian staff, through the great progress he witnessed in the quality of care, to the final involuntary separation of the Iran Foundation from involvement with the project, Janeway experienced both elation and deep disappointment. The final separation must have been painful. He moved, as a result of his immersion in this foreign culture, from the naïve belief that one could improve the health problems in a developing country by transferring American traditions, to a more realistic appraisal of the cultural mileau in which health care must function. At first, CAJ thought that Western-style medical education and high-quality medical care, similar to those that obtain in teaching hospitals in the United States, undergirded by basic and clinical research, and their sponsorship through the highest levels of government, could be applied to the Iranian experience. He evolved to a more realistic belief that these problems required a very long time frame and a more integrated approach involving many sectors of society, including education and community involvement as well as medicine, with a stronger "bottom up" community level approach.

He also learned that luck played a part in the process, and especially that a stable political situation was necessary. Iran, for all its apparent stability and wealth in the early 1960s, did not have this, and thus Janeway did not have the dollop of luck he needed to accomplish his aims. Iran was on the brink of revolution most of the time he was involved, although that fact was not apparent to most. The attempt to graft an American-style medical center onto a centuries-old traditional culture was bound to be difficult; just how difficult was not apparent in the early days of the adventure. Another complicating factor in America's involvement in Iran was the struggle with the Soviet Union for that part of the world. Dr. K.E. Livingstone told of the enthusiasm of the residents of Shiraz in general about the benefits of the medical care to be provided. But when asked about the effect of the whole U.S. Agency for International Development (US AID) program on the country, they responded pessimistically. The program had contributed to inflation without increasing the income of the poor, making the rich richer and the poor poorer. But if the United States withdrew from the program, Russian influence would undoubtedly take over by default.

Livingstone's answer to that option was no; he felt that United States military and foreign aid must be coupled with changes in the underlying instability in the country.[3] Thus the cold war and U.S. relations with the Soviet Union lay behind the whole enterprise, and especially the financial support of the American government, no matter how altruistic were the aims of the individual participants.[3]

Dr. Janeway was nothing if not an idealist. His commitment to the power of modern medicine, high-quality care, the American style of medical education coupled with research and, most importantly, the moral and ethical basis on which all that stood, was joined by his over-arching commitment to peace. At the time the cold war was heating up, he spoke eloquently of the role physicians could play in furthering peace through international activities. Given that commitment, the Iran Foundation and the Nemazee Hospital project appeared to be vehicles by which he might achieve his altruistic goals.

The story began in 1944 when Mr. Mohamed Nemazee, a wealthy Iranian businessman, returned from a period in the United States to his native city. Shiraz, a city in southern Iran with a population of about 150,000 people, is located about thirty miles from the ancient capital of Persia, Persepolis. Nemazee's father had built a public health clinic in Shiraz in the late 1930s which, because the elder Nemazee had bad financial luck, had deteriorated into poor quality and had been given by him to the government. Originally, Mr. Nemazee wanted to upgrade his father's clinic, but Dr. Torab Mehra, a physician and graduate of the Johns Hopkins School of Public Health, who now had a vision of how to improve health care for all of Iran, persuaded him to build a new hospital along the lines of an American teaching hospital, one that would change medical care and education in Iran in a way that had not been seen before or since in any country from Western Europe to the Far East.[4]

Nemazee was a generous, highly principled man. He hoped to set an example of wise philanthropy to other Iranians. He saw the need of a modern hospital combined with and financed by a necessary public health measure. No city in Iran had at that time potable drinking water piped directly into homes; Nemazee decided to build a public waterworks in Shiraz from artesian wells, sell the pure water to well-to-do families in Shiraz and, with the profits fund the operating expenses of the hospital, also paying for twenty-four outlets in poor districts of the city in order to improve the public's health. As it turned out, however, the scheme did not work as planned, for Nemazee found that he had to pay for the hospital's operating expenses as well.[5]

Nemazee recognized that to provide the excellent care he desired, he needed a high-quality staff for his hospital and a body to serve as a conduit for financial resources from the United States, much like trustees of hospitals in the United States. In 1948, he created a legal entity in New York City that he named the Iran Foundation, a tax-exempt entity that would advance health and education in Iran and develop a hospital and nursing school.[6] He also created a parallel organization in Iran, the Vaghf Trust, with an Iranian board of directors called Boyadiran, which gave legal status to the Iran Foundation in New York. The legal document creating the New York entity was drawn up in Farsi, the national language of Iran, and then was translated into English by Nemazee. The translation used the words "full control and authority over the Shiraz Medical Center," but also stipulated, in the same document, that "the Donor reserves the right to appoint or dismiss the director and staff of the center."[7] This document was received by the New York foundation's Executive Director, Dr. Bettina Warburg, in November, 1959; at the time, she also asked for a separate translation by an Iranian, Mr. Taba-Tabai, who, in a letter to Dr. Warburg, noted that the Farsi word similar to "control" had to be translated to include control, although the Farsi word does not explicitly mean that.[8] This note of ambiguity, present from the outset of the Foundation, was in later years to be a source of great problems. In several later communications, Mr. Nemazee also used the words, "Approbational Trustee" to indicate the role of the Iran Foundation relative to the several institutions created, although recognizing that these words did not exactly parallel those used in Farsi. This ambiguity was to be another source of dispute later.[9]

The Iran Foundation appointed a Medical Advisory Council, of which Dr. Janeway was chair from 1955 to 1958, and a Nursing Committee to develop the professional personnel needed until Iranian personnel could be trained in the United States to replace them. The Boyadiran, who were required by Iranian law, were composed of well-known and well-connected people; among the elite members of the

U.S. Iran Foundation were the honorary President, Hussein Ala, then Prime Minister of Iran, Dr. Claude Forkner of New York City and Cornell Medical School, the chair of the Foundation, who had been the physician of the Shah of Iran and other heads of state in the Middle East, as well as the King of Nepal. Forkner had explored with the Shah the possibility of an American-style medical school in Iran and had received some interest. The board also numbered three former United States ambassadors to Iran and several well-connected businessmen. The Medical Advisory Council consisted of senior, well-known largely academic physicians, such as Dr. Allen O. Whipple, former chair of surgery at Columbia University's College of Physicians and Surgeons, who had been born in Iran of missionary parents and was a life-long friend of the country and its people. He developed policies for the hospital, recruited staff, and, after Dr. Janeway became president of the foundation, resumed the chairmanship of its Medical Advisory Council. Dr. Whipple visited Iran at least on two occasion on the foundation's behalf, the last in 1959 when he was preparing a book on Arabian medicine. It was an extraordinary board.

The counterpart board in Iran had an even higher profile politically, most members being highly placed government officials, which was a help in obtaining funding from the Iranian government. However, most of these men lived in Tehran, 600 miles from Shiraz, and were very busy; thus, they contributed little to the effort. The plan called for creating a nursing school at the hospital, with the U.S. nursing committee recruiting staff and setting standards. In 1948, Mehra said that there were very few nurses in all of Iran, and only one school, that in Tehran, was of high quality. To staff a new American-style hospital it was clearly essential to have a nursing school. A vocational school, an eye hospital, and community outreach programs were envisioned for the enterprise and were, in fact, added later. One of the early strengths of the Nemazee Hospital was the recruitment of Dr. Mehra as its director. Mehra, a graduate of a U.S. medical school and school of public health, was a visionary who knew how to articulate the goals and directions in which he wanted the enterprise to go. He had outstanding leadership qualities, a charming personality, and maintained excellent relations with Mr. Nemazee and other leading Iranians. The hospital was to operate like any voluntary hospital in the United States, with in-

patient and outpatient services and clinical and laboratory departments. Patients would be charged in accordance with their ability to
pay. Such an organization, while seemingly commonplace now, was
revolutionary in Iran at the time, for it emphasized high-quality care
with education and research. The hospital opened in 1955 with only a
few beds available, but by 1957 there were ninety-nine and the hospital
had an average daily census of seventy-six patients. The hospital and
nursing school together became known as the Shiraz Medical Center.

Originally the Iran Foundation and staff envisioned building their
own medical school, proposing that the Rockefeller Foundation support it, but officials of that foundation were not enthusiastic. After it
soon became clear that the Iran Foundation could not raise the necessary resources for a new medical school, in 1957 a relationship with the
University of Shiraz and its existing medical school was developed,
with the staff of the Nemazee Hospital providing clinical education for
its medical students. In that year, the University of Pennsylvania began
a close relationship with the University of Shiraz; and it and the Iran
Foundation were able to obtain U.S. government help to supplement
the salaries of the American medical faculty. Relations between the
University of Shiraz, with its traditional (for Iran) medical school, and
the Shiraz Medical Center were rocky at best. The relationship resulted
in little but problems. In 1956, the first pediatrician was recruited to the
Medical Center; this was Dr. Campbell McMillan, who had recently
finished his residency at Boston Children's Hospital. Born in China, the
son of a missionary, Dr. McMillan was a perfect candidate, and his
wife, a surgical nurse at the Children's, was an ideal personal and professional companion. In a letter written at a later time, McMillan
would outline his views of the difficulty of engrafting a U.S.-type hospital on a culture so different as that of Iran.[10]

Another problem was that Iran had only recently attained political
stability, or so it seemed. Early in the twentieth century it was characterized by financial crises, riots and short reigns of various factions.
Only in 1906 was the first constitution approved, but fledgling democracy was suppressed by Russia. After a civil war, the Iranian parliament
was revived and in 1925 elected Reza Pahlavi as Shah. But he was a
ruthless dictator who early during World War II sided with the Ger-
mans. In 1941 he abdicated and his son replaced him as Shah. Struggles

for power between the Shah and the landed nobles continued, and in 1951 the premier Mohammed Mosadegh nationalized the oil industry; but the grip held by the foreign oil companies, aided by the U.S. Central Intelligence Agency, pushed him out and restored power to the Shah in 1953. The Shah then dissolved parliament and began a campaign of reform, redistributing land from the nobles, trying to eradicate illiteracy,[11] and making other long-needed changes, but progress was slow. Furthermore, Iran balanced itself between the Soviets and the Americans during the cold war, although the British-U.S. consortium enabled those countries to retain some control over Iran's greatest asset, oil, under the auspices of the National Iranian Oil company, an arrangement that produced over a billion dollars a year for Iran. Nonetheless, tensions within the country remained high, forcing the Shah to use secret police to help stamp out dissent. This created the inevitable resentment of the people of Iran as well as the wealthy landlords, and the rise of Muslim fundamentalism further eroded his power. Although the revolution that drove the Shah from power and brought about the religious autocracy occurred several years after the health initiative of the Iranian Foundation and Dr. Janeway, the seeds of revolution were being seen even then. The nation's political problems were to be major factors in the difficulties encountered by the Shiraz experiment.

Charles and Betty Janeway first went to Iran as part of their 1956 sabbatical to Europe and India, which occurred with the financial support of the Rockefeller Foundation. In their first stop, at the capital, Tehran, where the red carpet was laid out for them, they immediately saw the contrast between what wealthy Iranians had and the poverty of the general populace. They quickly became aware of the differences between the aristocratic Iranians who entertained them and the other ninety-five percent of the Iranian people. It was the beginning of their realization that all was not well in Iran. Charles entered into his diary, "What can one say . . . after a 3-day visit? Superficially: #1, need an income tax, to cut rich down to more common level and encourage giving."[12] He sensed that many things that were told to him were not the truth; that "Mosedegh was champion of people vs. Shah—present ruling groups King's party—but still making progress in fields of health particularly;" that as one gets away from Tehran, "one gets rumors of corruption in government from top to bottom." He especially liked Mr. Ala, the Prime Minister, and he felt that the Minister of Health was dynamic, with great courage and a capacity for getting things done. After this quick visit to the capital, the Janeways went on to Shiraz, where they were met by a large delegation, including Campbell and Florence McMillan. Among the attractions of the Nemazee facility was a cluster of homes for the staff and a swimming pool on the hospital grounds. While Janeway was kept busy at the hospital every day, he and Betty attended parties every night. They were beginning to see the complex nature of Iran: "Iran is a complicated country; politics weave their way in and out of every phase of life from absentee landlordism in the mud villages to bribery in high places. We're not in a position to know or judge, but it's not impossible to sense the undercurrents," he confided to his diary.[13]

When they arrived at the Nemazee Hospital they found a facility that had a potential 250 beds but only fifty of them were open, owing to a shortage of nurses and also to the reluctance of patients to come because of fear of costs. The contrast with the British Mission Hospital in Shiraz amazed them; that 89-bed hospital did 1,000 operations a year and the courtyards were filled with patients and families who were cooking and doing laundry. CAJ began to wonder whether the U.S.-style Nemazee Hospital was indeed needed in developing countries; however, the idea of the waterworks, providing both pure water as well as support for the hospital, was seductive. The importance of water to this dry land became evident wherever they looked. The Nemazee water works, which provided an abundance of good water to the whole city of Shiraz, was located in the spacious hospital compound. Its pipes led to homes in the good or new parts of the town and to thirty-five water points in the poor section, the latter being free but bills being sent to the former—"unfortunately, many of the bills are unpaid." When summarizing his thoughts about the Nemazee Hospital, Janeway recorded that he was "Impressed here that problems [were] no different from ours in the U.S., but more difficult to solve." He noted that there were hopeless problems with transport—things ordered from abroad took many weeks to reach port, yet "Takes 3–6 months to get from there to here with stuff stolen. To get anything through customs . . . requires bribes."[14]

Before leaving Shiraz, Dr. Janeway wanted to nudge Mr. Nemazee and Dean Gorban to support the American-Beirut type of medical education—small classes and less didactic work. CAJ, who was rarely devious, wrote to Nemazee instead of Mehra in an end-around play to ask what his plans for the school were, and "how we can help him."[15] The conflict between the old municipal hospital (Saadi) in the Shiraz Medical School and the new Nemazee Hospital was evident. At the end of the visit he made a number of recommendations to start to bring them together. Dr. Mehra was skeptical and concerned that the old, entrenched faculty at the medical school would undermine the efforts of the Nemazee Hospital to become a high-quality institute.[16] CAJ was unhappy with the old Nemazee clinic, which he found dirty, of poor quality, and providing purely symptomatic care,[17] but he got a lift at the Health Center, where he observed "young people, up and coming, doing a swell job—good place to use PM [preventive medicine] teaching."[18]

On the last day of his visit Janeway met with the entire staff to explain the goals and discuss the problems and the options, the upshot of which was that he determined to appoint committees to study two short-term problems: "1. How to cooperate with Shiraz Medical School to help without hurting the institution. 2. What needs to be done to develop emergency service."[19] Janeway's belief in participatory democracy seemed to go over well with the Iranian staff. Later he noted that one of the greatest needs was "to get rid of competition and idea of cutting your neighbor's throat. Hospital will do more to teach democracy and teamwork in action."[20] With the dean he agreed that the Iran Foundation would try to help recruit Iranian basic scientists, who would share appointments and salary in the medical school and the Nemazee Hospital. They agreed to have Claude Forkner "sell plan to Shah, Ala, etc., to get blessing and backing. Good day."[21]

Janeway was pleased with himself to reach compromises with various parties. However, he was overly optimistic; he failed to recognize the cultural willingness of Iranians to appear to agree when in fact there was no agreement or little ability to carry out agreements. In addition, the superior young Iranian staff that had been recruited to Nemazee Hospital was adamantly opposed to integration with the medical school, which it perceived to be a lowering of standards. CAJ's antenna picked up some of this. He noted that the staff felt that independence must be maintained at all costs.[22] At a party Janeway threw for Dean Gorban, he gave the dean a strong talk on how he could make or break his school through the appointment of preclinical faculty, that he would have to wait to find the right people, and he had to give them stable working conditions, noting that there was "No question of his intentions." But then he wrote, equivocally, "Maybe best policy lies between the opportunism which meets needs somehow and Iran Foundation policy of no compromise at any cost. But it remains to be seen how it will come out."[23]

Janeway was intellectually committed to only the highest-quality people, but emotionally he was a compromiser, especially in his work in developing countries, where he was beginning to realize that the best was sometimes the enemy of the good. "From the standpoint of public health it's [i.e., the hospital] an unrealistic flop—its excuse must be teaching and research—how to do things better."[24] This first, of what were to be many visits and enormous energy devoted to Iran, ended on a much more positive note than was to be the case as time went on. But Dr. Janeway was always buoyed up by what had been accomplished. On the way out of Iran, he and Betty flew to Abadan, where they were guests of the Iranian Oil Company. Their stay in a guest house, a palace with house boys waiting on Americans and Britishers, heightened the contrast between the rich and the poor, and continued to depress them.[25]

The next morning they flew to Karachi via Dahran, where they saw people with "Much Negro blood mixed in from slaves." It made Janeway "Sad to think of Walter K., former idealistic head of International Student Service, [who] had to announce at anti-slavery UN meeting that his government [the United States] would not sign or take position on slavery [oil lease with King Ibn Saud]—dirty business."[26] Janeway's liberal views were never far below the surface. It would appear that he was happy that he did not have to represent the United States in such a meeting and be forced to compromise his ideals. He summarized his observations upon leaving Iran:

Impressions on Shiraz Medical Center ? (1) Most beautiful hospital buildings and grounds in the world, (2) First-class staff, (3) having all problems we have during growth of Children's Medical Center, complicated by trying to implant Western medicine and ethics in a foreign culture where [a] few people are enormously wealthy and can pay more than it cost but hate to, and vast numbers of people have practically no money. Believe it has a fine future and will make a real contribution.[27]

These comments indicate Dr. Janeway's understanding of the cultural differences that would make it difficult to transplant Western medicine, and especially ethics, but which nonetheless typify his essential optimism: the Nemazee facility would "make a real contribution." CAJ went on to remark, "Although high quality medical care is urgently needed in Iran, the most important function of the Shiraz Medical Center is to provide education and training for Iranians in their own country, not only in the skills of medicine, surgery, nursing, and allied health fields, but in the concepts of self sacrifice, teamwork, and devotion to the patients' welfare which characterize the best in modern medicine in western countries."[28] He was mindful of the risks for the enterprise, which

> inevitably makes them a symbol of American technical assistance. The United States in particular, and the Western nations in general, have their necks out in Shiraz. If these institutions fail, particularly the Shiraz Medical Center, with its private, voluntary basis, upon which we have set so much store as a means of setting standards and exploring new and better ways of doing things, we shall lose face in Iran and provide the Russians with another argument in their persuasive wooing of the underdeveloped countries . . . We cannot let this institution fail for lack of funds just as it begins to fulfill the mission in medical care and education for which it was founded.[29]

Dr. Janeway's apprehensions were prescient. Failure was perceived almost from the start. In his annual report of 1957–58,[30] Dr. Mehra, observing that the hospital was only two years old, was pessimistic: "The year may justifiably be called a year of crisis." The expected revenues from the water works had not materialized; the government of Iran had delayed its payment; funds from the U.S. International Cooperation Administration (ICA) had been delayed; and revenue from patients was less than anticipated. The institutions survived that year with an advance from Mr. Nemazee of over $172,000, a grant of $108,000 from the Ford Foundation for the vocational school (originally developed by a gift form Mr. Nemazee's cousin), and surplus food and medicines from the United States. Despite the meager financial support from the Iranian government, Mehra praised Mr. Ala, the Court Minister, for access to the Shah and the Shah's interest and support of the enterprise.

The situation then seemed to improve. In the 1960 report, Mehra stated, "The year started out bleak but ended in successful achievement."[31] The Iranian government and US-ICA paid what had been promised. Mehra credited Mr. Ala with the success in obtaining funds from the Iranian government. "As before, it has been through the good offices of this great and dedicated patriot that we have been able to bring our pressing problems to the attention of His Imperial Majesty."[32] In Iran, clearly, the Shah's approval was necessary for everything. In addition to helping secure the ICA grant and another from the Ford Foundation, the Iran Foundation was instrumental in organizing transfers of donated supplies from pharmaceutical companies and raising small amounts from individual donors. The Iran Foundation's function, other than being a conduit for grants for U.S. institutions, was recruitment. Distinguished faculty, comprising physicians who had headed departments in the United States and were retiring, were among the Iran Foundation's initial recruiting successes. Drs. James Halstead and Hobart Reiman came in internal medicine, Drs. Monroe McIver and Robert Wise in surgery, and the first of the outstanding Iranians trained in the United States began to arrive with Dr. Mohsen Ziai in pediatrics and Dr. Jamileh Yeganeh in obstetrics.

Dr. Ziai was a perfect example of the sort of physicians Janeway wished to recruit to Shiraz. An Iranian of a distinguished family, his father and grandfather had been physicians; indeed, he was an eighth-generation physician. His father, well known in his home region and in the nation, had been a member of parliament; Ziai's uncle was a senator. Mr. Nemazee, as well as Mr. Asadolla Alam, who was to become the chancellor of the new Pahlavi University in Shiraz, were also close family friends. Ziai's grandfather had treated Mr. Alam's father and had cured him. As a result, he and Mr. Alam became close friends. Close family ties are a factor in organizations everywhere, but in Iran they were the essential factor in success or failure of a new enterprise. When Ziai was to come to the United States to attend college in 1948, Nemazee told him of his plans for the new hospital in Shiraz and encouraged him to come back there when he finished his training.

When Ziai came to the United States to attend college, Nemazee told him to talk to people at the Iran Foundation. Thus, he was preparing him from his earliest days in the United States for a career in Shiraz. After college, Ziai was accepted to Johns Hopkins Medical School, interned in pediatrics there, had a residency at Bellevue-NYU Hospital, and a senior residency and chief residency in pediatrics at the Children's, completing his training in what most in the United States would consider three of the most outstanding pediatric centers in the nation. He then spent a year as a fellow in infectious diseases at Harvard's famous Thorndike laboratory at Boston City Hospital. There could have been no more distinguished preparatory career to become chief of pediatrics at the new Nemazee Hospital, and he went there with a youthful vigor in 1957. This type of outstanding Iranian physician, well trained in the U.S., was to typify the first few recruits. Things were getting off to the start that Janeway had envisioned, and he felt optimistic because of physicians such as Ziai.[33]

In his introduction to the 1959–60 Iran Foundation report, Dr. Janeway voiced his optimism about the future of the project:

> To every organization and to each person who has helped in this cooperative effort to diminish the toll of disease and illiteracy in a great and ancient country, we wish to express our heartfelt gratitude. May you take pride in this record of accomplishment . . . may your imagination enable you to visualize in human terms the true significance of . . . this report. And may we all redouble our efforts to meet the challenge and to rise to the opportunities which lie ahead, as we participate in the great changes which we hope will lead to a better life and greater opportunities for the people of Iran.[34]

Nonetheless, by the time Dr. Janeway undertook his next trip to Iran, he recognized the almost insurmountable problems of grafting an American-style hospital and medical school on the Iranian health system. The graft was being rejected. As he left for this subsequent trip to Iran he wrote in his diary, "Why do I leave this smiling, green, pros-

perous, free and friendly country for a land of deserts, heat and personal power struggles, pride and individualism [?] I suppose the answer
is belief in the world. The brotherhood of man and the deep conviction that freedom of opportunity, and the four freedoms should be
available to all. Maybe this is something I can do to give a little shove to
peace."[35]

Dr. Janeway went to Iran in 1958 for one week as part of a committee of the Rockefeller Foundation that had been sent to Iran to survey
the need for an American-British style university medical school. The
committee first went to Tehran, where they met with very high officials, including the Prime Minister and the Shah. In his report to the
Foundation, Janeway articulated the difficulty of understanding the
nuances of a different culture when "one is unable to speak Farsi."[36]
Perhaps this comment forewarned him of the criticism that Mr.
Nemazee would later make on those who came for short visits and
recommended policy on that brief basis. Janeway noted that there had
been a tremendous increase in material wealth since his first visit. In
Tehran there was now "a magnificent airport, a great increase in the
number of cars . . . people better dressed, stores filled with a wider variety of goods [and] one could now drink water from the tap!"[37] He la-
mented, however, that with oil revenues of over $2 billion a year [at
that time], the temptation of the government to use it for current operation rather than invest in infrastructure such as potable water,
health care, education, and diversified industry was great. A development plan had been offered by the U.S. Tennessee Valley Authority to
do so, but its offer was never implemented.

Dr. Janeway was aware of the overriding importance of the political
situation to the success or failure of any enterprise in Iran. Despite
"the political situation which seems superficially stable, Iran is now a
benevolent dictatorship, with the king giving orders through his appointed ministers. His majesty impressed me as a very able, courageous and intelligent man. The worries arise from the Army, the real
source of power in a rapidly changing country."[38] In spite of his disappointment with the overall lack of success of the Iran Foundation's
grand vision, in Shiraz Janeway was pleased with the progress of the
hospital. Now 129 beds were open, medical students were being selected on aptitude, from over 600 applicants with 120 selected in the

University and forty in the medical school, thirty interns and residents were on staff, and several well-trained Iranians had been recruited successfully for the hospital, especially in the basic sciences. Dr. Janeway realized that the hospital was a turning point. The dean of the medical school wanted it to evolve into a university, and the thought that the Nemazee Hospital might become the university hospital rather than an affiliated institution was intriguing. As usual, however, lack of finances was the barrier.

The Rockefeller Foundation group met with many high officials who expressed their hopes that an American-style university could be created, "free from political pressure . . . free faculty selection, full time system, etc."[39] In his diary, CAJ reported that Mr. Ala said, "The real purpose of the plan [for an American university] is a model of private enterprise—to show how opportunities can be utilized as seed to open thousands of young men to do things themselves . . . to create confidence and hope."[40] At a meeting with the International Cooperation officials (the name was later changed to the U.S. Agency for International Development—US AID), Janeway determined that the Shiraz project got off on the wrong foot in several ways, the first being that Mr. Nemazee had "sent a sharp lawyer to beat people over the head at the ICA," and because of other misunderstandings and administrative errors. And while the new director of the ICA was good, he was in a difficult position being only an acting director. "Thus it was not only Iranian bureaucracy that was a problem in Shiraz but also US."[41]

Both Janeway and Mehra asked for funds from the Iranian authorities to expand the nursing school at Shiraz. They were reassured that the current budget of $129,000 per year was probably satisfactory but expansion was caught up in a jurisdictional dispute between the Ministry of Health and Ministry of Education. Nurses were not considered "professionals," creating a problem for the Ministry of Education to support. The detailed notes in Janeway's diary outline the discussions he had in Teheran over two days with many ministry people and the representatives of the Rockefeller Foundation about the needs of an American-style university, but none of this seemed to add to the support of the effort at Nemazee Hospital. He then proposed that the Association of American Medical Colleges organize a "public/private venture" with a broad-based group of young people from abroad in a

variety of health disciplines and also senior faculty (nearing retirement) to work for such a purpose. Given Iran's subsequent history, it
seems indeed a pity that such a vision was never carried out.

Janeway was impressed with an audience he had with the Shah, who
talked for about ten minutes about ideas of what a university should
be. "He spoke as if the University to be located at Shiraz was a fore-
gone conclusion without ever saying so."[42] This account suggests that
Dr. Janeway was not immune to the grandeur of the Shah's setting and
style, although he personally never exhibited anything we would recognize as grandeur or ostentation. Later, in discussion with Mr. Alam,
it was clear that Shiraz was not necessarily to be the site of the new
university; but CAJ was also enthusiastic after a two-hour discussion
with Alam, who ended it with, "We may consider ourselves engaged,
but not married."[43] Janeway wrote, "most exciting 2 hours—proud to
be an American."[44] Was he taken in by the rhetoric and the red carpet
treatment? Perhaps. The Shah and the Rockefeller Foundation authorities were more interested in the entire university, whether or not
affiliated with Nemazee Hospital. CAJ and Mehra were first and foremost interested in the hospital but saw that it could only succeed in the
long run if it was part of a major Western-style university. The two vi-
sions did come together for a time.[45]

On his final day in Iran on this visit (which was the Shah's birthday
and so featured large celebrations), CAJ and Mehra spent all of it writing reports and applications to the ICA, although at its end, he concluded his diary entry for the day with the comment that his Iranian
dinner companions felt unrest, "nobody knows what is going to happen."[46] In his typical outline fashion, Janeway ended his 1958 Iran diary
with a list of the factors present for success as well as the problems existing at Shiraz. After seeing the world through rose-colored glasses following his audience with the Shah, he had returned to reality and was
committed to try to solve the problems because he felt this experiment
was so important and because "The stage [was] now set for development of Shiraz University Medical Center with the whole teaching
hospital complex . . . around the Nemazee Hospital."[47] In his report to
the Iran Foundation of his visit, he noted that "both Dr. Gorban and
Dr. Mehra have agreed to stop any further developments in either institution until a joint committee . . . has a chance to make a ten-year

plan for a University Medical Center."[48] He recommended that a request be made to the Rockefeller Foundation to support an "outstanding person to come to Shiraz for a period of three months" to develop the plan. The failure of this vision, that of a major university to be developed around the Nemazee Hospital, was yet in the future.

In the 1960–61 annual report of the Iran Foundation Dr. Janeway took note of the continued financial problems but acknowledged new support from the Iranian Oil Consortium, the name for a group of affiliated oil companies. He also reported that this year saw two engagements with the public that enhanced the reputation of the medical center at Shiraz. First, a terrible earthquake occurred at Lar, 200 miles south of Shiraz, killing over 10,000 people. Within an hour the hospital cleared its ground floor and received over 100 patients, all of whom survived.[49] As Mehra said, "This great challenge, which tested our personnel and the character of the organiztion, gave reliable, positive proof of the growth and maturity of our institution." Illustrating the resentment of many towards this new entity, Mehra went on, "Even the worst propaganda of the feudalistic gentry could not mar this achievement."[50] Unfortunately, the Red Lion and Sun (the Iranian Red Cross) failed to pay the extra cost incurred by the hospital for the care of the earthquake victims. The hospital's action was a public relations success but a financial failure.

The second event was a move both Janeway and Mehra had envisioned from the beginning: the hospital would begin to work in the community. One slum section of Shiraz was visited regularly by medical and nursing students, who gained experience about the needs of the poor and about public health activities. In the same vein of service to the community, an educational program, titled "Adult Night Classes," was opened for Nemazee Hospital employees who had completed the equivalent of a sixth-grade education. Staff at the hospital were moving away from the original concept of a tertiary care hospital on the American model to work at the community level as well, a model much talked about in the United States but still rarely implemented there. By this time Nemazee Hospital was largely an Iranian institution. It had grown to a staff of 427 personnel; only six of the twenty-two physicians were American and there now were thirty-two interns and residents.

A measure of the changed times is reflected in a letter from Mr.
Nemazee to the Boyadiran. He pointed out that he was no longer supporting the expenses of the Iran Foundation office in New York.
Nemazee stated that he ultimately wanted the Boyadiran to take the
responsibility of managing the whole medical center, albeit for a variety of reasons that time was not yet ripe. Therefore, he "temporarily
endorsed the trusteeship of the Shiraz Medical Center over to the Iran
Foundation."[51] This letter was the first time the word "temporarily"
was used, and CAJ underlined the word in his copy. Nemazee specified
that the Iran Foundation would act as purchasing agent for the medical
center, the water works, and the vocational school, "for which services
these shall pay an appropriate remuneration." In a six-page attachment, Nemazee spelled out the several functions to be provided by the
Foundation in order to set policy and manage the Shiraz Medical Center until the Iranian counterpart, the Boyadiran, could take it over.[52]

Dr. Janeway had repeatedly warned Nemazee that the Iranian counterpart, composed of prominent Iranian citizens, was a problem. First,
he pointed out, "we can't have two boards . . . one in the US and one in
Iran both giving orders to Dr. Mehra."[53] Later, in several letters, he
pointed out that the Iranian board comprised high government
officials who lived in Teheran and had many other responsibilities that
precluded close oversight of the Shiraz Medical Center. As a result, the
responsibility for almost daily operations lay with the U.S. foundation,
for which CAJ as president felt responsible. It was characteristic of him
that he felt that with extra work he could do the job. The organizational structure, in retrospect, was so ungainly that it was bound to create problems in addition to those caused by the political instability of
Iran. One of Janeway's failings was that, as a modern manager, he was
often remiss in delegating responsibilities, but one of his endearing
characteristics was his optimistic attitude that, by giving himself totally to any project, what might seem to be overwhelming problems to
others could be solved by hard work and high ideals.

At this remove, more than forty years later, it is difficult to understand how Janeway could be expected to accomplish all these functions
as a part-time executive in Boston rather than in New York, where the
Iran Foundation's offices were located, in spite of the presence there of
a very good executive secretary, Dr. Bettina Warburg, and the help of

the various advisory committees. All of this responsibility was in addition to his main job, head of one of the largest pediatric departments in the United States. The correspondence between all these parties alone was voluminous. It was also difficult to put together a full budget of income and expenditures for the whole operation, but records show that in 1960 Dr. Janeway obtained a loan of $60,000 from a bank and received $13,600 from friends to help pay this back. If this was all the New York office had to work with, times were difficult there indeed, as well as in Iran. Also in 1960, and perhaps as a result of the financial conundrum, CAJ drew up two tables of organization to illustrate possible ways the Iran Foundation could function. One, which he felt was the way they had been operating, was for the Foundation to be responsible for all three of the operating entities in Iran: Shiraz Medical Center, which in turn was composed of the Nemazee Hospital, the Khalili eye hospital, and the Nemazee School of Nursing, the Nemazee Vocational School; and the water works. The other scheme, which is what he felt that Mr. Nemazee now wanted, was for the Boyadiran to run the water works and the vocational school, while the Iran Foundation managed only the Shiraz Medical Center. Lack of clarity on this central issue plagued the combined operations for the next six years and, combined with the cultural divide between American and Iranian views of the operation, helped to decrease the Foundation's effectiveness.[54]

Want of adequate funding was also a major continuing problem. With Mr. Nemazee decreasing his commitment and the Iranian government delaying or avoiding payments, the Iran Foundation turned to fund raising in the United States. In the 1961–62 report, Dr. Mehra observed that such fund raising in the United States had begun with the production of a film of the medical center and a fund drive that had added more than 1,000 members to those giving, but had resulted only in total contributions of $40,678, highlighting Mehra's assertion that this was unlikely to be a large or reliable source of support.[55] Mehra compared the amount to the $145,800 secured from US AID to pay salaries of the American staff, and the contributions of the Iranian oil operating companies and the Iranian government. Some additional funds were being raised in Iran from private sources. It is no wonder that the Iran Foundation and Mehra had to seek government support, knowing that it brought with it considerable baggage and risk.

Dr. Janeway's third trip to Iran, in December 1961, included stops in Athens and Ankara, as were mentioned in a previous chapter. He compared the Haceteppe Hospital in Ankara, which was developing well under the leadership of Ihsan Dogramaci, with the problems he was facing in Shiraz. He attributed the differences to three reasons: Turkey had undergone a social and governmental revolution many years before; Heceteppe Hospital was in the capital city; and, finally, there had been one leader, Dogramaci, in Turkey who was politically astute and had money of his own to put into the enterprise, which had allowed him to solve the financial and political problems as "no one possibly could in Shiraz."[56]

Dr. Janeway acknowledged that his analysis of the situation in Iran was superficial but nevertheless was essential in planning for the future of the Shiraz program. Inflation had been halted, but at the price of high unemployment. The contrast between the extreme wealth of the few and the desperate poverty of the many was still very apparent. He added, "Corruption, particularly in high places, is at least the subject of far more frequent and bitter journalistic comment than on my previous visits," and he commented further on the restive students, warning that "It is a race against time."[57] He wondered whether the government of Iran could institute the essential fiscal, administrative, and tax reforms, particularly the latter, in time to satisfy the restless intellectual groups. He sensed that revolution could occur in Iran.

Janeway's detailed notes reveal his concern for all phases of the Iran Foundation's operation, including the water works and the vocational school. The medical center remained his major concern, however. In addition to the constant problems with underfinancing, he now recognized that the administration was overburdened. Mehra continued to provide superb visionary leadership and had played a large role in developing plans for the new institution, Pahlavi University, to be the name of the old University of Shiraz. He had bought up small pieces of property that, all together, allowed the university to have sufficient land to develop. He supplied outstanding direction, but administering the day-to-day details of the center was not his forte. Janeway strongly recommended that the Iran Foundation find an experienced administrator for the center. In addition, he advised that since the government of Iran was such a vital part in the success of the Shiraz endeavor, an office devoted entirely to the Foundation's interest be established in

Teheran. Mehra had been performing this function in addition to all his other activities, but CAJ believed that Mehra would soon have a major role in the new Pahlavi University and would not be able to continue his previous activity on behalf of the Iran Foundation and the facilities in Shiraz.

Dr. Janeway conducted interviews with almost all of the staff in private and received an earful of grievances.[58] In addition to participating in several lectures and case conferences, he also saw several children in consultation, making for extremely busy dawn-to-late-night days. He was not discouraged, however, for among the many interviews he found several of the staff doing what he had hoped: "This man makes me feel good. He has no preconceptions. He's working. After one year he wants to evaluate the situation here with his own objectives."[59] He also met with the director of engineering for the water works and went into details of needs, such as "5 million Rials—Connections and pipes—might be cut in half by using Iranian asbestos and cement pipe."[60] This, as well as similar details of plant management and expansion, and the fact that Janeway, with little knowledge of engineering, felt it necessary to go into such detail, demonstrate that the management of the hospital left much to be desired in the details. On the trip home, a stop in Teheran found him busy with visits to the Prime Minister, the Minister of Health, and the head of the US AID mission. CAJ was distressed to finally understand why the Rockefeller and Ford foundations were reluctant to fund Shiraz. "They won't play officially—because must serve the whole country, not one university." He wondered who would carry the ball; he felt that they couldn't find the right Iranians in Teheran for the Boyadiran; so he wrote a letter to Ala, warning him of the dangers to the university if a bad group inserted a few trustees at this point.[61]

As if the stress of the problems in Shiraz were not enough, the trip home was a nightmare: delayed flights, passports taken in Bagdad, plane to London delayed, kept in a "dungeon." Janeway was clearly upset when he made entries in his diary. Nonetheless, Janeway's diary reflected his view that the trip was worthwhile after all. He was glad he had made the trip, although he felt that he had been away for years.

The gulf which divides most of Iran from the US is not years wide, it is centuries wide, but it's worth it. There are fine people in this coun-

try . . . They are fighting a long, tough battle for human brotherhood. Their job is infinitely tougher than mine. If I can help them,
it's worth while, because nationalism, in the political sense, is the
bunk . . . It's a long tough battle, in which all men are in the same
boat to find happiness, serenity and a feeling of unity with men of
good will that I have found, in Ankara, in Athens, in Teheran and in
Boston. I've found selfishness and nastiness in all these places. The
world is our country and it's a fascinating and inspiring one to be in.[62]

He praised several people by name and ended: "We belong to the human race." This is as good a statement of his world view as any he ever
made, wrote, or published. It is a vision that all of us can aspire to today and that our leaders would do well to follow.

Relations with Shiraz University had deteriorated, however. In his
report to the Iran Foundation, Janeway pointed out that a dissident
group of professors had unseated the chancellor, Dr. Gorban, and
wanted to revert to the old traditional Iranian school with its large
classes and mainly didactic teaching. His diary recorded that a bright
spot was the recruitment of a "Fine man, Dr. Rahmatian, Professor of
Pathology," who had come from Teheran as chancellor and had
brought people together. He had arranged a luncheon in Dr. Janeway's
honor, which the Governor General and the commanding military
general of the region attended, as well as deans and faculty. As an example of Dr. Rahmatian's diplomatic ways, CAJ noted that he "gave
credit to both the old professors" and the "new young teachers."[63]
Janeway then, in his official report, discussed the new Pahlavi University, the history of which we will now briefly review.

The University of Shiraz Medical School operated a nearby hospital,
the Saadi, which had 213 beds. The faculty of medicine had been established in 1946 and was one of the oldest of the major parts of the University, being incorporated as part of Shiraz University in 1957, making
it only one of five such medical faculties in Iran at that time. The medical school's class size was small; thirty-nine physicians were graduated
in 1956. Janeway considered the Chancellor, Dr. Gorban, "to have vision and dedication to the American system of medical education."[64] It
was natural for the physicians recruited to Shiraz Medical Center (*i.e.*,
the Nemazee Hospital) to want to teach there and for the Shiraz Medical School to want them, as there were only twenty-eight faculty in all

of the clinical departments. As usual, money was the problem. The medical school owned the Saadi Hospital and paid one-third of its total budget for the care of indigent patients in this hospital in order to have teaching material. There was little left for the faculty of the Shiraz Medical Center, who, by teaching students, had less time to care for patients at their own hospital and improve the finances of that institution. As noted above, the Iran Foundation had considered originally establishing its own medical school but did not have enough money to do so. Dr. Janeway acknowledged that "turning our back on the current Shiraz Medical School, which is less than half a mile away, and which does have government support, would be unwise."[65]

In 1959, the Shah became interested in developing a modern university based at Shiraz, as mentioned earlier. In 1960, a team under the chairmanship of the president of the University of Pennsylvania made an exhaustive study of higher education in Iran and recommended establishment of an independent university, that is, an institution supported by government funds but supplemented by independent sources. Among the recommendations was the need for diversity among the units of higher education, as was practiced in North American institutions. The recommendations pointed out the strength of such diversity compared to the monolithic structure in Iran, where all schools of higher learning were of one mould and were administrated by the Ministry of Education. The report also recommended freedom from political influence.[66]

In December 1961, just before Janeway's visit, such a university was formed. The Shah was honorary chair of the Board that was chaired, in fact, by his close associate, Mr. Ala, Minister of the Court (i.e., Prime Minister). The new institution departed from the usual Iranian university in that instead of being controlled by the Ministry of Education, it was to have independent legal status as embodied in its Board of Trustees.[67] The University of Pennsylvania entered into a relationship with the University of Shiraz and its name was changed to Pahlavi University, after the family of its patron, the Shah. The name of the medical center was also changed to Pahlavi Medical Center. This allowed extension of the contract with US AID ($250,000 in 1962) and the promise of an outstanding academic institution. Dr. Janeway was enthusiastic about this development.

In early July of 1963 the president of the University of Pennsylvania and a committee reported to the Pahlavi Board of Trustees. They noted a number of problems affecting the medical center, including some arbitrary decisions by the Chancellor. One of these was the closing of 120 of the 200 beds of the Saadi Hospital, thus throwing on the Nemazee Hospital a huge burden for the care of the indigent. Other problems included the lack of trained faculty at Saadi hospital and a disruption of cooperation between the various components of the Pahlavi University Medical Center.[68] The effort at Pahlavi University was a remarkable blueprint for a modern university, emphasizing as it did the need for independence from political interference, the marriage of the college of arts to prepare a broad-based professional group, and a modern organizational structure. The report also pointed out a number of problems that Pahlavi University now faced in Shiraz.

However, these educational reforms and the financial burden of needing to provide free care for indigent patients had also created severe problems. Dr. Janeway would point out in the Foundation's 1962–63 annual report that those years had brought about a great political change in Iran, provoked by "continuing drought and consequent hardships . . . the water works has devoted all of its income to drilling new and deeper wells."[69] But despite these problems, as Janeway proudly pointed out, the Nemazee Hospital now had 200 beds open, as well as an extensive educational program, ambitious community services, and basic research programs. Noting in the report that this combination of objectives had made the Nemazee Medical Center a medical lighthouse in that part of the world, director Mehra told that the medical center had moved into the community, as had been his dream. In slum areas, 10,000 people at a time were being rehabilitated; cesspools were being filled in; drinking water was being supplied from taps installed on the streets; windows were being put in houses; courtyards were being paved; and trees were being planted. In addition, other projects dealing with nutrition, sanitation, clothing, education, and civic improvement were being implemented. Much good was being done. But on a darker side, Mehra reported that the center had by then incurred debts of over $1,000,000, and neither the community programs nor the hospital were generating adequate funds to pay for the services. As a result, a crisis erupted in early June that would have serious consequences.

The crisis was precipitated by a letter that the Foundation received from Mr. Nemazee on June 4, in which he pointed out that there had never been adequate budgetary control over expenditures, especially for various expansions. Nemazee noted that director Mehra's virtues constituted faults; he was inclined to expand and commit himself before obtaining authority from the Board or assuring himself that adequate funds were available. Nemezee stated that he blamed himself, in part, as treasurer for not restraining Mehra. The bottom line was that the Shiraz Medical Center was now $2,000,000 in debt. He proposed several steps to solve or check the problem, including making the Boyadiran responsible for approving budgets. He proposed a lesser role for the Iran Foundation, suggesting that it be limited to "interesting American citizens to assist Iran, not by donations to meet deficits, but by way of technical advice as well as services (doctors, nurses, technicians, etc.) or donations of equipment."[70]

This sudden news resulted in a series of letters passing between Dr. Janeway and Mr. Nemazee. Janeway wrote to Nemazee after the June meeting of the Iran Foundation's board, remonstrating him that the severe crisis in financing was the result of the Iranian government not paying its promised share for indigent care, as well as debts incurred in the completion of the plant and equipment and deficits from past operating losses. In one of the last of these letters, CAJ, for the first time, rather bluntly told Nemazee that part of the crisis was his own doing. Mr. Nemazee was demanding repayment for capital expenditures that he had felt were necessary and for which he had given the money, but which the Iran Foundation had assumed were gifts, not loans. As CAJ put it, "Whatever was in anybody's mind when these operating and capital expenditures were made, both governments and private contributors are now bound to feel, when they learn, as they are sure to do, that the staff house and waterworks revenues are paid to you rather than to the hospital, that they are being asked to extricate you from a philanthropic endeavor of which you have now repented."[71] These strong words from such a mild-mannered person are indicative of Janeway's sense of honor to meet commitments. He felt betrayed. He ended his letter with the comment, "Such an impairment of the public image of one who deserves so much respect and affection from the country would deeply grieve those of us who have had the privilege of working with you to bring to fruition a great idea." He went on to warn that, unless adequate resources could be found, the Iran Foundation would "be forced to take drastic action, even to the extent of closing most of the hospital."

In mid June, Bettina Warburg had been dispatched on an emergency fact-finding trip to Iran, which included discussions with Nemazee; she delivered her report of the situation there at at meeting of the Medical Advisory Council of the Iran Foundation on June 24.[72] In discussions that followed, it was determined that the Foundation did not consider Nemazee's initial proposal to be a viable option. According to the terms of the Foundation's incorporation, as well as the agreement of 1960, its officers believed that they had what was known as "approbational trustee status." Therefore, they felt, by law, responsible for determining overall budgets and administrative direction of the institutions in which they had become involved. While conceding that the Foundation's goal was to assist Iranians in organizing and ultimately operating those institutions, in their opinion that day had not yet come. In their view, the emphasis of the Shiraz Medical Center, unlike most Iranian institutions, was upon quality rather than quantity. They felt that Mr. Nemazee had, from early 1957, arbitrarily decided that what the Foundation considered contributions to the hospital building and operation became debts payable to him, and they informed him of their view. The Executive Committee of the Iran Foundation met on July 22 to review a reply from Nemazee, in which he disagreed with some points in the Foundation's resolution and demanded that Dr. Janeway come to Shiraz to work out the problems.[73] But at a meeting of the Board of Directors on July 25, CAJ said that he would not go.

Janeway wrote to Nemazee in early August and outlined steps he thought necessary to preserve the center.[74] But in the end, he changed his mind and made a fourth trip to Iran, from August 19 to 26, 1963. His ultimate change of mind, or heart, may have been influenced by a cable that Dr. Mehra sent to the Iran Foundation on July 31: "Our financial situation hopelessly desperate. Please send thirty thousand immediately."[75] Janeway's records show that he sent a Foundation check in that amount with a note that this came as a loan from an anonymous donor. It is not clear where the money came from, but the 1962–63 annual report records several donations from Janeway's family and friends, including $1,100 from himself; and in a letter to his brother

Edward about this time, he asked for a donation to help meet the crisis.[76]

So it was that in August 1963 Dr. Janeway again visited Shiraz. He began his diary with the note, "Mission—a tough one,"[77] aware of all of the difficulties that lay ahead. When Janeway came face to face with Mr. Nemazee following his arrival in Iran, he found the philanthropist angry because he felt that Janeway should not have been so honest with Mr. Ala and Mr. Alam when he said that the experiment was a failure if the government did not pay on time. CAJ did not appreciate the cultural differences in Iran, where one did not blame the government, especially if it wanted its support. Janeway found that the same problems as before continued to exist at Shiraz Medical Center. Some of the American medical staff felt that it had not sold itself as a center for community service to the well-to-do. The start-up of Pavlavi University had complicated the picture. While the university desired to support the hospital, it was short of money also and substantial rivalries had developed between the Nemazee staff and the staff of the university hospital. At a dinner Janeway was complimented by one Iranian for grasping Iranian psychology, his point being, "You are dealing with crooks. Americans too decent. British much better."[78]

On this visit, Janeway and Mehra inspected the site of the planned university. They were impressed with the site, but were dismayed that, with significant money available, construction had not begun. Yet, the university was an operating organization, and, in medicine, was operating the old Saadi Hospital and medical teaching hospital even while it was sending too many seriously ill patients to the Nemazee Hospital. At the end of his trip, CAJ made a number of recommendations: maintaining high standards; cutting a number of beds; working toward a caseload of two-thirds indigent and one-third private patients; drawing up an agreement of cooperation with the University; cutting expenditures and submitting a regular financial statement to the board of the Iran Foundation, with no capital outlays without approval of the board and making every effort to increase support. At a meeting back in Teheran, at which he again met Nemazee, Ala, the Prime Minister, said that the Shah wanted the indebtedness settled. And, at an apparent later meeting with Nemazee, Janeway noted that Nemazee was willing to forego his claim for expenses he had paid for, adding, "but didn't like how he said it."[79] When he called Mr. Ala the next day, Janeway was told that as soon as the man from the bank came, he would arrange payment. To CAJ this sounded like "the check is in the mail," but at a later meeting with other government officials he learned that he was right to be concerned. It was likely that the chancellor of the University of Teheran desired to let Shiraz wither on the vine; there was still concern that the Shiraz program was too expensive; and Janeway found it "tough to sell a quality idea."[80]

Back in America, Janeway found that once more the financial crisis had been forestalled but by no means solved. The Shah had issued an order to take over the debt of the medical center and send additional sums for the care of indigent patients and expansion of the nursing school, but these payments were late and never for the full amount. In the summary report of his visit that he prepared for the Iran Foundation, CAJ was much more optimistic than he was when making diary entries.[81] Dr. Janeway also wrote a position paper for the Iran Foundation Board in which he went over the history and many of the details and problems that they had reviewed there, citing the difficulty of breaking down the walls of a traditional feudal agricultural society and trying to build a tradition in the Nemazee Hospital and in the Shiraz community that reflected the dignity of the individual, a sense of cooperation and self-help, and civic responsibility.[82]

All of these events were taking place in a climate of social and economic revolution in Iran. The Shah had begun land distribution, alienating some of the wealthy; he had also initiated programs to increase literacy and emancipate women, both of which goals challenged centuries of tradition. This was extremely true in the province of Fars, in which Shiraz was located and where 800,000 people were nomads. With land distribution, once-wealthy landlords could not, or believed they could not, pay for Nemazee Hospital care. There had been riots, and the hospital had cared for a number of people injured in them; but fortunately, there had been no damage to the buildings of the medical center. And, as was so common with the enterprise, the pledge of the Shah to free up money did not result in its immediate release; only after some five months of further pleas by Mehra were emergency funds transferred to Shiraz. Another problem was the government's relationship with the University of Pennsylvania, which did not share Jane-way's vision of a close relationship with the Nemazee Hospital. CAJ had written, as a goal of this trip, "Must make Penn realize that SMC [Shiraz Medical Center] and PUMS [Pahlavi University Medical School] are one, not warring factions."[83]

The years 1964 through 1966 were critical for the Iran Foundation's role in Shiraz. The financial problems of the medical center continued to be worrisome, as the Iranian government's payment was not received. Even the New York office had to be reduced in staff, and only "another generous gift" allowed it to continue. In his 1963–65 presidential report, Janeway related that in 1964 Mr. Ala had died and Dr. Mehra had resigned.[84] When tendering his resignation, Mehra had complained that "his principals [sic] had been compromised and may cease altogether, I no longer wish to be associated with this center."[85] Mehra's departure had come as a blow to Dr. Janeway, who had found in him a visionary soul mate. After Mehra passed from the scene, Dr. Ziai, as Acting Director, presented the financial crisis to the Shah. In response, eighteen million rials were advanced and the salaries of the center's personnel were included in the budget. With the Shah's intervention, the chancellor resigned and Mr. Alam assumed his position. If one could get to the Shah, and the Shah was interested, things happened. However, the deteriorating political situation often made it impossible to get the Shah's ear or to establish a permanent subsidy from the government.

A number of problems arose in 1964 after Alam became chancellor of Pahlavi University. A particularly troublesome one surfaced after Mr. Alam made appointments to the Nemazee Hospital staff without consulting the authorities of the Iran Foundation, causing Mr. Nemazee to appeal to Dr. Janeway to have the Foundation exercise its duties as "approbational trustee" to defend the interests and integrity of the hospital.[86] While Janeway responded that he thought they at the Iran Foundation should resign as trustees, since they could neither exert any influence of serve any useful function,[87] he nonetheless persuaded the foundation's board to continue for a period of six months to see what might be done. He was not quite ready to call it quits; he had too much invested in the enterprise to do that. At a meeting of the board on November 16, 1964, after several members stated that the Iran Foundation should resign as trustee, CAJ, ever the peacemaker, and because the Americans had started and helped develop the Shiraz institution, again argued that they should not walk out because "the people in the Hospital are in real trouble and asking for help, and that we should give it to them if we could." After much discussion, calm heads prevailed and the members of the foundation agreed to "hold off resignation at this time."[88]

An ominous note soon was heard when Mehra, who was now chancellor of the university at Gondi-Shapur in Ahwaz, Iran, as well as serving as roving ambassador for the Iran Foundation, reported that anti-American attitudes were now prevalent in Iran. Indeed, the Ford Foundation had seen fit to close its Teheran office for lack of cooperation. In late December, Ms. Dorothy Sutherland, chair of the Nursing Advisory Committee, visited Shiraz and reported to the Iran Foundation that the nursing school had made good progress, but that morale in the hospital was low.[89] Following Mehra's resignation, Mohsen Ziai, who had shared the duties of acting director for a time, found the pressure intolerable and left to return to Johns Hopkins to direct pediatric ambulatory services. Ms. Sunderland also reported conflicts between the staff of the Nemanzee Hospital and the team from the University of Pennsylvania, as well as general discontent on the part of the university's medical students. As the situation in Shiraz continued to deteriorate, with no resolution of the impasse in sight, Janeway in June 1965 resigned from the presidency of the Iran Foundation, although he continued to chair its Medical Advisory Committee. Claude Forkner, who had started the whole project in the late 1940s as a result of having been a consultant physician to the Shah, had resigned from the board of the foundation the previous November. Following these events, the Iran Foundation gradually turned its attention away from the Shiraz Medical Center to other aspects and problems of Iranian society, culture, and life.

In 1986, Dr. Campbell McMillan, the first American pediatrician to go to Shiraz, communicated to one of the authors that his experiences in Iran were incredible, and he listed many diseases he had never seen before going there. "And yet," he went on, it was clearly evident that the experiment was beset with some faulty assumptions . . . the incongruity between what we were demonstrating and what the people of Iran could assimilate and use was simply too great . . . After all, medicine as we know it is a middle class enterprise and Iran had no real middle class . . . in retrospect the countdown for the fall of the Shah had begun while we were there. Many of these problems were not clear to us then, and that includes Dr. Janeway, whose incredible goodness often bordered on the naive.[90]

Charles and Betty Janeway concluded their 1965–66 tour of Asia with a visit to Iran on the way back home. Their curiosity to know what was going on there could not be quashed. They arrived in Shiraz at the end of January, where, as evidence of his interest in the entire university, CAJ met first with the dean of engineering and the chair of the mathematics department before attending a staff conference at Nemezee Hospital, which, he noted, had grown greatly, although its underpinnings appeared to have weakened. On the following day CAJ went to the university to discuss how the Iran Foundation could help. His diary notes that the dean wanted several visiting professors to come for three months each, and asked for help in placing people who were going to the United States and for assistance in teaching research (through visiting professors). At midday, Dr. Janeway gave a lecture on the development of immunity to a full house and noted that the audience were attentive, asked questions, and "seemed to enjoy it."[91] In the afternoon he toured the Nemazee Hospital, remarking on everything from maintenance to a cobalt irradiation machine. He met with the nursing staff and heard a number of complaints, particularly about a lack of administration and clear division of responsibility, and that they were experiencing the same flight of their faculty to the U.S. as the doctors were.

Dr. Janeway concluded that Pahlavi University needed Iran Foundation support and help but it had to "clear relations with Pahlaui University and Mr. Alam." He summarized his impressions: "Peace reigns under Mr. Alam and money is coming. Basic sciences have moved ahead. Clinical [care] may have slipped, but situation more stable. Nemazee Hospital O.K. but weakness in administration and clear cut lines of authority, with doctors doing too much."[92] His recommendations included the need for pediatrics to have a convalescent facility, more money for nursing, and the need to get research going.[93] The visit to Nemazee Hospital had been reassuring to him, although the medical center was not up to his dreams; however, the chances of a top rating were not available in a developing country.

Before going on to Teheran, the Janeways paid visits to a few other places of interest, one of them being the new school of medicine at Gondi-Shapur in the oil-rich area of Ahwaz, where his friend Torab Mehra was playing a leading role. CAJ was particularly pleased to find that a few of the nurses at Ahwaz were from the Nemazee school.[94] In May 1966 Dr. Warburg and Dr. Mehra spent two weeks surveying Iran to ascertain the feasibility of further Iran Foundation services in Iran. They returned with a number of possible projects, They were especially impressed with the need for welfare and health programs in the Persian Gulf region, where some of the oil companies seemed interested in investing in projects. CAJ's purpose in Teheran, where they arrived on February 5, was again as consultant visiting a new hospital. Some of the Iranians he had trained in the United States worked there. He noted that it was "A first class hospital . . . organized beautifully . . . Good care at every level . . . Sorry we don't have these men at Shiraz . . . Doing what Nemazee Hospital set out to do."[95] The problem was that Shiraz was still looked upon as provincial, and the school at Gondi-Shapur had money from the oil companies. In Teheran, Janeway had an opportunity to see Mr. Nemazee and report on Shiraz. He also visited with Mr. Alam who "doesn't want Mr. Nemazee interfering with hospital."[96] To Mr. Alam, Janeway emphasized the development of the Shiraz Medical College and the need for administrative coordination, a clear budget, and authority. He recommended an administrative survey of needs and the necessity to have a channel of communication from Pahlavi University to the Iran Foundation via the dean of the University.

Although the Iran Foundation had by this time given up management of the Shiraz Medical Center, Janeway was still emotionally involved with the project. He wanted it to succeed under the management of the university and was prepared to help it do so. He was welcomed by the Iranians who were then in charge. CAJ's ongoing commitment to Shiraz Medical Center was characteristic of the man: once he was involved with anything, he never let go. It was also true of the faculty he trained and the friends he made, as well as the international institutions he worked so hard to establish. This seemed to be the last chapter in his deep involvement in Shiraz, however. Mehra, in a summary of the history of the Iran Foundation's involvement in Shiraz, said, "Although the Iran Foundation had in the past aimed at high standards in Shiraz, it had become evident that in certain ways the infrastructure of the country had not been ready to accept this type of American thinking and organization. Therefore the foundation was now turning its interests to a people-to-people approach."[97]

Although this was the end of the Iran Foundation's involvement in Shiraz, it was not the end of the enterprise. In 1968, Chancellor Alam convinced Dr. Ziai to return as director of the hospital. Ziai did so reluctantly, for he recognized the almost insurmountable problems. After one year, he left, and, as arranged by Alam, assumed the presidency of the University of Meshed in northern Iran. He stayed at Meshed for one year and then returned to Teheran as dean of the medical school. He returned to the United States in the late 1970s, was chief of pediatrics at Rochester General Hospital, affiliated with the University of Rochester, and then moved to Virginia where he ultimately retired as chief of pediatrics at Fairfax Hospital in 1999. He reported recently that the Nemazee Hospital is an integral part of the University Medical School and that, while it does not function at a high level of expertise as was originally envisioned, it has been a force for improving medical care and education in Iran. Even though many of the physicians recruited to Shiraz later left that city, they brought a higher level of care to other areas of Iran. Ziai sees the experiment as having achieved some, if not all of the original goals. The glass is at least half full, in his view.[98]

Charles Janeway made a final visit to Iran in 1975, the visit taking place between April 19 and 25. He met his daughter Barbie in London following a trip to the Cameroons, and they proceeded to Shiraz. His terminal illness had by this time so progressed that either Betty or Barbie accompanied him on international visits. Charles and Barbie were housed in one of the new luxurious villas in Shiraz, leading CAJ

to write in his diary, "Mr. Nemazee's tomb to left of hospital entrance
. . . when you see what he created (with Torab's help), a great man, but
he must have been mad at the end."[99] Symbolically, perhaps, the sumptuous villas reflected the final dissolution of the Iran Foundation's role.
Janeway must have been annoyed that the Shiraz center, which had endured such financial problems, should at the end have received such a
luxurious gift not directly related to its central mission of patient care
and education. Dr. Janeway attended a congress at Shiraz, which presumably was the reason for his visit, for the Iran Foundation had long
ceased its involvement. He presented a lecture, toured facilities, and
was impressed with, in addition to the nursing care, the good medical
records and the Clinical Research Center. He also noted that people
wanted to come to the hospital, in contrast to former feelings.[100] Yet,
many of the problems of the past still remained. Young Dr. Garib, son
of Dr. Ziai's father-in-law, was concerned that students were "not curious, don't have drive to do research, and [because it was] hard to get
good residents."[101]

Janeway saw much progress evident in Iran on his 1975 visit. However, he did not see the impending revolution. In 1978, the Shah imposed martial law to end violent anti-government demonstrations; the
oil industry was shut down; and the Ayatollah Khomeni appealed for
labor strife to overthrow the Shah, which was accomplished within a
year. There is no record of what Dr. Janeway thought of the revolution. Perhaps he, like Ziai, saw so many aspects of the Shah's regime as
blemished that he welcomed a change; in any case, he did not live long
enough to see the harmful aspects of the revolution. Ziai and others
still believe that the noble experiment in Shiraz left a beacon of hope, a
vision of what good medical care could do to promote good health
that has survived all the terrible consequences of the revolution. Indeed, the experiment in Shiraz was a revolution in medical care. Like
most revolutions, it was needed, but for the time swung too far. A recent commentator has observed that the American revolution is the
only one that has not, in time, been overturned.[102]

As the cliché has it, hindsight is always 20/20. From the high hopes
in the beginning to the more realistic but somber ending of the Iran
Foundation's involvement in the Shiraz project, it was a roller-coaster

ride. Janeway and his colleagues on the Iran Foundation's board had highly principled reasons to start this program. Mr. Nemazee was contributing his wealth to build and sustain a modern American-style hospital in Shiraz that would not only help improve the health of the local residents but would also be a beacon to change medical education for Iran and the entire Middle East. Charles Janeway and his colleagues found an outlet for their desire to improve the health of the world's poor and, in Janeway's case, fulfil the belief that in doing so he would contribute to the peace of the world.

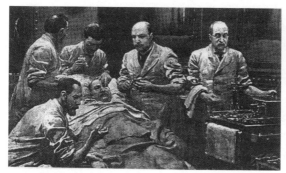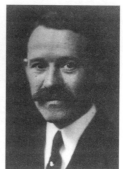

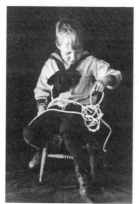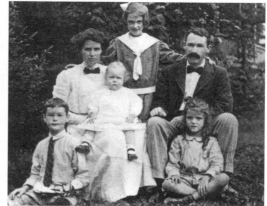

Illustration 1. *Above:* left, Edward Gamaliel Janeway (lower left) as consultant at the operation of President Clevelend on a boat on the East River, New York, 1895 (reproduced, with permission, from *Pharos of Alpha Omega Alpha,* summer 1995); right, Theodore Caldwell Janeway, about age 40 (courtesy of Alan Mason Chesney Archives, Johns Hopkins Medical Institutions). *Below:* left, Charles Janeway, age five, dressed in a sailor suit, untying the Gordian knot, on entry to Calvert School in Baltimore, September 1914; right, The Janeway family, 1910. Seated at front, Edward and Agnes; center, Eleanor Alderson Janeway holding CAJ, and husband Theodore; in rear, Eleanor (called Nora).

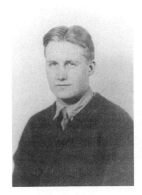

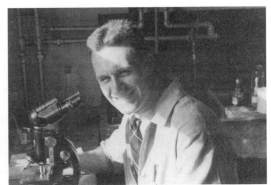

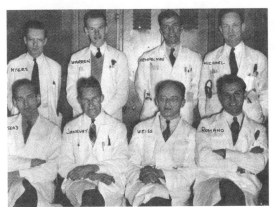

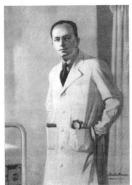

Illustration 2. *Above:* left, CAJ, age 18, as freshman at Yale, 1927; right, CAJ at microscope in Hans Zinsser's laboratory, Harvard Medical School, ca. 1938. *Below:* left, Peter Bent Brigham Hospital Department of Medicine, 1940. First row, left to right, Drs. Stead, Janeway, Weiss, Romano; second row, Drs. Myers, Warren, Hempelman, Michael (reproduced from *Pharos of Alpha Omega Alpha,* summer 1996); right, oil painting of Dr. Soma Weiss, 1939, by Martin Mower.

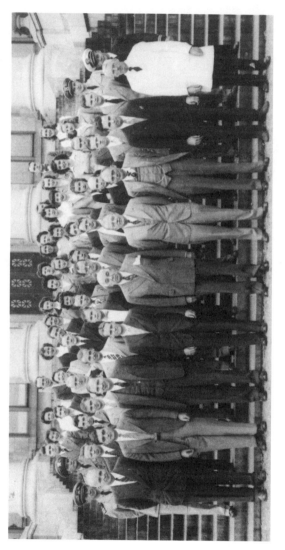

Illustration 3. Members of Protein Laboratory, Department of Physical Chemistry, Harvard Medical School, 1944. CAJ is in front row, fourth from the left, with Edwin Cohn in the center next to him, and John Enders is seventh from the left, with Franc Ingraham (white coat) at the end of the row.

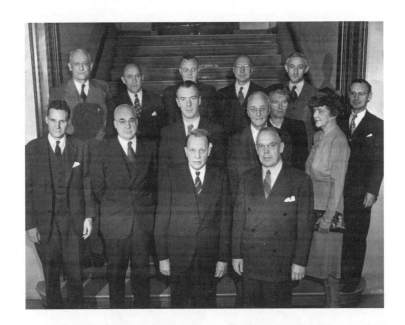

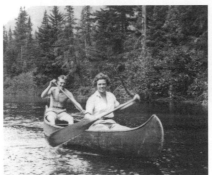
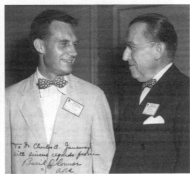

Illustration 4. *Above:* Meeting of the Executive Committee of the American National Red Cross Advisory Board on Health Services, Washington, D.C., November 20, 1946. Front row, left to right, L.H. Weed and H.R. Viets; second row, CAJ, I. Hiscock, A. Christie, E.A. Graham, M.W. Sheahan, R. Emerson, C.G. King; Third row, E.A. Strecker, M. Fishbein, E.L. Stebbins, K.F. Maxey, and A. Wolman. *Below:* left, CAJ and Betty canoeing, probably in the Adirondacks, ca. 1940; right, CAJ with Basil O'Connor, president of the American National Red Cross, Atlantic City, New Jersey, at the time Janeway chaired the Committee on Blood and Blood Derivatives for the Red Cross program.

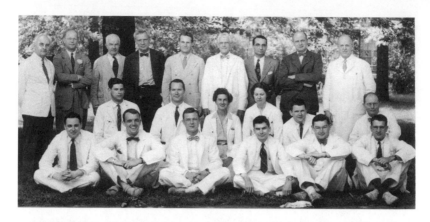

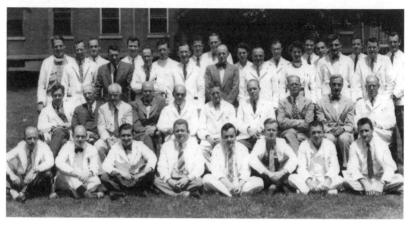

Illustration 5. *Above:* The Children's Hospital Pediatric Department in 1944–46, at the time of CAJ's appointment as chair. First and second rows (seated), unidentified residents; last row, Drs. William Lenox, Randolph Byers, Bronson Crothers, James Gamble, CAJ, Richard Smith, Louis K. Diamond, Charles Lowe, John Davies. *Below:* The Pediatric Department of Children's Hospital Boston,1946–47, CAJ's second year as chief. Front row, left to right, Resident staff, including Drs. Jack Metcoff (second from left) and Thomas Weller (sixth from left); second row, Drs. Clement Smith, Louis Webb Hill, Bronson Crothers, Charles Lowe, R. Cannon Ely, CAJ, Charles May, Randolph Byers, Harold Stuart, John Davies; third row, Drs. Harry Schwachman, Sydney Gellis, William Wallace, unknown, Stuart Stevenson, William Berenberg, Gretchen Hutchins, Fred Moll, unknown; back row, residents and fellows, left to right, unknown, Drs. Charles Lowe, John Eliot, John Kennell, unknown, Alexander MacDonald, Elizabeth French, unknown, unknown, James Wolff, T. Barry Brazelton, unknown.

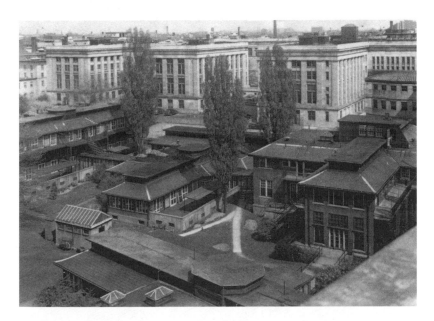

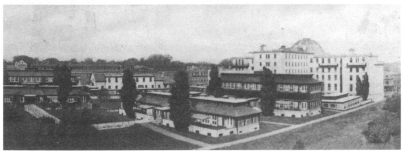

Illustration 6. *Above:* Children's Hospital cottage quadrangle, 1944, with the buildings of the Harvard Medical School in the background. *Below:* Another view of the Children's Hospital cottage quadrangle, 1944, with the domed Hunnewell structure in the background. The cottage complex now is, in part, the Prouty Gardens.

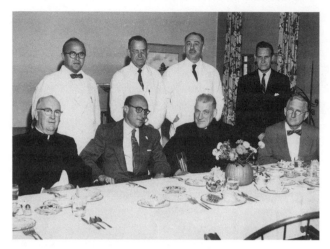

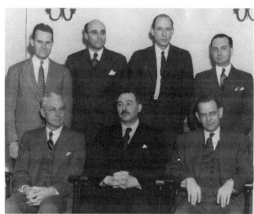

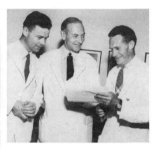

Illustration 7. *Above:* Luncheon for Archbishop (later Cardinal) John Cushing at the Children's Hospital, October 20, 1954. Seated, left to right, Msgr. Dalton, Guy Brugler, Archbishop Cushing, Mr. Wheeler; Standing, Drs. William Berenberg, William Green, Sidney Farber, CAJ. *Below left:* Executive Committee of Children's Hospital, 1951. Front row, left to right, Dr. Franc D. Ingraham (Chief of Neurosurgery), Dr. Sidney Farber (Chief of Laboratories and Pathology), Dr. William T. Green (Chief of Orthopedics); back row, CAJ (Chief of Medicine), Guy Brugler (Hospital Director), Dr. Edward B. Neuhauser (Chief of Radiology), Dr. Robert Gross (Chief of Surgery). *Below right:* St. Mary's (London)-Boston Children's Exchange Resident at the Children Hospital in 1953. Left to right, Drs. Henry Giles (Exchange Resident from St. Mary's Hospital, London), Reginald Lightwood chief of pediatrics of St. Mary's staff, and CAJ.

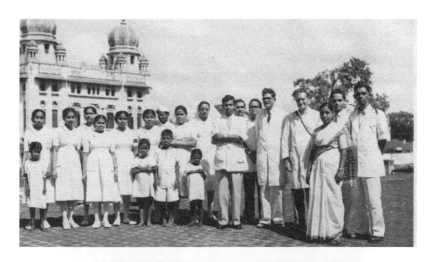

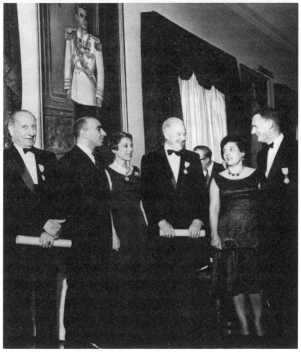

Illustration 8. *Above:* Staff of the Pediatric Department at the Madras, India, Medical School during Dr. Janeway's sabbatical in 1956. CAJ is fourth and Dr. Achar is fifth from the right; Mrs. Susila is to CAJ's left. *Below:* Dr. Janeway (right) at the Iranian Embassy in Washington, D.C. on the occasion of awards given by the Iranian ambassador to officers of the Iran Foundation. CAJ received the Order of the Taj from the Shah of Iran.

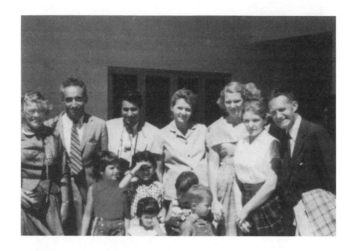

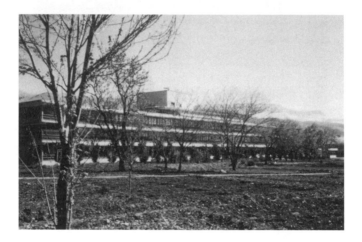

Illustration 9. *Above:* CAJ (far right) and Betty (far left) bidding farewell at the airport in Shiraz, Iran, in 1957. Others in photo are, from left to right, Dr. Torab Mehra, Dr. Ghademi, Mrs. Mehra, Mrs. Ghademi, and Mrs. Florence McMillan (wife of Dr. Campbell McMillan, pediatrician from Boston at the Nemazee Hospital). *Below:* Main section of Nemazee Hospital, Shiraz, Iran.

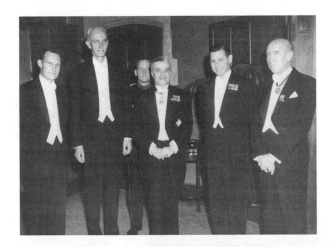

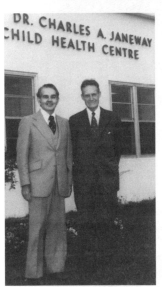

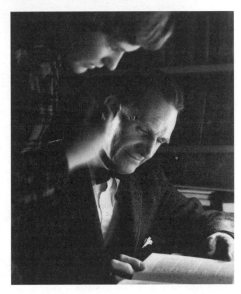

Illustration 10. *Above:* Dr. Janeway (left) at the combined meeting of the United States, Canadian and British pediatric societies held at Quebec City, Canada in 1959. CAJ was president of the Society for Pediatric Research at the time. Others pictured are to CAJ's left, Dr. A. E. Washburn, president of the American Pediatric Society, the Hon. G. Fauteux, Lieutenant Governor of Quebec, Dr. R.L. Denton, president of the Canadian Pediatric Society, and Dr. F.M.B. Allen, president of the British Pediatric Society, with Fauteux's aide-de-camp, Col. J.F. L'Esperance, in background. *Below:* left, CAJ (right) with Dr. E.J. Kelland, Executive Director of the Charles A. Janeway Health Centre, St. Johns, Newfoundland, Canada, in 1960; right, Dr. Janeway and his daughter Barbie in 1962.

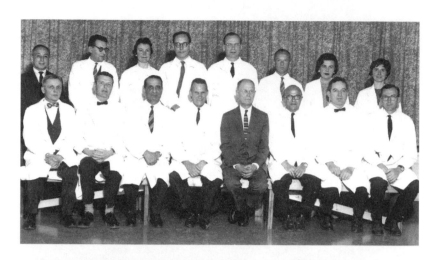

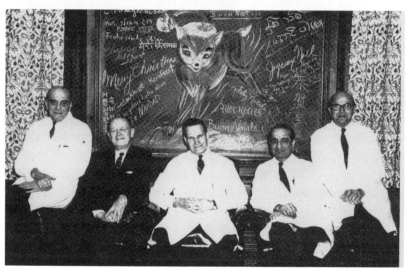

Illustration 11. *Above:* Pediatric Department faculty, 1963. Front row, left to right, Drs. Harry Mueller, C. Davenport Cook, Louis K. Diamond, CAJ, Randolph Byers, William Berenberg, John Crigler, Robert Haggerty; Back Row, Drs. Al Frank, Caesare Lombroso, Audry Evans, Alan Crocker, Park Gerald, Francis Fellers, Anna Mitus, unknown. *Below:* Image from a Department of Medicine holiday card, 1963, "Merry Christmas" written in many languages on the blackboard to the rear. Left to right, Drs. R. Cannon Eley, Randolph Byers, CAJ, Louis K. Diamond, and William Berenberg.

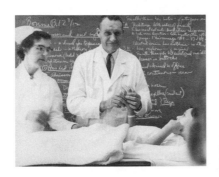

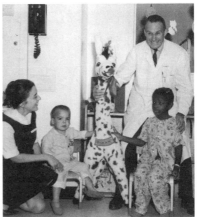

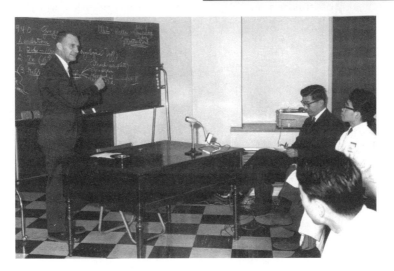

Illustration 12. *Above:* left, CAJ with head nurse at Childrens, Ms. Brooks Barnes and unidentified patient, January 14, 1964, with typical recordings of findings on the blackboard in Janeway's handwriting; right, CAJ in hospital with patients. His normally reserved demeanor was almost never evident in the presence of children. *Below:* CAJ lecturing at St. Lukes Hospital, Tokyo, 1965. His masterful use of the chalkboard was legendary, even in international circles.

10 INTERNATIONAL WORK AFTER 1966 AND DR. JANEWAY'S INTERNATIONAL LEGACY

CHARLES A. JANEWAY'S passion to improve pediatric medicine and the health of children abroad, especially in the underdeveloped areas of the world, continued uninterrupted during his final years as chair of medicine at the Children's Hospital in Boston; and the many travels he made overseas during this time, while sometimes including skiing and other vacation activities, had as their main focus the same altruistic interests on behalf of the underprivileged of the world that had been paramount to his thinking in the past. In March 1967 Dr. Janeway's international outlook took him on a trip to Europe in conjunction with a meeting of the board of the International Children's Center in Paris (about which we will have more to say later). And in February and March of 1971 Dr. Janeway undertook another journey overseas to attend a board meeting of the International Children's Center, this time in Senegal, at which time he was also to be the representative of the International Pediatric Association at the IPA congress that occurred in Senegal about the time of the ICC meeting.

Charles and Betty's first stop on this journey was at Dakar, Senegal, where they found that their luggage had become lost. That occurrence prompted him to tell his diary "NEVER AGAIN" and to resolve to put everything in the future in carry-on luggage.[1] Charles and Betty had to buy such necessities as clothing and toiletries, after which the airline located their luggage. Thereupon, in true frugal Janeway fashion, CAJ "returned clothes" to the store where he had bought them![2] The sights of the city offered a panorama of new experiences. Janeway, ever the observant and interested traveller, was amazed at local dress, customs, and obvious signs of unemployment such as disabled people begging and men selling "the same useless things."[3] One place in Dakar made a profound impression: the visit to Goree Island. The old slave market saddened Charles and Betty as they realized that a large number of slaves exported to the United States had passed through its one tiny building.

The IPA conference began on the third day of their trip. Janeway reported detailed papers on iron deficiency anemia among children with malnutrition. His previous criticism of IPA papers seems to have been muted; perhaps the papers were better, but Janeway may have come to accept the realization that papers from developing countries were the best the physicians from many countries could do at that stage of their development, and further, that these should be encouraged. Later in the meeting he also noted that Professor Fanconi of Switzerland gave an impassioned speech against building "big fancy hospitals in favor of health centers, controlling population—a dramatic change from his earlier interest only in rare cases. He has grown."[4] While Betty went on a visit to a rural Maternal and Child Health Center, Charles wrote his congress paper. That evening they had dinner with the American Ambassador; on another evening they enjoyed dinner with the French Ambassador; and as a grand finale, enjoyed a performance by the Senagalese National Dance Troupe and had a dinner that led CAJ to comment, "we've eaten and drunk a good part of the government's health budget for 1971."[5] He offered little comment about the content of the IPA Executive Committee issues, as he had done at previous congresses.

Dr. Fred Robbins had arranged with the president of the Firestone Tire and Rubber Company, which had rubber plantations in Liberia, for the Janeways to use the Firestone guest house in Monrovia, Liberia, their next stop (March 7–8). They did not discuss politics with the manager of the guest house, a Texan who told them "one black face was just like any other."[6] Charles and Betty must have kept their resentment under wraps. The visit to the Firestone Hospital was especially interesting to the Janeways because it had a high-risk pregnancy program that admitted mothers from regional health centers to a "Belly Ward" until they delivered. Although Janeway was impressed with the regional health center and the easy referral to the central hospital, he commented, "over 65% of money spent [on] amenities for the staff plus high pay."[7] At the airport on their way out of Liberia, they met a "former Colby College boy who had taught at Rivers [Country Day School] and had taken a year off to write on how two cultures could live side by side . . . he gave us an article he'd written on Liberia on basis of 11 day stay."[8] To such seasoned travellers as Charles and Betty Janeway, it must have sounded jarring to hear someone boast that he would be able to understand a foreign culture in eleven days.

The Janeways' next stop was Acra, Ghana (March 8–9), where they were greeted by a former resident at the Children's, Dr. Nkrumah, the son of the then dictator of that country. Janeway's friend, Bo Vahlquist, was also on this leg of the trip as they visited rural health centers. The Janeways and Vahlquist were impressed with the organization, the emphasis on family planning, and the evaluation efforts and involvement of medical students. Much of CAJ's later plan for the Cameroon venture that we will discuss shortly seems to be a mirror of what they saw in Ghana. The university hospital was restricted to babies under six months of age and referral cases, in order to keep the patient load manageable. On this short visit to Ghana Janeway was shown several unusual cases, which he enumerated in his diary.

Their next stop was Nairobi, Kenya (March 10–16), where they received a warm welcome from Dr. Alan Ross and his family. Dr. Ross was the former chair of pediatrics at McGill University in Montreal and a close friend. The early part of their visit was devoted to the impressive tourist sights of Kenya, but soon, at the hospital, which had a Canadian contingent of visiting faculty, Janeway went on student teaching rounds with Drs. Donald and Elizabeth Hillman. Here he saw severely ill patients with preventable diseases, such as measles, tuberculosis, gastroenteritis, and tetanus, but, "measles vaccine cost 5 shillings and health budget for Kenya [is] 7 shillings per year" (per person) .[9] In his diary CAJ listed several "problems for investigation; 1. Cellular immunity in patients with kwashiorkor, 2. Measles like diseases, 3. Coxsackie, in immunized children."[10] On this trip, as on every trip that Charles and Betty Janeway took, it is impressive to note how they arranged to meet old friends for lunch, dinner, or lodging, and were always making new friends at parties and airports, as well as keeping detailed accounts of expenses, dividing them between personal and professional. They were a meticulous pair. They were also wonderful American ambassadors of good cheer, representative of the best of American travellers.

In autumn of 1971 Janeway made another trip abroad, which, according to his diary, indicates that he was "a short term consultant to Center for Social Pediatrics, University of Antiqouia, Medellin, Colombia."[11] He travelled alone. When he arrived at Bogota there was no one to meet him, and problems continued: "Now I'm patiently waiting for a call to Medellin, which I put through in 5 minutes from Boston, but has been 30 minutes so far."[12] Janeway must have contacted someone, for early on November 1 he took off for Medellin, arriving after a harrowing approach to the airport through high mountains on each side of the plane.[13] Confusion continued at Medellin; no one was there to met him, either. Eventually, after several calls, Janeway was paged by a Dr. Solorzano, who briefed him on his duties as consultant: "four two hour sessions, some ward rounds and visits to clinics etc."[14] His host explained that the day was a religious holiday, which explained why no one had answered his telephone calls. CAJ learned, however, that another reason was conflict between the university's rector and faculty—many faculty had been fired and students were on strike.

His visit went ahead, however. His tour of the Children's Hospital included the surgical wards, which he described as "impressive, well organized," and the medical wards were "good . . . infectious diseases with cubicles . . . wards full of parents who love children and don't reject handicapped."[15] The social pediatrics unit attended to a population of 60,000 at a health center. He liked the plan whereby, after internship, all doctors would go to rural areas together with an older, supervising physician. Often during his visit he was told about the political situation confronting the University and the nation; the leftist university faculty and rightist rector, at loggerheads, mirrored a larger dynamic in Colombia. Two "girls" from Harvard Medical School (he seemed to call women medical students "girls") had spent time in these clinics. Whatever else he might have thought about the situation in Colombia, he notes that these individuals "got a marvelous education."[16] Janeway's lecture the next day on Infection and Immunity was well received, "except a start 25 minutes late. We only got through half the lecture so leave the rest till tomorrow."[17] He met with the dean, who was anxious to have exchanges with U.S. schools.

Dr. Janeway liked to walk about cities, the better to become more familiar with them. One afternoon, he look a long walk and described in detail funeral homes, which fascinated him because caskets were put in a wall with nameplates on the outside. He noticed numerous book stalls, and, in the latter, "plenty on Marxism and socialism, Trotsky, dialectics predominate. Absolutely no books in English."[18] On another day he was taken to visit the leading artist, Maestro Gomez. CAJ was much impressed with Gomez as a man, "a light in his eye, and an enthusiasm for life and a kind of creative vigor you feel."[19] The next day, he and the artist visited one of the university buildings, where was located one of Gomez's huge murals. Janeway was moved by "the atomic bomb scene and its effects on youth and phases of Colombian myths . . . at the bottom in stark white [was missing] the head of a man which the students didn't like so they cut it out. What sacrilege!"[20] Although Dr. Janeway was a liberal, certainly politically to the left, student revolts that destroyed art or damaged university property appalled him. He was a true academician in that he believed in the transforming power of education; to witness the willful destruction of facilities intended for education must have cut to the quick of his sense of values.

During most of his visit, Janeway's hostess was Dr. Piedrahita, who had spent two years in Boston with Dr. Francis Fellers in nephrology. Janeway's pride in what his institution had helped to accomplish was almost palpable: "The more I see of her the prouder I am that we gave her 2 years in Boston. She's intelligent, balanced, dedicated and knows everyone."[21] He was always especially happy to see people who had been at the Children's doing well. His vision of what Children's could be to the rest of the world was confirmed.

A familiar complaint surfaced when CAJ made ward rounds: "Noticed nobody washed hands."[22] This was anathema to Janeway, who washed his hands between every patient on rounds anywhere, in any hospital, in any part of the world. He described a number of seriously ill children and commented that one with agammaglobulinemia and pneumonia, who was not doing well, "had not been given loading dose [of gamma globulin] and I think I helped on that."[23] Later, at dinner, Janeway and his hosts discussed the future of Colombia. He reported that "all seem convinced a lot of things have to change and a revolution [is] likely."[24] The next day, after his lecture and lunch, "came the best of all . . . [a visit] to a district Hospital . . . The most impressive thing was the well worked out regionalization of health services . . . for the whole district . . . Rio Negro."[35]

On CAJ's final evening in Medellin, he met with several students, who came from several countries; each talked about her or his country. His trip home included a stop in Cartagena, Colombia, with description of the area. The diary concludes with a note about ethnicity in Colombia,. He observed that he had seen "few Indians—people are either Spanish stock descended from Conquistadors or Negroes who were brought as slaves. In general the rich are light, the workers dark. It is not possible for dark skinned industrialist to get into fancy clubs."[26] The fact that he wrote about this indicates that he disapproved of the ethnic segregation. He also disagreed that violence was a way to end it, however. He described a final conversation with Solarzano, who felt the university would not allow rich conservatives to force their views. Janeway appears to have been disturbed at the tenor of the conversation. "I put in the strongest pleas for non-violence and tolerance. I should send him the declaration on rights and responsibilities from Harvard."[27]

In many situations Janeway worked to compromise a seemingly intractable problem debated by opposing advocates. This was also true at the Children's and in the IPA. Now that he saw first hand the potential destruction of a university by ardent advocates from the right and the left, he was even more secure in his belief that compromise was the only way to resolve conflicting human affairs. His narrative ends with the name and address of a pediatrician in Medellin, with a note, "Told him he'd have the Beverly job unless it's gone on return."[28] (The Children's frequently placed foreign fellows in the Beverly, Massachusetts Hospital until they learned English and became acculturated to the U.S.) This was one more example of CAJ "bringing home another foreigner in his suitcase," as the residents liked to say.

The following year (March 1972), Dr. Janeway journeyed to Egypt. There were two reasons for the trip: CAJ was project officer for a

"Study of Genetic Anomalies in Egypt," a grant between the National Institute of Child Health and Human Development and Ain-Shams University in Cairo, and he went to assist in a project of the Harvard Maternal and Child Health Service on "Detection and Treatment of Inborn Errors of Metabolism Which Impair Mental Development." Janeway's host was Dr. Namet Haskem, who had been so hospitable to Betty and him on an earlier trip.

Janeway's visit to the dean of the Ain-Shams medical school to talk about medical education was followed by a visit to the old children's hospital, "with a mother or grandmother in every bed with the child. In the OPD they saw 400 to 800 children every day!"[29] Dr. Haskem was the geneticist with the grant. Her unit was "Clean, neat, charts on wall—not fancy but perfectly adequate."[30] He visited a postgraduate course and was surprised to hear the professor tell the students about dextro-maltose to be added to milk for babies' formulae but added, "but if you can't get it, take powdered milk and spit on it!"[31] Presumably this would add enough bacteria to break down the complex sugars into more digestible ones! Janeway was taken to the bazaar and to the main mosque, which was said to contain the tomb of Hussein. After viewing all the ill people touching the brass rail around the tomb in the hope of a cure, he wrote, "I emerged with my wallet, deeply impressed that religion had this much meaning to so many."[32]

Back in Dr.Haskem's office they discussed the grant and the need for a human investigation committee. Dr.Haskem felt that such a committee would be hopeless "Because jealousy would keep members from approving others' work. 2, Prevailing climate of only serving patients and not doing research. [She] wonders whether we can work it so our committee [i.e., at Children's, Boston] screens projects."[33] Janeway was concerned that some of the studies did not come under diagnosis and therapy and would need some type of approval. After more meetings CAJ felt "A committee here would be a disaster and we could take responsibility. In fact a more formal tie-in with HMS genetics Program would be good both ways."[34] After meeting with the dean and hospital director, Janeway realized the difficulties that Dr. Haskem was having with the rivalries and bureaucracy. He later met with the head of obstetrics, who was part of the grant. "He agreed with Namet that the Committee was important and satisfied me he understood ethical problems and would not do things that were questionable."[35] It is questionable, however, whether Janeway understood the cultural differences thoroughly and was therefore lulled into agreeing with the omission of an ethical committee review for this grant. It was difficult to know when CAJ was shrewd or when he was merely being agreeable so as to make things happen in the developing world. At any rate, his recommendation resulted in the project proceeding without a review committee.

After meeting with Dr. Haskem's staff he opined, "Residents may be best group, like ours. Must remember genetics here [is] like CHD [congenital heart disease] when I was in medical school."[36] Such vignettes testify that CAJ took his visit seriously and with insight. He examined the budget and visited the laboratories, looking at problems they had with starch gel and pH gradient work and other technical problems. At the final meeting with Dr. Haskem, he and she discussed the details of the grant: "Tried to tell her not to keep trying to compete in basic research, but do uniquely Egyptian things—think she tries to do too much but knowledge and determination are admirable."[37] Before leaving, Janeway toured the "Fever Hospital" and found the work to be an "impressive example of best form of tech cooperation."[38] (Several of the people had trained in the United States.)

In 1973 Dr. Janeway was invited to be the Felton Bequest Visiting Lecturer to the Royal Children's Hospital, Melbourne, Australia. Fulfilling this invitation led to a five-week (August 29–October 7) journey around the globe. Betty accompanied him, even though she was experiencing what proved to be the onset of serious neck pain.[39] Before arriving in Australia, Charles and Betty travelled to Ankara for a Middle East Pediatric Congress, where Janeway presented a number of papers and was wined and dined by Professor Dogramaci at a lavish dinner party. CAJ danced "first with the Governor's wife then Ayser [Dogramci's wife], who said I was the first person who ever got her to dance," Janeway wrote, recalling several incidents that had occurred earlier in 1956.[40] At that time CAJ began to hear more about the animosity of the Muslim world to U.S. support of Israel. The wife of the foreign minister of Turkey told him, "Since Dulles we couldn't depend on the morality of American foreign policy."[41] And a young immunologist told him that the "U.S. looks totally the villain to Arabs . . . with our total commitment to Israel."[42] Betty wore a neck brace much of the time. (Ultimately she required a sectioning of her trapezius muscle.) After the last dinner party she was sick and limp all the next day. She continued to feel unwell after the closing ceremonies; CAJ reported that "Bet collapsed but pulled herself together for a pleasant small party."[43]

The next leg of their trip would have been trying for anyone, but at sixty-four, both Charles and Betty were not quite as resilient as in the past. To reach Australia, Charles and Betty flew from Ankara to Istanbul, to Bierut, to New Delhi, to Bangkok, and finally to Singapore, where they spent a night before flying on to Perth, Australia. There they spent two days of sightseeing and CAJ made rounds at the hospital. Then it was on to Melbourne, to the Royal Children's Hospital, the largest children's hospital in the southern hemisphere.

A printed program in Janeway's files lists the nearly two-week (September 10 to 20) stint as visiting professor. This involved lectures once or twice daily, as well as rounds. Australians work their guests very hard, and CAJ's trip was no exception: in his diary CAJ comments, "a busy schedule it was, particularly for the first five days . . . More lectures than I've given at HMS in last 5 to 10 years."[44] Something had to give: "Betty complained to me and the doctors complained to H. Williams [their host] and it was relieved a good deal the second week."[45] It took a lot for Janeway to complain of overwork. As always, Betty was protective and CAJ was probably beginning to show the effect of age and the beginnings of his chronic illness.

Janeway commented on the hospital organization, noting that each consultant had his own ward and even the chair of the department at the university had only one twenty-bed ward, a practice very different from U.S. children's hospitals but similar to the British system. His lectures included the familiar "Current Concepts of the Development of the Immunological System," and "Immuno-deficiency Diseases," but also some new ones such as "Problems of the Affluent Society in Relation to Child Health" and "Children and Television." His final lecture was "The Pediatrician, the Family and Community." It is a pity that we cannot find manuscripts or notes of these latter lectures, which are so different from his previous ones but are so in character with his broadening interests in the ecology of childhood. At the final, sumptuous dinner, Janeway reported, his host, Howard Williams, raised a toast and said "there were two outstanding Bequest lecturers [James Spence and me]. I blushed and stammered, 'I learned from Spence and Williams.[46] Janeway undoubtedly was embarrassed, but the fact that he related the story suggests that he was not above enjoying accolades.

The two weeks in Melbourne were followed by a three-day visit to Sydney, followed by travels to Brisbane, Cairnes, and the Great Barrier Reef. Charles and Betty then left Australia and continued on to Port Moresby, New Guinea, where, as in almost every place CAJ visited, a colleague, Dr. John Biddulph, met and hosted them. He toured the area and hospital, and presented a case. From Port Moresby, Charles and Betty flew to Goroka, in the highlands of New Guinea. There they were met by Dr. John Rooney (it is not clear from the narrative whether CAJ knew him) and expatriate colleagues who, before taking the Janeways to visit the hospital, took them to a "Sing Sing" and a pig roast called a "Moo Moo." Janeway appears to have been fascinated; here they watched group dancing, in which "All dancers basically naked, but covered with paint, feathers, shells . . . It was the real McCoy."[47]

Dr. Gregory Lawrence was in the village to study "Pig Belly," a devastating disease that was usually fatal and consisted of "distention, severe toxemia, very little diarrhea, usually comes on after a pig roast and finds many clostridia in bowel wall."[48] In the village hospital, as in most of the developing countries Janeway visited, he remarked at the presence of mothers and grandmothers in the beds with sick children. He further remarked that there was very little allergy or asthma, a finding now corroborated and thought due to the multiple early infections these children have.

The trip back to Melbourne, before returning to the United States, sounds terrible. CAJ and Betty encountered pilot and electronic maintenance strikes, endured broken navigational aids, cancelled flights, lost luggage, changed plans many times, and finally took a long bus ride from Sydney to Melbourne, a journey of 500 miles and a fifteen-hour trip. They also were caught in a power blackout. Much of the difficulty owed to strikes against the new Labour government, which, in the opinion of some of his hosts, had given in too much to some unions and thus had created demands from others. Janeway, inherently a liberal, wanted to side with Labour, but wrote, "It has made me realize that when you have private sector as employer vs. Labour, Gov't can intervene on behalf of people, but when Gov't itself is employer, then what can represent the public? Food for thought!"[49] In the airport at Melbourne, Charles and Betty chanced to meet Dr. Helen Caldicott and her husband, who had been residents at the Children's. Helen later became one of the leading opponents of atomic bomb testing and a leading figure in the anti-war movement. The Janeways and Caldicotts apparently had a stimulating discussion, "We talked a lot about medicine. He thinks current Australian Medical Association responses to pian of government for National health scheme is acting just like our AMA . . . advising against scheme instead of working constructively . . . on best program for all."[50] Janeway was against labor using the strike power to disrupt public services, but very much in favor of a national health insurance or service plan. Like many, he was not entirely consistent in his political views.

After all their travails, including forty-eight hours without sleep, Charles and Betty arrived in Honolulu. The respite was beneficial; experiences such as they had undergone on their way back from New Guinea were enough to cure any but the most intrepid traveller of future overseas excursions, but Charles and Betty were so interested in all cultures that they were soon to set off again in spite of failing health on the part of both. One factor that made their travels so exhilarating was the many friends and colleagues they visited and the many new ones they met along the way. Throughout the diary of his trip around the world, as well in other diaries, Janeway mentions people he talked with on the plane and at the innumerable dinner parties. Most were listed in the back of the diary with names and addresses, and in the pages of the diary were detailed reports of what he and Betty and their visitors talked about. The Janeways liked people and were energized by meeting and talking with them. On many occasions he made notes about certain persons as being good for a particular position at Children's Hospital or for further training in Boston. On the final page of his around-the-world diary, labelled "Incidental intelligence and reminders," the first entry reads, "Mel Avery appt as my successor in Honolulu papers on Oct. 5." He was finishing the most gruelling trip of his many and was pleased that it was ending with the appointment of a successor for whom he had such great admiration.

This global trip had taken Charles and Betty to five continents, dozens of pediatric hospitals, and exposure to most of the leading pediatricians in the world; CAJ's views on research and patient care, and his warm personality, had enlightened hundreds of people, from parents of sick children to the highest national leaders. From the sophistication of Paris to the remote highlands of New Guinea, "Dr. Janeway" was known, admired, and, in most cases, loved.

The Cameroons Project

In 1973, Charles Janeway became a participant in an ambitious program somewhat akin to the Shiraz project that was intended to directly improve medical education and health care in a vastly underdeveloped region of the world, with Harvard University also taking part in the venture. Although his commitment here was not nearly as difficult and long-lasting as was his task in Iran, Dr. Janeway undertook this burdensome assignment in the face of advancing age and deteriorating health. He would incorporate into this undertaking many of the lessons he had learned in Iran and not repeat the mistakes made there. This last ambitious third-world venture in which he became involved, his "swan song," so to speak, became known as the "Cameroons Project."

Cameroon is an agrarian state, about the size of California, in west equatorial Africa. It comprises the former United Nations Trust Territories known as the British and the French Cameroons, one Anglophone and one Francophone.[51] In 1961, the two territories were unified under a democratically elected government with a president and a unicameral legislature, but it quickly became, in effect, a one-party governed country. Diseases typical of equatorial Africa—infections and parasitic problems, especially malaria and protein-calorie malnutrition—were highly prevalent, and population growth and infant mortality were high. In 1963, recognizing a shortage of physicians and other health personnel, the government requested the World Health Organization to study the feasibility of developing a medical school there. A new medical school was begun in 1969 with forty students and a faculty of seven, with Dr. Monekossa, a Cameroonian who was professor of medicine in Nigeria, being appointed its first dean.[52] In the summer of 1970 the US AID agency commissioned Dr. Steven Joseph, formerly a pediatric resident at Children's Hospital Boston, to go to the Cameroons to determine whether support from the United States would be useful; in 1973, Joseph, while visiting four American medical schools to seek interest and collaboration, selected Dr. Janeway and Harvard University as the project director and the lead institution in US AID support of such an initiative. Subsequently the AID agency asked Janeway to organize the American effort.[53] Janeway, who was nearing the end of his time as chief at the Children's, accepted Joseph's proposal. CAJ acted initially as Campus Coordinator to get the program launched, and served on the project for about five years before illness overtook him and forced him to relinquish it.

The salient feature of the Centre Universitaire des Sciences de la Santé, as the effort was known, was an education program to prepare personnel to meet the health needs of a largely rural population. It was designed to train physicians for that purpose rather than to copy the medical schools of the industrialized world. It was to achieve its overall goal through a three-fold institutional building effort entailing support in teaching, direct patient care, and research directed toward maternal and child health as a major part of community health, with a large dose of preventive medicine added in. Implementation of the Harvard-sponsored plan envisioned a teaching team composed of a pediatrician project director, an obstetrician, a midwife and a pediatric health nurse and other personnel from the West, working in collaboration with a counterpart team from the Cameroons, with an investment in institutional continuity envisioned.[54] The aim was to initiate a program in maternal and child health with gradual withdrawal of foreign personnel planned as the program progressed and local Cameroonian professionals could take over. Dr. Janeway's initial duty, getting Harvard Medical School to give appropriate appointments to American staff, proved difficult, but he was able to recruit nine people initially, five from the United States and four from Canada. Dr. Joseph, who later was Health Commissioner in New York City and thereafter Deputy

Secretary of Defense for Health, was team leader in 1972 and 1973; Dr. Noel Guillozet succeeded him and was leader until 1976.

The focus of education was a teamwork approach, with emphasis on community public health. The physician was to be the planner, the teacher and supervisor of a large group of allied health personnel, prepared to carry out preventive services as well as being a consultant physician. The plan was exemplary, but turned out to be difficult to implement. The Central Hospital at Yaounde, a former French military hospital built between 1929 and 1939, which served as the University teaching hospital, had a skeleton physician staff. In the pediatric area as many as a dozen critically ill infants, most of whom had preventable diseases, might arrive for admission each day; and in the first years of the Harvard project the new staff had to assist in the care of these children, however impatient they were to develop the preventive programs that were the prime goal of the program. An added difficulty was the hospital's organization that strictly separated out-patient and in-patient staff, preventing the development by the Harvard staff of an integrative service program with the same personnel providing both preventive and curative services. As had been the case in the Iran project, CAJ was finding it difficult to make the plan focus on the whole community and on prevention. As Dr. Joseph later reported, the deficiencies were immediately recognized. Students there had no exposure to preventive medicine or general medical care out of hospital.[55]

The medical school curriculum in the Cameroons consisted of six years of study following high school graduation. Graduating students were obliged to provide ten years of service at whatever location the government wished to send them, many of them isolated, and forced to be responsible for all aspects of medical and surgical care as well as public health. Dr. Robert W. Chamberlin, who was later recruited to be staff pediatrician, told that he encountered language problems from the beginning, since Cameroon was officially a bilingual country.[56] In addition, students who were used to British pronunciation had difficulty understanding Chamberlin's American English. Conducting ward rounds was another challenge. A ward setting often found a child with meningitis or hepatitis next to a child with diarrhea and malnutrition next to another with pneumonia, with no separating curtains between them. Further, the sinks were stopped up; one could not wash his or her hands between patients. In the hospital, family members who sat next to a child's bed carried out much of the bedside care, with mothers often cooking, washing, and looking after other children in outdoor adjacent areas when not attending their ill children. Nor were wards equipped for such procedures as lumbar punctures, which had to be carried out under primitive conditions in view of all in the room. There was a shortage of incubators, often resulting in several infants being placed together in one.

Teaching primary care in the rural clinic was challenging. When the team arrived, they found a throng of mothers with infants who were to receive immunizations; the children were weighed and measured and examined and treated for fevers and other illnesses. The general policy adopted was to treat any child having a fever with an anti-malarial drug. Dr. Bernard Guyer, then a medical epidemiologist from the Center for Disease Control in Atlanta, was stationed in the Cameroons as a smallpox coordinator; but since there was no smallpox present, he concentrated on the prevention of measles, polio, and other vaccine-preventable diseases.

Given the state of education and clinical care, Dr. Janeway determined that, in contrast to his experience in Iran, where they had first built a teaching hospital modelled on the Harvard hospitals, the first building in the Cameroons would be a preventive outpatient and community-based facility. While curative medicine could not be ignored, he determined that such care should be integrated with a practical preventive medicine program, and not be allowed to dominate the program. By late 1974, the proposed team system was in place. With these personnel on hand, active service programs in family planning, tetanus immunization of pregnant women, and a high-risk pregnancy clinic were established. Dramatic changes in health statistics ensued. The perinatal mortality fell from 41.3 to 31.2 per 1,000 live births from 1973 to 1975.[57] The arrival of the obstetrician and nurse midwife in the second year of the Harvard project was well timed. The significant number of surgical abortions performed previously, together with the poor clinical state of pregnant women, made family planning a high priority for the new clinic. In its first nine months, over 1,000 patients were served, the most popular child-spacing method used being the intrauterine device. But getting women to accept family planning was initially a problem; for until they came to see that most of their children would live, they were not sympathetic to any pleas to curtail their reproduction.

Dr. Janeway travelled to the Cameroons in 1973–74, but no diary of this trip has been found.[58] He made a difficult trip once more to Yaounde in the spring of 1975, difficult because he did not feel well, was sixty-five years old, and was in the early stages of the chronic disease that would eventually kill him. He wanted to assess the progress that had been made in the program since his prior visit and look over the new University hospital that was under construction.[59] After arrival in Yaounde with four hours' of sleep, he was up for "Hospital Rounds." He was impressed with the accomplishments of the staff, but uncovered some resentments and lack of communications in the team.[60] He tried to deal with the latter in open discussions, during which his diplomatic skills were tested severely. With the multiple nationalities and disciplines involved, and working in a different culture, he felt it understandable that tensions should arise.

Bernard Guyer accompanied CAJ on a visit to the new University hospital. He reported that upon learning that the pediatric unit was to be located on an upper floor accessible by elevators, and knowing that electricity frequently failed in Yaounde, Dr. Janeway questioned how mothers would look after their children on the ward when they had limited access to the out of doors where they often cooked, washed, and looked after their other children. This caused Guyer to comment that CAJ "was a very astute observer."[61] After only three days, Janeway was off on a small plane to a town, N'Gaoudere, about 300 miles north of Yaounde, where he saw a wide range of cases: "terrible burns, fractures, infections." He liked the interne, "in spotless white. Was good. Knew his patients and was happy . . . Nice French puericulturist from their peace corps treating the children and teaching the mothers."[62]

Before Janeway left Yaounde he had a long meeting with Dean Monekossa, who later became regional director of WHO for West Africa. Monekossa was considered by Janeway to be very able and to have a clear vision of where the project would go. He and CAJ agreed that the need for equal academic recognition of preventative and curative medicine, the central concept of the project, was a major goal even though it was difficult to achieve. Monekossa was in favor of more emphasis on public health and regionalization of care, which accorded perfectly with CAJ's emerging vision.[63] Janeway met a missionary nurse who solidified his growing belief in the importance of public health and preventive medicine. In the rural area where she worked she recognized that the first priority was clean water and had taught villagers how to prevent contamination of springs and introduced health education into twenty primary schools. "Fascinating woman who shows what an effective person can do," was his brief comment.[64] And at a final meeting with the sixth-year students, he concluded that the program had met some of its goals: notably, one student did not want to go to America and had done a good research project by himself on why measles was so much more serious in Yaounde than in America. "He's probably the best student in class, but I was impressed with his motivation, work and knowledge."[65]

Much was accomplished during the first five years of the project that Janeway helped initiate. The new hospital was built and running with two ambulatory clinics. A number of local clinicians had been trained to take over most of the teaching roles. An African-oriented family planning manual and a community nursing textbook had been written by staff members and had been published. Teaching rounds were established. A family health clinic had been organized and was operating, and it became well established and functioning with local professionals and well attended by patients. It provided good on-the-job training to students who previously had been taught only by lectures, to mention but a few of the pluses. All in all, and near the end of his life, Charles Janeway had served as a beacon signal to all who are committed to help others in the developing world to have a better life with a greater chance for peace. He was remaining faithful to his vision.

Charles A. Janeway remained an internationalist all his life. This passion persisted even into his final illness, for some of his later travels were made after he was diagnosed and was suffering from the effects of his disease. It is no wonder that late in his life he was being referred to as, "Pediatrician of the World." Janeway himself believed that not only he, but the Children's Hospital, had responsibilities far beyond the limits of metropolitan Boston.[66] He made major commitments to India and Iran only a decade after assuming the chair at Children's, and, as we have just observed, he made a similar commitment to the Cameroons project late in his career. The latter part of his career was a panoply of other international involvements. One of these involvements, however, was largely involuntary. In 1966, a hospital in Canada was named after Janeway; however, this was an accolade that Janeway did not seek (he never sought honors of any kind) and which, we suspect, he would have liked to avoid.

The "Janeway Hospital" at St. Johns, Newfoundland

The story of how an old U.S. military facility, Pepperell Air Force Hospital at St. Johns, Newfoundland, became the Charles A. Janeway Child Health Centre is interesting. The original hospital was part of the "Destroyers for Bases" agreement between Britain and the U.S. in 1940; in 1960 it was abandoned by the U.S. Air Force. It was a very well-built structure, located just outside of St. Johns and was, in fact, the first military hospital built by the U.S. outside the United States and its territories and possessions. President Franklin D. Roosevelt took a personal interest in the plans, perhaps because of his summer residence at nearby Campobello Island. The fact that the facility ultimately was named for Janeway, however, was one honor that CAJ did not think he particularly deserved.

The organizer of the affair was an ambitious former pediatric resident from Montreal who spent 1953–54 at the Children's, Dr. Clifton Joy. After that year in Boston, Joy returned to his native city, St. John's, where he built a large practice. He was an excellent clinician and recognized very early that children with asthma had significant amounts of inflammation in their bronchial tubes; he treated his patients with corticosteroids at a time when it was customary to treat such children with only bronchodilators. His success in treating such children gave him a wide following of grateful patients, which stood him well when he aspired to political office. Joy was impressed with the high infant mortality in Newfoundland and made an assessment of child health, demonstrating the poor health of Newfoundland children and the inadequate facilities for their care. It was Joy's dream to have a children's hospital in St. Johns.

In his history of "The Janeway," the short name used by local residents for the hospital, Kelland, the director of the hospital, wrote, "not a few doctors had reservations about the need to build the director a separate hospital for children."[67] Joy used an epidemic of *E. coli* diarrhea among the children of St. Johns in 1962–63 to advance the project, and invited two distinguished Canadian pediatricians, Drs. Harry Medovy of Winnipeg, Manitoba and John Rathbun of London, Ontario, to St. Johns. In a public news conference he asked them if St. Johns needed a children's hospital. They agreed. Joy then invited Janeway to visit as a consultant to plan a new hospital; while visiting, Janeway was asked if the old Air Force hospital might make a good children's hospital. Janeway had no alternative but to say yes. Joy then ran successfully for Parliament in Newfoundland, convinced the Premier to support the project, and in 1964 succeeded in securing legislation to convert the American hospital to a children's hospital; he gave it prestige by naming it "The Dr. Charles A. Janeway Child Health Centre," without asking Janeway's permission.

In 1966, a report of a commission chaired by Lord Brain of Britain suggested that the children's hospital be the first part of a postgraduate medical school to be developed in St. Johns. Controversy continued, however, when in the same year another commission that recommended establishment of a medical school in St. Johns "Strongly criticized the government's decision to establish a children's health center at Fort Pepperrell."[68] This opposition was overcome, and "The Janeway" was officially opened on August 9, 1966. Several long articles appeared in St. Johns's newspapers.[69] Janeway spoke at the opening and congratulated the organizers for "combining private and government" funding with an independent board of governors: "Here we see the literal accomplishment of the age old longing which has become a necessity ('beat swords into ploughshares'). Here part of our war machine . . . [is used] to building of the future generations' constructive [efforts]."[70]

Betty told us said that Janeway had wished the hospital to be named for Eleanor Roosevelt. It is clear that the hospital would not have happened without the vision and initiative of Joy; whether Janeway was as positive about it as the dedication implies is not clear, however. Richard Goldbloom, a distinguished Canadian pediatrician and later depart-

ment chair at Dalhousie University, Nova Scotia, felt that CAJ was always somewhat embarrassed by having his name attached to the hospital, since at that stage of his career he was concerned that children's
hospitals were not sufficiently oriented to prevention and the community to really affect the health of the total population of children, but
he accepted the fact with grace when he was invited to its inauguration.[71] Janeway's vision of what the hospital should be has subsequently been recognized by the hospital board, which has created an
outreach-oriented service program for all the children of the widely
dispersed population of Newfoundland. One of the concerns voiced
by many was that the medical school and the rest of the clinical departments were in the city of St. John's, while the children's hospital was
several miles out of town. However, in recent years most of the other
clinical departments have moved to sites adjacent to "The Janeway."

In 1976, Dr. Donald Hillman was appointed chair of pediatrics at the
medical school and chief at "The Janeway." He and his wife, Elizabeth
(both had been residents at Children's), director of the ambulatory services at the hospital, invited as their first academic guest, Dr. Janeway,
who visited them September 18–24, 1977. In their words, his "visit to
St. John's will long be remembered . . . A beautiful copy of Dr.
Janeway's portrait welcomes you as you enter the Janeway Child
Health Centre. We went out to the airport to meet Dr. Janeway, where
two small girls asked if we were meeting our auntie—when we said we
were meeting Dr. Janeway, the children laughed and said, 'The
Janeway is a BUS!' The BUS labelled Janeway still travels Newfoundland Drive to the hospital many times a day."[72]

The story of this hospital reminds one of the saying, "A Prophet is
not without honor save in his own country."[73] This does not apply to
Dr. Janeway entirely, for surely he is honored in the United States. Even
so, neither hospital nor bus line is named after him here. One of us
(FHL) was amused when, as a visiting professor at the Janeway, he
asked a taxi driver, "Who was Dr. Janeway?" The driver replied, "I believe he was a famous American general that the Canadian government was honoring!" This would have rankled Janeway no end; he was
the most unmilitary person most of us have ever known.

By 1977, Janeway's health was not good. Trips to Newfoundland,
Europe and India were all completed in spite of his need to undergo

plasmapheresis and blood transfusions for his Waldenstrom's hyper-gammaglobulinemia. Dr. Janeway was an uncomplaining person, but after the New Delhi Congress, on April 3, 1978, he wrote to Ihsan Dogramaci and enclosed the paper he had given at the congress for publication in the IPA *Bulletin*.[74] When apologizing for missing the Paris meeting of the Council of IPA after the India meeting, he related,

> I am afflicted with the mildest of the lympo-proliferative diseases, namely Waldenstrom's Hypergammaglobulinemia, which is a good disease to have, but after returning from India, I was really exhausted and my doctors have started a new regime [*sic,* meaning regimen] of treatment, so I have been cutting down on activity until this is over. I feel fine when I get up in the morning, but by the second half of the day, I have got very little energy left. Now I am on a regime of weekly plasmaphoresis and an attempt to get my hemoglobin level which sticks stubbornly between 50–60% up to something which will enable me to be more active for longer. Everything else is fine. It is really not a malignancy, but the macroglobulin.[75]

We suspect that, even then, Dr. Janeway was sicker than he was allowing others to know. Certainly, his days of international travel were over.

CAJ's Work on Behalf of the International Children's Center, Paris

When, in March 1978, Dr. Janeway was invited to the thirtieth anniversary reunion of the International Children's Center in Paris, to be held the following year, his commitment to that organization was of nearly thirty years standing. He had been appointed to its board in 1949, soon after the ICC had been founded. That appointment and his role in the 1947 International Congress of Pediatrics were the earliest manifestations of his commitment to international pediatrics. Robert Debré, long time professor of pediatrics in Paris and a friend, was founder and president of that institution. The core of its activities was to do practical research and teach child health in the third world. Janeway's command of the French language was quite good, which made him a very useful talent on its behalf; he remained on the Administrative Council of the ICC until 1977, a year before Debré's death on April 20, 1978.

In an 1989 interview with the authors,[76] Professor Michel Mancieux, a leader of French social pediatrics and a member of the ICC board, noted that he had interviewed Professor Debré about Dr. Janeway's participation in ICC, and he told that Professor Debré had remarked that Janeway's comments were always full of good advice and good guidance, but that he (Debré) had hoped that in putting CAJ on the board he would become a greater advocate in the United States for the Center, that he would raise money and interest on its behalf, and that the Center would become a type of WHO for children.

This is an interesting concept because the International Pediatric Association has always suffered from lack of a strong presence in WHO and UNICEF (which was presumed to be children's advocate within WHO) and was never able to fulfil this role because it was designed to meet emergencies. The need still exists. Mancieux also noted that he especially remembered Janeway's talk to the IPA in 1960; it was at the height of the Cold War, and for an American to propose peaceful solutions for the world's conflicts, as a way to work for all children and to diminish conflict between the U.S.S.R. and the U.S., was especially attractive to Europeans. Mancieux observed further that Janeway "was always very interested in pediatric and social issues," and that "Janeway was really a wise man."[77] CAJ was especially interested in one ICC project, a longitudinal growth and development project in Senegal, and visited the project on one occasion, as we have noted earlier.

Although Dr. Janeway praised many of the activities of the Center, his major criticism was the European orientation of the Executive Board. Noting that, of the ten members, "8 are from Europe, and one each from North America and the Soviet bloc," he named eight pediatricians from the developing world whom he would recommend for the board.[78] This advocacy for representation from Asia, Africa and South America was consistent with his similar recommendations for IPA. He suggested that the Center's programs could be more effectively diffused if there were "comparable regional programs."[79] Surprisingly, given his investment in the large international congresses of the IPA, he noted, "In the U.S. . . . [in] this day of big organizations and huge congresses, the only effective meetings are small ones."[80]

Pierre Royer, a prominent French pediatrician and later director of ICC, remembered fondly his meetings with CAJ at the Sick Children's Hospital in Paris. "It was a pleasant surprise for us . . . to see this great scientist was also a marvellous clinician, interested in each sick child and his family . . . By his example, he showed us that it was possible to develop different levels of medicine to very high levels: scientific research, attentive and humane treatment and strong concern for public health issues, particularly in developing countries."[81] There is no record of Janeway's attendance at Professor Debré's memorial service on April 29, 1978, nor that he actually made the trip to the ICC's thirtieth reunion a year later, despite the fact that there exists an undated handwritten letter in French from CAJ to Professor Mancieux confirming his attendance and requesting a hotel room for himself and Betty. Poor health had by this time completely overtaken him.

Charles A. Janeway's International Legacy

Charles Janeway had changed markedly from the 1930s, when he first began to treat patients with the new antibiotics and later spent so much time doing research on rare disorders of immunology. In his later years his main concerns were population growth, adequate nutrition, and prevention rather than cure. But it was all of a piece: thoughtful, dedicated, constantly growing and evolving wisdom, with intense application of his remarkable mind and his dedication to the human race to improve mankind.

As additional evidence of CAJ's commitment to international pediatrics, Mrs. Mildred McTear, his secretary for many years, remembered that the Lab Study in the research building (Dr. Gamble's laboratory) had a conference room with a large blackboard at the end. She felt that the blackboard was extremely important to Janeway because it allowed him to have foreign visitors place "Merry Christmas" in their own language on that board.[82] In today's world, when political correctness frowns upon mentioning "Christmas" in the presence of non-Christians, such a practice likely would be disparaged. But Dr. Janeway had a deeper understanding of "political correctness" than perhaps we have today; he wished to include all cultures in a common celebration, and thus to celebrate the common human desire to reach out to one another. Today he probably would have asked visitors to write "Happy Holidays" instead, but in those naive days there never was heard any criticism from those of different religions about this event; indeed, most thought it was another indication of his inclusiveness. Janeway knew how to make friends, to open his arms, figuratively if not literally, to all that he met and welcome them to his world.

His world view included the importance of "one world," of the interdependence of the nations of the world, in the cultural contributions that countries could make to each other. He did not believe that the United States is the sole paragon of virtue that some, then and now, espouse. He advocated peaceful resolution of international conflicts, which, among other things, meant support of family planning as the way to allow a country to develop and prosper, coupled with health care and education; and he thought that U.S. tax dollars should support such endeavors.

One's personal library is one measure of one's interests. In CAJ's home library were several copies of *World Health,* the journal of the World Health Organization, but also technical reports on family planning, the American Society of Agronomy's publication on "World Population and Food Supplies, 1980," "Malaria Control and Population Pressure in Ceylon," and a variety of publications on health services in Norway, the United Arab Republic, and the Soviet Union, as well as a number of publications of the American Universities Field Staff Reports on South East Asia, Argentina, Persia, and North Africa. One wonders how many other pediatricians were reading publications such as *Man, Food and Land,* one of the books in his library. This literature illustrates his view of the inter-relatedness of population control, adequate food, economic development, education, and medical care as the keys to better health and community development.

Many international and local honors accumulated for CAJ over the years. In 1956, as part of his Indian sabbatical, he was appointed Visiting Lecturer on Pediatrics of the Government Central Hospital in Madras, India, a consultant *pro tempore* at St. Mary's Hospital, London, and received honorary memberships in the pediatric societies in Britain, Czechoslovakia, and Korea. In 1964 he received the prestigious Von Rosenstein medal of the Swedish Pediatric Association, and in 1965, a medal from the Cultural Center of the Philippines. In 1973 he was the Felton Bequest Lecturer at the Royal Children's Hospital, Melbourne, Australia.

In 1969 Janeway was given an honorary degree and membership in the French Pediatric Society. In his acceptance letter and speech, written and delivered in French, he noted the need for developed nations to help developing ones and the need for men and women of good will to understand "social injustice, war, poverty and overpopulation . . . as [part of the] multiple causes of diseases . . . and the concept of comprehensive, or social, pediatrics" as the future of pediatrics.[83] In 1973 he received the Samuel Z. Levine Award of the Foundation for International Child Health in recognition of his long-time commitment to the improvement of the health of children everywhere in the world. In 1974 he received a medal from the Children's Hospital of Krakow, Poland, celebrating the 600th anniversary of that city. The Children's Hospital in Krakow, built by a donation from Project Hope, has a plaque honoring Janeway. In his files is a reprint of the narrative by Dr. Josef Stroder and signed by him, "For Charlie with cordial regards 25–4–77." Stroder must have given it to Janeway when CAJ went to Krakow to dedicate the new Children's Hospital. There is also a three-page personal letter from Stroder to "Mein lieber Charly."

Many of Dr. Janeway's memberships were awarded at the time of a major lecture he gave at a society's meeting. In 1957 he received a letter of congratulations from P.M.S. Blackett, head of the department of physics at the Imperial College, London, thanking him for his remarks made at a lecture by Blackett to the British Association, in which CAJ complimented him on expressing the view that scientists must take into consideration the social consequences of their science. He also remarked that powerful nations must provide international aid; if they did not, it would lead to despair and doom.[84]

It was natural that someone of Janeway's stature in world pediatrics, and especially for his renown in supporting international pediatrics, would be asked to serve on international health bodies. One was the World Health Organization, for which Janeway served as a consultant to the U.S. delegation to the World Health Assembly beginning in 1953, and on the Expert Advisory Panel on Maternal and Child Health, beginning in 1964. In a letter written many years later, the secretary of the Panel noted that she had not heard from Janeway but wanted to reassure him that if he desired appointment for another three years to the Panel, it would be renewed.[85] There is no record of CAJ's acceptance, perhaps because he was then in one of the difficult periods of his illness. In December 1978, the new Chief of Maternal and Child Health of WHO, Dr. Goran Sterky, asked him, as a member of that advisory committee, to "draw on your experience . . . on what have been the milestones in development in the past 30 years and what is likely to happen in the next 20 years." Sterky asked for a response to this formidable request within a month's time. Again, however, there is no record of CAJ's response. One additional testimonial to Dr. Janeway's international reputation was his membership in six foreign pediatric associations: British, Finnish, Irish, Korean, Mexican and Czechoslovak. He was also a member of a national medical body, the Korean Medical Association.

In 1986, at the time of the IPA International Congress meeting in Hawaii, one of the authors (RJH) organized a reception in Betty's honor for friends of Dr. Janeway, most of whom Betty also knew from her travels with him and from hosting them in her home. More than 100 people attended, comprising individuals from many countries that the Janeways had visited and from pediatricians who had some training at the Children's. Typical of the warm response was that of Dr. Gustavo Gordillo of Mexico, who, although unable to attend, said, "Please give Mrs. Janeway my warmest regards, since I was a research fellow in 1952–54 and I keep a very pleasant remembrance from Dr. Janeway."[86]

From these rich international experiences Janeway constantly expanded his view of the world and of what was important in child health. Although he was always an internationalist, his first major immersion in international child health was to lead the Iran Foundation to build a "modern" medical center based on the Western medical model. He also had the traditional Western medical view that care of the individual patient was the heart of what medicine should be. While he never gave this up and continued to believe that superb care of the individual patient was one of the most important qualities that Western medicine could teach the world, he began to see that this approach was insufficient to improve the health of populations. He recognized that effective care of a child with severe diarrheal disease was important, but if something was not done to help the family and thereby give this child good nutrition in a hygienic environment, the child would soon be back in hospital with a recurrence. He began to see the relation between family size and health, thus his interest in family planning, industrial development, family education, and improvement of the physical and social environment as necessary components of health. He became a public health doctor while maintaining his superb clinical skills. He believed that clinicians in the developing world would accept the population or public health approach more quickly if taught by someone who was manifestly a superb clinician, as he was.

Dr. Janeway's opposition to the Vietnam war was in part a reflection of his belief that war is the most severe threat to the health of children, not only directly causing their increased mortality and morbidity but also taking huge resources that could so much better be used to support education, nutrition, and health. He would have agreed with George Kennan, the former U.S. foreign officer in Russia, who said, in an address to the National War College in 1946, as the Cold War was beginning, "I would be happier, and I think on sounder ground, if we had things that were constructive to offer people in fields besides military."[87]

It may appear that CAJ's international work had major influence on him and his ideas. However, it was a two-way street. His contribution to the world should not be forgotten. In his masterpiece "Pediatricians for Peace" lecture (and subsequent paper), he said that of the three things that had improved health one was the dedicated personal and skilled care of individual patients, but the other two were improvement of the environment and improved socioeconomic conditions. If Janeway learned public health from his overseas experience, the thousands of faculty and students he saw in every country that he visited learned from him that superb care of the individual was equally important. He lectured, usually with a blackboard as his only prop, to demonstrate his reasoning about the pathology in each patient. His sheer brilliance as a lecturer, and his interpersonal warmth with each patient, must have left an enduring impression on all who saw him in action. He extended that brilliance in his "Pediatricians for Peace" paper, which captures better than any other his vision of an international body of pediatricians, from developed and developing countries, enriching both and helping the children of the world to achieve better health.

Dr. Janeway's commitment to bring pediatricians in training to the United States, usually to the Children's, for what he considered better scientific training to prepare them to enhance the health of children in their own countries was a major contribution to the health of the world's children. Although he believed that there was a need for more research to understand the basis of illness and so to lead to its rational cure or prevention, the exposure to other cultures that he experienced when he travelled abroad, and the exposure that foreign physicians received at Boston taught him by example that research was only part of what pediatricians needed to improve children's health.

The thousands of students he taught at home and abroad are what led to the common question asked whenever any of us from the Children's went to other schools in the United States or abroad, "How is Dr. Janeway?" The affection, even many years removed, was palpable. This aspect of CAJ's life was his most enduring contribution to the many students he taught throughout the world. His humility and interest in others made him less a missionary than one who saw the reciprocal benefit of international activities. He ended his "Pediatricians for Peace" paper by writing that pediatricians who participate in exchanges and international activism "will have an infinite variety of cultural adaptations which make humanity so fascinating, and will enjoy the great satisfaction of having played an essential role in the creation of one world, which technology has produced and that politics has not yet appreciated. In addition, they will have made lasting friendships with fine colleagues in other parts of the world."

Janeway's legacy to international child health is found more in the transformation of attitudes among his students from all over the world than in any single model of service that he created. This commitment to international child health was predictable from his other personality traits—altruism, integrity, high ideals, willingness to work very hard for anything in which he believed, a willingness to work for peace, to find peaceable solutions to controversies at home as well as abroad; he was a gifted teacher who was anxious to share his knowledge of modern medicine with the world, but also willing—indeed committed—to learn from others, especially in the developing world. He was a man of vision. He became committed to internationalism early in his career, but this does not mean that he was rigid in persisting in his original vision. This was especially true for his involvement in Iran. His original vision was that the establishment of a Western-style teaching hospital would spark a wave of imitators. As we have seen, several events intervened and prevented this from happening: unrest and eventually revolution in Iran as well as the difficulty in transforming a centuries-old landed aristocracy to support the new hospital. But, more profoundly, Janeway changed his model. He recognized that a Western-style teaching hospital did little to improve the health of the public; he carried out this realization in the Cameroon project, where his transformed vision was to create rural health clinics first and use them for teaching to the next cadre of medical students the value of preventive medicine first. Here too he showed some naivete, failing to recognize the political pressure of the government to have a showplace teaching hospital in the capital. Rural health centers were not visible enough for leaders of a new country seeking bragging rights.

In addition to his naivete (which was part of his attraction to students and colleagues) was his belief that through hard work—very hard work—problems could be overcome. In many ways great difficulties were overcome, but in retrospect it was almost foolhardy of Janeway to think that he could preside over an organization that was developing and that he could run a teaching hospital 8,000 miles away in a country that he did not fully understand. For a man who could work effectively twenty hours a day nothing seemed impossible. Travel to Iran was long and time-consuming. In spite of his many trips there, none were for more than a week or ten days in duration. To have expected to understand and lead such a complex endeavor was certainly naive on Janeway's part. In his heart of hearts he could not believe that the physicians whom he had recruited so carefully would have such difficult times readjusting to their native Iran, nor could he admit that they would be so involved in power plays in Shiraz and were at the same time working to find a way to return to the United States.

By today's standards, Janeway was not a good administrator. He did not delegate authority sufficiently and he did not build the type of administrative structure that would have been necessary for the Iran initiative to succeed. He failed to recognize at first the impossibility of a shared administrative structure of the United States-based Iran Foundation and the Iran-based counterpoint organization, Boyadiran. The pragmatist would have seen the difficulties in trying to change Iran or the Cameroons; the pragmatist, perhaps, would have done nothing. That was not Janeway's way. His early interest in being a missionary was part of his personality. In his view, nothing was impossible if one believed in a goal and worked hard for its attainment.

Added to the other problems were the cultural differences in education, which were tremendous. In North America the emphasis is on teaching principles and basic science rather than rote learning; on problem solving rather than didactic methods; and on incorporation of the laboratory into diagnosis and therapy. It was difficult in a culture of authoritarianism to change to the open, questioning American style of education (it must be admitted, however, that these ideals of education are not achieved entirely in the United States either). Janeway's honesty and dedication made it difficult for him to understand others' human failings. These difficulties in Iran and the Cameroons were not apparent in India nor the many places Janeway served as visiting professor because his role in those situations was different; as an educator and model clinician in these settings he left behind a powerful legacy, remembered by all who saw him behave as the consummate clinician.

In Janeway's letter to the Rockefeller Foundation (see chapter 8) his last reason for going to India was to further the cause of peace by being a good ambassador. There is no doubt that he and Betty were good ambassadors; wherever they went, people must have been left with a better image of the United States. CAJ certainly counteracted the stereotypical image of the "Ugly American," but was it simplistic on his and Betty's part to think that they could further the cause of peace in the world? Probably. Even so, throughout the ages peaceful movements have begun with a single person dedicated to the cause. During the period covered by Janeway's international activities, war and peace were mega issues: the Cold War, the American involvements in Korea and Vietnam. the beginning of the Israeli-Arab conflicts—these were obstacles no one person could overcome. Nonetheless, Janeway made hundreds if not thousands of us who were touched by him better persons. He made us see the goodness in everyone and led many of us to pursue international activities that, in aggregate, did some good. The measure of success for a man who wanted to improve the chances of peace in the world cannot be judged by whether there is peace today but rather by his influence on the activities of the many people he did touch, and what their activities did to edge, in a few places at least, the world toward a more peaceful existence.

Janeway's greatest legacy, in the international field as in the United States, was his students. He left behind a host of young physicians who saw him take a patient's history, do a careful physical examination, and apply patho-physiological principles to reach a diagnosis in patients with complex medical problems. And they saw a compassionate physician who treated each patient with dignity and respect. It was these characteristics that all who were in contact with him remembered and which led them to ask all of us who followed in his footsteps around the world, "And how is Dr. Janeway?" Perhaps he was naive and, as some said, naively saintly. He believed with passion that doing good would somehow promote the cause of peace; that being a role model would leave behind a legacy among the many students who were in his presence. The authors received so many letters from those who saw him in this role, remembering with vividness his teaching rounds, that it is clear this legacy persisted in their minds for years. What better use of man's energies, vision, and faith can one imagine?

11 CHARLES JANEWAY'S EDUCATIONAL LEGACY

EDUCATION, ARGUABLY, was Charles Janeway's greatest contribution to pediatrics. The teaching he did and encouraged at the Children's was disseminated throughout America and the world by those whom he trained. More importantly, he promulgated an attitude, based in a scientific approach leavened with compassion for others, that his students, in turn, passed on. Janeway's formal portrait at the Children's shows him full length in a white coat in front of a blackboard. In all of the countries he visited, the most enduring memory of those who saw him and learned from him was the image of Dr. Janeway using the blackboard to outline a patient's problem, after examining the child with a careful but compassionate physical examination, and then using the Socratic method to elicit from the audience a diagnosis based upon the patho-physiology rather than on an empirical syndrome name. He coupled this with an insistence on always having the patient present; at such encounters he would demonstrate his careful physical examination and, above all, his empathic communication between doctor and patient.

There was a strong Janeway tradition of teaching the scientific basis of illness. For CAJ's grandfather, it was pathology; for his father, physiology. However, his own international associations, notably his work with the International Pediatric Association, added an emphasis on prevention and medical education. At his first IPA congress in 1947, which met in New York, Janeway presented a paper on controlling influenza and measles.[1] At the next IPA congress, in Zürich, CAJ participated in a symposium on teaching pediatrics. Prior to the Japan IPA congress in 1966, a study group on pediatric education was formed by the IPA; Janeway was a participant in this symposium, and sessions on education were thenceforth a part of most subsequent congresses. As a result of meeting with pediatricians from throughout the world, we believe, Dr. Janeway evolved his tenet that clinical medicine is best taught at the bedside, starting with a patient, emphasizing the careful history and physical examination, and linking the patho-physiology in the individual patient with the psychosocial aspects of illness. He was critical of the then traditional European tradition and its lecture format, and was reinforced in his belief of the virtue of the Socratic method with active involvement of the students. But he learned from his contacts with other cultures that application of science to whole populations of children required additional educational experiences. He was impressed in his visits to other countries, especially developing ones, of the importance of physicians working in communities, usually in health centers, where several disciplines worked together, and where the importance of environmental health programs, family planning, outreach, and home visiting could be learned by doing. Janeway tried to implement these lessons "back at the ranch," at the Children's, first in the Family Health Care Program with greater or lesser success, and in his daily rounds and conferences.

Although Dr. Janeway wrote articles for the education of the general physician in review articles for *The New England Journal of Medicine* as early as 1939,[2] and fourteen textbook chapters in the early 1940s, which he continued to do both throughout his career, and even spoke in a radio broadcast to the general public,[3] his first published article focussing on medical education appeared in 1957, at the conclusion of his first sabbatical in India.[4] Ten years later he published an article dealing with deficiencies in medical education in Western countries.[5] In both articles he outlined the problem of inadequate numbers of physicians and lack of training in general medicine because of medical education's emphasis on sub-specialization, a point he drove home with particular force in the latter paper:

> University medical schools have become so engrossed in the extraordinary successes of the medical sciences in overcoming the life

threatening and crippling diseases which are concentrated in our teaching hospitals that they have failed to pay adequate attention to the overall health needs of the community. They have also failed to examine scientifically the ways in which medical knowledge can most effectively be applied to the health of our people.[6]

Also in 1957 he published his famous "Pediatricians for Peace" article in which he discussed ways in which physicians trained in the West could contribute to physicians from developing countries. Such experiences for physicians from developing countries in Western medical institutions could be very helpful, he believed, "provided they were sufficiently mature to adjust to the far heavier case load and more limited facilities that they must inevitably face upon their return."[7]

Janeway had become convinced that one role he could play in the health of the world's children was to provide education for physicians from the developing world and spend time himself abroad bringing the best of Western medicine to those who cared for the majority of the world's children, as well as being an advocate for more training in general medicine. In the last fifteen years of his career, he added medical education and health policy at home and abroad to his repertoire; the experiences in developing countries seemed to galvanize this expansion of his mission. In his writings he emphasized the need for teaching the social and emotional aspects of medicine while children were in hospital, probably because of the serious physical illnesses of those admitted, many of them attributable to preventable causes, causes that were often social in nature. However, he continued to emphasize the patho-physiological aspects of disease as well.

Throughout his writings and talks, Dr. Janeway's philosophy of education was consistent. Medicine was not a spectator sport, he used to say. It must be learned by doing, under some—but not intrusive—guidance, but mostly by precept. "Do as I do, not only as I say" was his unspoken motto. He opposed rigid requirements of outside bodies that sought to impose a cookie-cutter approach to all education; he thought that departments should be encouraged to be innovative, and was strengthened in this thought by his work in foreign countries, where he was opposed to the standard curriculum imposed in many former colonial nations. It is likely that he would be worried about the increasing regulation of residency training, although many of the newer requirements such as continuity clinic and community, behavioral, and adolescent medicine experiences were among those he was responsible for initiating. He would have preferred that others do these things because of his example and the conviction that they were essential, rather than to satisfy outside requirements. He became active in the Association of American Medical Colleges (AAMC), participating in several symposia and in his later years publishing several papers on education. In the report of a talk he delivered at one such symposium he wrote,

> What are the characteristics of a really effective teacher? There isn't any one characteristic, but the scholarly attitude and the degree to which the teacher [can] make the student an active participant is important. Even as a lecturer the teacher can make the student a participant just by the drama with which he may be able to present his subject. Inspiration and enthusiasm, once you have the intellectual content, are very important.[8]

In Dr. Janeway's files at home were two large folders labelled "Pediatric Education;" these contained letters from other department chairs in response to his request for information about their schools' curricula. CAJ asked them about changes in medical education as a whole at their schools; he inquired as to how they taught pediatrics to medical students; he wondered about changes in teaching programs for residents; he was curious about changes in postgraduate programs (*i.e.*, continuing education for practitioners). All of these inquiries seemed to be in preparation for one or more symposia at the AAMC meetings, but they also influenced his international teaching.

In his Department of Medicine Annual Report for 1969, five years before his retirement, Janeway articulated four core principles of effective medical education.[9] Firstly, he believed that "teaching above all must be by example," carried out in "a training program in which service is an integral part." He went on to say, "we are training people to be doctors, and service is the hallmark of our profession." Secondly, increasing clinical responsibility was important: "Our student and house officer training programs are designed to give as much responsibility to them as they can take for their patients, while at the same time maintaining close supervision so that the child gets the best possible care."

Thirdly, he believed that effective education occurred through the solving of problems rather than through rote learning: "The essence of education is to learn habits of thinking that would be applicable to new problems in the future." Fourthly, he believed that "teaching must be as relevant as possible to the demands of society in the present and the future." In summary, he held that the best medical education occurred in the context of service, with increasing responsibility under the direction of the faculty and with a focus on problem-solving skills relevant to the patient and societal needs.

In a keynote address at the State University of New York in 1959[10] and in his annual report for 1966,[11] Janeway outlined his views on medical student education. In the first two years of medical school, he pointed out, "the student learns the basic body of knowledge with which he has got to work for the rest of his life." He saw biochemistry as the basic science of modern medicine. Even in these preclinical years, he noted, "teaching must have relevance to the human experience . . . biochemistry can be taught with clinical examples." As a precursor to the educational pedagogy of today, Janeway observed that "in research the sciences are constantly overlapping one another, and this has led to a concept of integrated teaching, an attempt to bring disciplines to bear upon the understanding of a biological or physiological process." He warned, however, "we have to remember you cannot integrate the student. He has to learn material and integrate it in his own mind if it is going to mean anything to him."

Dr. Janeway taught a clinical correlation demonstration for first-year medical students, employing this philosophy. It is interesting, however, that students later remembered more his kindness to patients rather than the integration of basic and clinical sciences. We feel certain that he would not be opposed to the recent development of early exposure of students to clinical experience, but we think he would have worried about the possible neglect of the basic sciences that might ensue. As an overarching principle of the clinical years, CAJ stated, "our objective is not to teach pediatrics completely but rather to train students to use their knowledge of medical sciences in the prevention and diagnosis of diseases of children . . . You cannot teach every thing you need to know in medical school. We have given up trying to turn out the finished general practitioner after four years of medical school."

During his more than twenty-eight years as chief of a department of medicine, Dr. Janeway developed the concept of medical residency to a significant degree. At a meeting of pediatric department chairmen in 1964 he reflected on the process of successful education during residency: "You have to catch a resident's interest during the first two or three years of training by facing him with the responsibility of taking care of very clear cut, definite, serious illnesses. In a sense it is the very first year called internship (now called Post Graduate Year 1—PGY1— or Pediatric Residency Year 1) which is the critical one in establishing habits of work, thought and attitudes in caring for sick patients."[12] (We should note here that CAJ never "caught on" to the need to be more gender neutral in his writings, despite his personal behavior and complete acceptance of women in medicine. In fairness, however, we must point out that he lived in a period when these were not the major considerations that they are today.) In reflecting on the transition from residency to practice, he went on to say, "in a sense we need a bridge between residency training and practice." Reflecting on the clinical exposure of residents who served in the military, he observed that, "often they [the residents] come back for a third year of residency and get more out of it." (This was said at a time when pediatric residency lasted only two years.)

As a precursor to current debates, Dr. Janeway in 1965 stated that "internship and residency are the last vestiges of the apprentice system in which one learns by doing under the supervision of a master."[13] After warning against the dangers of overemphasing rote learning at the expense of "theoretical aspects of the educational experience" as well as abuse of the resident by an overemphasis on service, he went on to say that "service is the goal of medical practice and a clinical education that does not include a large measure of responsibility for the care of patients is an empty program." He felt that the hospital is the best institution to entrust the educational experience of residents, "because it offers exposure to patients in sufficiently large numbers to provide a concentrated exposure for the resident." Finally, as a precursor of today's continuity clinic exposure, in his presidential address to the American Pediatric Society in 1971,[14] he reflected,

In the early 1950s I became convinced that extensive training in the care of seriously ill children alone was not enough for a profession with an increasing obligation to keep children well. In fact, health supervision, the prevention of disease by immunizations and hopefully by anticipatory guidance and the minimization of disability by early recognition of potentially serious illness have proven themselves to be far more effective than hospital treatment of advanced disease.

These concepts were formalized in teaching and practice in 1955 in the Family Health Care unit at the Children's, one of the first formal continuity clinics in the United States.

As we look back on the residency program we knew, it almost seems as if we are in a time warp. Prior to 1946, house officers' titles were relatively simple: the junior men were called "Medical House Officers," the senior men, "Residents." Women became residents in the early war years. In Janeway's era the nomenclature changed at Children's to include the designations of Intern, Junior Assistant Resident, Assistant Resident, Senior Resident, and Chief Resident. The first three designations corresponded to the PGY I, II, III terminology used commonly in residency today.

The size of the house staff peaked in the Blackfan era at twenty-five. It fell markedly during the years of World War II, but then began to rise again in Janeway's era, reaching twenty-eight by 1951, from thirty to forty by the 1960s, and more than fifty by the end of his tenure in 1974. In 1952 there were eight Senior Residents, twelve Junior Residents, and four Interns. The reason for so few interns was that CAJ urged young physicians going into pediatrics to intern in another area such as pathology or internal medicine and then come in as junior residents. By 1968 there were eight Senior Residents, fourteen Junior Residents, and fourteen Interns, reflecting the fact that the pediatric internship was now fully operational. Today, most residents proceed through in the same program, starting the year after medical school. We suspect that Janeway might be saddened by this uniformity and concentration solely on pediatrics, in light of his own beginning in internal medicine.

During Dr. Janeway's tenure there were five different types of residency programs. Four of them began during his chairmanship. The traditional medical residency lasted three years. The resident served twelve months each year in a program that involved inpatient care, the emergency room, clinics, and community hospitals. This residency was similar at the Children's to residencies all over the United States, although the third year was not uniform everywhere until the mid-1960s. Early in his tenure, Dr. Janeway introduced the second residency concept, the Medical Outpatient (MOPD) resident. The first candidate was Alexander (Sterling) McDonald, appointed in 1947. MOPD residents served for one to two years and were responsible for outpatient clinics and community hospitals. Many of these were physicians returning from military service and headed for community practice.

The third type of residency program was for "affiliated residents." These residents rotated into the Children's from such institutions as Massachusetts General Hospital, Roger Williams Hospital in Providence, Rhode Island, and others, as well as out from Children's, to work in various affiliated community hospitals, mainly in the medical outpatient clinics. The first appointment of affiliated residents occurred in 1951; their curriculum also lasted one to two years. The fourth program was for "coordinated residents." This program evolved out of the large number of residents coming from other countries to the Children's, a practice that was so very typical of the Janeway years. It was formalized in 1969 and was run by Dr. Barry Adels for foreign medical graduates. These individuals rotated to outpatient clinics and community hospitals; their curriculum, like that of the MOPD and affiliated residents, lasted one to two years.

Coordinated residents who were especially talented entered either the MOPD residency or the traditional residency. A goodly number moved on to fellowship positions. It is interesting to note that Dr. Janeway was ahead of his time in terms of increasing the flexibility of residency to make life easier for those who were married, perhaps remembereing his own experience. He thus created the part-time residency; a number of individuals served in this capacity. Finally, Janeway introduced the St. Mary's Exchange with his counterpart, Dr. Reginald Lightwood, in London. The exchange residency involved an exchange, or trade, of senior-year residents from each of the two institutions. The exchange lasted, for each resident, for either six or twelve months. The program commenced in 1951 and ended in 1976; thirty-six Children's residents rotated to St. Mary's Hospital over the twenty-five years that the program lasted.

One of the exchange residents, John Tuthill, had an experience familiar to many of us who learned from and worked with Dr. Janeway. Tuthill had been recruited from Babies' Hospital in New York City to head the outpatient department. Soon after he arrived, he was called by Janeway to go to London for six months exchange when CAJ received a cable that the first registrar (the British term for resident) from St. Mary's was about to arrive in Boston. Janeway had forgotten about it, or perhaps had procrastinated a bit too long. As similarly occurred with CAJ's invitations to dinner or the movies, he made such decisions often at the last minute, perhaps in view of all the other details he attended to every day. Tuthill's experience did not mean that the exchange residency was less important. Certainly the program with St. Mary's was a high priority for Dr. Janeway, who talked often about the advantages that accrued to pediatricians of both nations. Later, Dr. Samuel Katz, a former chief resident at Children's and exchange resident with St. Mary's, initiated a similar exchange with Oxford when he chaired the pediatrics department at Duke University. In 2002, a fiftieth anniversary meeting was held in London, with a good number of English and American participants present from both programs. All praised the experience.

Clearly, one of Dr. Janeway's unique contributions to residency was his willingness to train individuals from foreign countries and then send them back to their countries to assume leadership roles. They, in fact, did exactly that, and many of the outstanding contributions to world health occurred as a result of Janeway's preference and desire to view pediatrics from a global perspective. He did this despite some rather significant concerns and even objections from his own faculty, who felt that this endeavor might dilute the high quality of the training program at the Children's. Janeway persisted, however, and believed that in the bigger picture of pediatrics, the contributions that these individuals made were most significant. Many of the coordinated residents, however, admitted that they felt to a certain degree like second-class citizens. The coordinated residency program lasted only three years, however, before it was discontinued in 1971; the feelings of inferior citizenship caused the demise. However, Dr. Janeway brought pediatricians from other countries for a variety of experiences at Children's Hospital, both before and after this formal program.

Looking back now, it seems a shame that the doubters of this training program for foreign physicians could not hear some of the tributes paid to Dr. Janeway by the physicians who went through the program, many of whom later assumed high positions in their own countries. One such former resident, Dr. Francisco Tome from Honduras, told one of us (RJH) that he arrived in Boston without an ECFMG (test required of foreign residents wishing to come to the United States) and was unable to speak much English. Showing the flexibility of designing these experiences to fit the needs of the participant, Janeway arranged for Dr. Tome first to be an observer in the hospital, then a student at the Harvard School of Public Health, and finally a fully integrated member of the residency staff. Tome later became head of the Children's Hospital in Honduras, chaired the Central American District of the American Academy of Pediatrics, and was a member of the Standing Committee of IPA. He attributed his success to the training he received in Boston, training that would not have happened without Dr. Janeway's personal interest.[15]

The post of chief resident evolved rather markedly over CAJ's twenty-eight years; forty-six chief residents were appointed during that time. The first two were Frederick C. Robbins, Jr., in 1947 and Robert J. McKay, Jr., in 1948. In some years there was only one chief resident; in others, Janeway appointed as many as four, two on the inpatient service and two in the Medical Outpatient Department. Most chief residents served for one year only. Janeway, however, duplicated the example of James Wilson, who served for a number of years as chief resident for Dr. Blackfan in the 1930s, by appointing Sherwin Kevy to the role of chief resident, and ultimately, Assistant to the Physician-in-Chief, for a total of seven years. One of us (FHL) served for four years, the first two as chief resident and the latter two as Assistant to the Physician-in-Chief. Many of Dr. Janeway's chief residents went on to serve in faculty positions at the Children's and ultimately in positions of stature in academic medicine throughout the country. All but one of his chief residents were male (see table at the end of this chapter). One of the joys of being chief resident, and one reason why so many ended up in academic careers, was Dr. Janeway's way of involving chief residents in planning curricula, hospital policies and resident experiences. They were active participants in the educational process.

In an article that he wrote with one of the authors (RJH), Dr. Janeway noted that among a cohort of 152 residents, 56% pursued practice and 33% pursued academic medicine.[16] The high percentage pursuing academic medicine continued to rise in the eras of Drs. Avery and Nathan, with 80% pursuing fellowship.[17] During the period of the Boston Combined Residency Program in the late 1990s, the number pursuing fellowship fell only slightly, to 75%. These figures represent career choices immediately after residency. If one tracks these individuals, the percentage in academic medicine falls to approximately 65% to 70% but is still significantly higher than in most residency programs.

Many of Dr. Janeway's philosophies about residency are worth noting. During the Blackfan era, residents lived in hospital. If they were off at night, they had to be back by midnight. At the beginning of Janeway's era, residents were on service every other night and every other weekend. By 1974, increased flexibility had been so established that residents were on duty every third night and every third weekend. They also lived outside of the hospital. They were given more responsibility and authority for the organization and nature of the residency program during Janeway's time. Significantly, CAJ supported the creation of the House Staff Association, which began in the mid to late 1960s and had matured remarkably by the end of his tenure in 1974. In addition, Janeway supported an adequate salary for house staff, as was noted in an earlier chapter. In 1964 he stated:

> House staff salaries, or lack of them, have been based on the notion that hard work itself and the educational experience working in an outstanding hospital are sufficient reward. This philosophy has become outmoded. Interns and residents are not students of medicine, but are productive members of society. They ought to receive adequate compensation, comparable to that earned by other young professionals at the start of their careers. One result [of higher salaries] is that fewer applicants now turn down an offer of a rewarding position at Children's Hospital Medical Center.[18]

The Medical Staff Executive Committee Minutes also show that Dr. Janeway strongly supported increased salaries for house staff in the 1970s. This was a time of considerable ferment and agitation for better living conditions and salaries for house staff. The Housestaff Association, led by Dr. Jan Breslow, strongly lobbied the Medical Staff Executive Committee. According to the Minutes of the Medical Staff Executive Committee, Janeway supported fully the importance of increasing house staff salaries. In addition, the Annual Reports of 1964 and 1970 provide a clear insight into Dr. Janeway's philosophy of training. In the 1970 report, concerning the issue of responsibility, he said, "Since most of our house staff will be engaged in hospital service and teaching and activities during the rest of their professional life, responsible participation in planning, evaluation and improvement in hospital programs is as much a part of their training as the actual care of patients."[19]

Dr. Janeway cared about many issues affecting residents other than salaries. He recognized the value and special circumstances of many women residents; the Annual Report of 1964 is indicative: "An interesting phenomenon of recent years has been the growing group of young women, whose medical career has been interrupted by marriage and the raising of young children, returning to complete pediatric hospital training on a part-time basis. We are pleased that it has been possible to introduce sufficient flexibility into our educational program to meet the needs of an able group of future physicians, whose obligations to their family must be met simultaneously."[20]

Janeway's understanding of the learning process was profound, and was, in our opinion, related to a flexibility and willingness to change that threaded through his entire professional life. In his 1970 report he remarks about the issue of critical analysis of a clinical program: "the give and take of daily rounds and the heavily attended Chief of Service Rounds all emphasize the critical analysis of clinical problems. The atmosphere is a far cry from the authoritarianism of much old world medical teaching and often surprises our foreign visitors."[21] In the matter of outpatient training, it is useful to note that Dr. Janeway saw emergency room care as fragmented care. He was instrumental in developing outpatient consultation clinics that ultimately found fruition in the Fagan Building of the hospital, through a number of subspecialty oriented floors. Continuity clinic as a formal part of the residency began in 1968, through the efforts of Dr. Melvin Levine and others, although it had been a central part of the Family Health Care Program (FHCP) since 1955. CAJ was instrumental in fostering and supporting this idea. Finally, he supported family health-care training for residents and supported the care of children as part of family care. He urged residents to attend their continuity clinics and the FHCP.

At the heart of Dr. Janeway's view of training was his affinity for the practitioner in the field, the doctor who used to make house calls. This affinity resulted in affiliations with North Shore Children's Hospital, Beverly Hospital, and other community-based rotations for residents. In point of fact, during his era there was tremendous growth in affiliations with outside hospitals. The Executive Committee Meeting minutes show that the hospital's Board of Trustees supported such affiliations firmly, but they were initiated by Janeway and he took advantage of them in an educational sense to be certain that house staff rotated as often as possible into these units, which included, besides the North Shore and Beverly institutions, Beth Israel Hospital, Mt. Auburn Hospital, Roger Williams General Hospital, Springfield Hospital, the U.S. Naval Hospital, and the Wellesley Convalescent Home.

Not all of these rotations to community hospitals were received warmly by the residents. When one of us (FHL) was chief resident, I noticed that things were beginning to break down a bit at North Shore Children's Hospital. The residents were not willing to do what some of the attending physicians wanted them to do. The residents had a tendency to make comparisons with the faculty at Children's Hospital, and it finally resulted in a disagreement that reminded me of a classic donnybrook. One night the house staff sat on one side of a table, the North Shore attending doctors sat on the other, and Dr. Janeway sat in the middle. CAJ listened to both sides, albeit with the most pained expression on his face as the charges went back and forth. He did a masterful job at the end, calming everyone down and raising the discussion to a higher level. This was another instance wherein I saw that, while Dr. Janeway did not like confrontations and conflicts, he was a master at resolving them.

His enlightened views notwithstanding, the chief was not flexible in everything. He had definite, traditional ideas about what a resident physician should look like. Dr. Fred Robbins, who later shared a Nobel prize with Drs. Enders and Weller, told an interesting story about Dr. Carlton Gajdusek, a later Nobel prize winner himself, when he was a house officer. Gajdusek never wore a necktie, but "Charlie insisted that he wear one. Carlton was poor at obeying, partly because he would forget, and it became something of an issue. Finally, we in the lab got Carlton a slip-on tie, and either saw to it before he left the lab that he had it on or put it in his pocket. It did bother Charlie's sense of the appropriate physician behavior [to be without a tie]."[22]

Dr. Julius Richmond, successively chair of pediatrics and medical dean at Syracuse, chief of child psychiatry at the Children's, and later Surgeon General of the United States, noted Dr. Janeway's strong commitment to medical education. At an AAMC teaching conference in 1958, CAJ "was an excellent discussion leader," according to Richmond. At the White House Conference of 1960, Richmond saw Janeway as "a statesman, with a broad view of the needs of children. He had a genuine generosity to younger people." Richmond, who was himself instrumental in bridging pediatrics and child psychiatry, stressed that Janeway "was a major force in nurturing the Child Development Program at Harvard that Dr. Brazelton ultimately ran. Dr. Janeway felt that it should be based in pediatrics and have a strong research component."[23]

Faculty development was another of Dr. Janeway's interests. The late David Smith told us in an interview several years ago that he thought "Janeway's main contribution was his emphasis on people," that "the main resources of any institution lie primarily in its people." Smith went on to speak of his discussions with CAJ as he (Smith) was about to leave for the chair of the pediatrics department at Rochester. "Life will change for you now," Janeway warned him. "You have been the person giving the talks, reporting laboratory data; now you will have to learn to step aside and get your thrills from seeing the growth of people around you."[24] In recognition of Dr. Janeway's impact on education and his excellence as a teacher, the Charles A. Janeway Award was initiated at Children's Hospital in 1978. Establishment of the award was spearheaded by Dr. Arnold Smith, who in turn became a highly regarded academic physician at the University of Washington in Seattle. Twenty-eight people have received the award. Dr. Smith was the first, in 1978; Dr. Berenberg received the award in 1979; and one of us (FHL) was thrilled to receive it in 1981.

With regard to fellowship training, fewer data are available, both in the annual reports and in departmental records, to summarize completely the programs Janeway initiated at the Children's. It is clear, however, that fellowship training as a concept began in a limited number of pediatric institutions throughout the country, including the University of Cincinnati, Johns Hopkins, Columbia, and the Children's soon after World War II. Dr. Janeway made good use of fellows and attracted many highly talented individuals from throughout the United States. He also trained a number of very important individuals from foreign countries, many of whom went on to attain high stature at an international level. One simply needs to look at the roster of Blackfan lecturers during CAJ's time and note that the individuals he selected to give these lectures invariably were those who went on to great achievements in pediatrics in their various countries. Notable examples would be Niilo Hallman, of Finland, Charles Scriver, from Canada, Bo Vahlquist, of Sweden, among many others.

Dr. Janeway began fellowship training almost immediately after assuming his position as chief in 1946. The first appointments of fellows were in the divisions of hematology, led by Dr. Diamond, and metabolism, led by Dr. Gamble. By 1948 there had been up to fifteen fellowship appointments; by 1951 there were thirty-five; by 1957, forty-two; by 1960, sixty-seven; by 1964, sixty-six; by 1967, sixty-eight; and by the 1970s, seventy to seventy-five per year. By 1957, appointments in cardiology, adolescent medicine, neurology, neonatology, family health care and oncology were added. By 1960, fellows in nutrition, respiratory medicine, endocrinology, child health, and psychiatry were added to the list. By 1967, fellowship programs in allergy, infectious diseases, and renal diseases had joined the others.

A rich history of accomplishment has supervened since the founding of the many new divisions at the Childrens Hospital and the appointments of fellows therein. The impact of the programs has been immense in the United States and around the world. The fellowship programs remain large and very strong, standing as an enduring legacy of Janeway's accomplishments. Physicians who trained under CAJ have amassed some of the most prestigious awards and honors offered in the discipline of pediatrics. More than sixty have gone on to chair departments of pediatrics; many more became heads of divisions or hold other responsible positions. There are four Nobel awardees in medicine, and at least ten E. Mead Johnson awardees in research and nine Howland awardees from Dr. Janeway's former faculty or residents. In addition, a number of former residents went on to distinguished careers in surgery and pediatric surgical subspecialties after one or more years in medical pediatrics. There is no way to count all the residents from other countries who returned to chair their departments or research institutes. This list of acknowledged awardees should not understate the importance of the over 1,000 pediatric practitioners in the United States who benefited from their education at Children's under Janeway and made their contribution as excellent community practitioners. Many have said that his greatest legacy was the people he trained. Dr. Janeway exemplified perfectly Sir William Osler's aphorism: "Through your students and your disciples will come your greatest honor."[25]

Postgraduate education (or continuing medical education, as it is now called) was an important investment for Dr. Janeway throughout his tenure. The hospital also invested in postgraduate education—a careful reading of the Executive Committee minutes documents regular review of postgraduate activities. Efforts in continuing education were led by R. Cannon Eley and were supported strongly by CAJ. The programs began following World War II in offerings of refresher courses to train physicians for practice in the United States and abroad. Dr. Janeway assisted the effort by introducing a Wednesday afternoon conference designed for general practitioners, who would come to Grand Rounds, have lunch with hospital physicians, and then attend the Wednesday afternoon conference. This was important to CAJ; he enlisted his chief residents often in support of the endeavor. In addition, throughout most of his time, he led and supported an important postgraduate course, a five-day offering that involved the entire faculty of the hospital. Individuals came from throughout the country for this course, which always ended with an award dinner in Boston for the attendees. In Janeway's later years, Barry Adels, Sherwin Kevy, and others led this postgraduate course, which continued to be highly successful for a time but began to lose its following in the late 1970s. We suspect that competition from other institutions, some nearer to the attendees' homes, affected its attendance and popularity. As part of his commitment to continuing education, Dr. Janeway allowed for a number of initiatives within divisions for postgraduate training. These included courses in adolescent medicine, infectious diseases, immunology, and other areas. In addition, through Dr. Thomas Cone and Dr. Melvin Levine, outpatient refresher courses were offered for physicians in practice.

We have often been asked, "What was it like to learn from Dr. Janeway?" Both of us had the immense privilege of learning to be doctors under his tutelage. We use those words deliberately: we learned much more than intellectual, technical, and professional skills; we also learned about compassion, caring, and responsibility for the children and families we served. These qualities underscored everything Dr. Janeway did; we absorbed them by doing as he did. The experiences of one of us are illustrative.

As noted above, I (FHL) served as Dr. Janeway's last chief resident. I fulfilled that role for four years and was immensely privileged to do so. The duration of chief residents' appointments were a reflection of CAJ's Hopkins traditions and the attendant tendency to select chief residents for more than one year. A longer duration of chief residency allowed for a closer relationship with the chief and some continuity in programmatic development. From this vantage point I was able to view Dr. Janeway's relationship with the training program. At that period of time (1970–1974) there were thirty-five to forty residents as well as a large number of "affiliated" residents. Dr. Janeway depended heavily on Drs. Berenberg, Cone, and Kevy as his main advisors for resident affairs. Drs. Kevy and Berenberg had major responsibilities for the inpatient services, while Dr. Cone lead the outpatient department and the "affiliated" programs. Dr. Janeway was in his early to mid 60's during this period of time; nonetheless, the degree of energy he committed to the residents and the residency program was remarkable. A number of elements of his leadership stand out.

Senior Rounds were daily presentations by senior residents to the senior faculty to review the cases admitted the night before. Dr. Janeway attended these rounds regularly; often, Drs. Berenberg and Kevy were present as well. We all enjoyed immensely the mornings when the chief was present. We learned a tremendous amount from him, but perhaps benefited most from his clinical wisdom. Understandably, given his strong scientific background, Dr. Janeway always felt that pathology teaching was extremely important; he believed that a strong understanding of the pathologic consequences of clinical diseases allowed for a far better understanding of those diseases. He maintained, therefore, that pathology was central to diagnosis. Pathology rounds occurred in the Pathology Department from 4:30–5:30 p.m.; Dr. Janeway was always present, as was Dr. Farber. CAJ expected the house staff to be there. In the later years the house staff placed less value on pathology rounds and consequently were somewhat reticent to attend. Dr. Janeway made it very clear to me, as chief resident, that he expected them to attend.

Among the great joys of being a resident were Dr. Janeway's weekly ward rounds. The chief resident would select a patient to be presented by one of the other residents. The rounds occurred on the floors at the bedside, from 4 to 5 p.m. Hand washing always proceeded and followed the examination of patients. The first half hour would involve Dr. Janeway's careful taking of the history and performing the physical examination, during which he would often talk to the parents and demonstrate thoughtful questioning in doing so. He regularly determined the setting in which a child was growing up and related it to the child's illness. He was unfailingly gentle and tender with the patients. The last half hour involved a discussion of the disease entity. CAJ never knew ahead of time what patient would be presented, yet he always was able to wax most thoughtfully, and eloquently, about the disease process. At 5 p.m., irrespective of where he stood in the discussion, he would leave; Betty was coming from her work at the Boston Lying-in Hospital to pick him up, and he was always on time to meet her. We learned much from this.

Grand rounds were more informal than today. They often included patients. The patient would be brought in and there would be a brief moment of history taking and physical examination, followed by thoughtful discussion about the disease and the patient in front of 100 or more assembled house staff, faculty, and practicing pediatricians from the community. At student rounds, on the other hand, Dr. Janeway made good use of his opportunity to teach clinical skills to medical students. This occurred on Mondays, from 12 to 1 p.m.; Harvard medical students on rotation at the Children's would attend. CAJ alternated weekly sessions with Dr. Diamond; Brooks Barnes, as head nurse, was always in attendance. A patient was invariably presented. What stood out was Janeway's meticulous recording of the history and physical examination on the blackboard. A thoughtful discussion, appropriate for the medical student and centered around diagnosis, was the major focus of these rounds. Dr. Janeway's manner and technique were Socratic, but in a gentle way. He probed the student's knowledge base; he offered broad factual information; he was always thoughtful and informative. The students loved it.

Chiefs' rounds occurred at 4:30 every Thursday afternoon. CAJ always attended, and he expected as many of his division chiefs as possible to be present. In contrast to today, when in many institutions chiefs of subspecialty divisions rarely attend when patients outside their specialty are presented, the chiefs at Children's were expected to attend this session; they sat in the first and second rows, and Janeway called on them often to reflect on a given point. The room, which held approximately seventy-five people, would be packed; house staff would often sit on the stairway in the middle of the classroom. We suggested that it might be more comfortable if we had a larger room, but Dr. Janeway did not accept that suggestion; he felt that a community of physicians gathered in close proximity to each other, and talking to and with each other, was the best way to have a great teaching session. He did not necessarily believe that there had to be subspecialty experts at every session. In fact, he often encouraged reflection and thoughts about a given case from the fellows, residents, and students in attendance. At times the house staff were concerned that discussions were too anecdotal, but Janeway responded to this concern and encouraged the faculty to draw from both their own experiences as well as the literature. We noted at times that he could be quite tired and would appear to fall asleep. We, in fact, were certain he was asleep, but then he would suddenly rise with five minutes remaining and reflect eloquently on the case and what needed to be done.

Dr. Janeway was very involved in the process of selecting interns, as were his most senior staff. The chief resident kept the list on the blackboard. The chief looked for a balanced group, that is, he wanted scientists and academic physicians, but he also wanted future practitioners. Most remarkable was his willingness to take a chance on the less traditional resident. He would often argue that a given individual might not make the best resident but if that person had great potential for the future, he or she was worth the investment. Dr. Janeway maintained his commitment to international pediatrics and the training of physicians from other countries. If a given individual had performed well in the "affiliated" program and in the Medical Outpatient Department, he was very anxious to include her or him on the house staff. He would give considerable credence in making these selections to faculty members whom he knew, and who had written in a given candidate's support. He knew whom he could count on, and an enthusiastic endorsement from such an individual influenced him greatly in the selection process.

Dr. Janeway held a meeting of division chiefs in his office once a week. He would invariably sit at his desk; the division chiefs would surround him on chairs to engage in thoughtful and collegial discussions. Those of us who were privileged to sit in on these often freewheeling academic discussions came away with deeper understanding of the dynamics of day-to-day academic pediatrics, particularly of the interrelatedness of the many subspecialties that were by that time prevalent. Most remarkable to a young chief resident was to hear the likes of Alexander Nadas calling the chief, "Dr. Janeway," never "Charlie," as most people called him when he was not present. This left an indelible impression.

Even in his mid-60's, Janeway made a valiant effort to attend social events offered by the house staff. If he could not attend, he always wrote a note expressing his apologies for his absence. He always went to the House Staff shows, an annual bit of theatre whereby the younger faculty could enjoy themselves with humor about their work and their teachers, and he intrinsically loved it when the house staff would mimic him. CAJ's long, flashing eyebrows were his trademark, and every resident competed avidly to be the best "Janeway."

Late in his career, Dr. Janeway espoused primary care and Family Medicine as important ways to provide care to all. He believed that one of the major contributors to the decline of the generalist was medical education that was "almost entirely biased toward producing specialists." He advocated an education that would produce family pediatricians and family physicians: "adequately trained for his job in providing health care to society's basic unit, the family . . . He should be trained as a specialist in people rather than in disease or organ system."[26] An article CAJ publishd in *Pharos* in 1974, which he had begun to write as far back as 1957, demonstrated an emphasis in his writings, notably after 1971, that represented a profound change, especially for one who had based his teaching and the development of his department on the integration of basic biomedical research with good clinical care. By the time the article finally appeared in *Pharos,* however, he had come to feel that one of the unforseen consequences of the Flexner Report was a denigration of primary care. He advocated that medical education provide training in primary care in the best academic institutions but with a strong health services research unit, blending "scientific sophistication with its intelligent and humane concern," which presented a great challenge, "particularly in medical education."[27] Although he wanted to change medical education, he wanted to do it as a scientific enterprise, not, as so often happened in many institutions in the 1970s, as purely an educational activity. At the same time, he was talking about the need for Family Medicine. "I must put in a plug for my pet project, 'family medicine' or 'family pediatrics' as a field that is not just an art learned by accident but which is a special branch of scientific medicine."[28]

He was even more explicit about Family Medicine in 1974: he noted that Harvard, "needs to be represented in its educational offerings" in family medicine "to serve as teachers in this field," and, "it has provided a field laboratory for the study of family health problems and health and illness in the community."[29] This sense of balance was characteristic of the man: he saw that the need for education of generalists to meet the needs of the public must be balanced by the need for it being based upon solid research.

In the aggregate, Dr. Janeway provided a wonderfully integrated learning experience for a young physician. His knowledge was both broad and deep. His physical-examination skills were wonderful to observe. He spoke as eloquently about family issues as he did about scientific issues. There was a profound balance of wisdom, clinical concern, and warmth. His demonstrated example was as strong as his spoken word.

Twenty-eight Years of Medical Chief Residents
Under Charles A. Janeway

Year(s) Served	Name(s)
1947	Frederick C. Robbins, Jr.
1948	Robert J. McKay, Jr.
1949–1950	Charles D. Cook
1951	John D. Kennell
1952	Leonard Apt Edward A. Mortimer, Jr.* Harrie R. Chamberlin*
1953	John R. Hartmann Alexander Blum*
1954	Maurice M. Osborne, Jr. Charles V. Pryles*
1955	Robert J. Haggerty Willard B. Fernald*
1955–1956	Mohsen Ziai Samuel Katz Lewis B. Anderson* Philip Adler*
1956–57	Peter A. Auld John Whitcomb* Seymour Zoger* Lisbeth Hillman*
1957–1958	Charles Andrew Rigg Michael Braudo* Richard L. Lester, Jr.* William London
1958–1959	Sherwin V. Kevy James N. Montgomery*
1959–1960	Sherwin V. Kevy John P. Eckert* Walter S. James*
1960–1961	David H. Carver A.A. Douglas Moore*
1961–1962	Robert A. Goodell Joel J. Alpert*

Year(s) Served	Name(s)
1962–1963	Thomas Adams David A. Smith
1963–1964	John L. Green James R. Hughes
1964–1965	M. David Atkin Myron Johnson
1965–1966	Sherwin V. Kevy**
1966–1967	Sherwin V. Kevy** Michael J. Maisels*
1967–1968	Sherwin V. Kevy** Robert Rosenberg*
1968–1969	Sherwin V. Kevy**
1969–1970	Sherwin V. Kevy** Robert Reece*
1970–1971	Frederick H. Lovejoy, Jr. John W. Graef*
1971–1972	Frederick H. Lovejoy, Jr. John W. Graef* Roger Ashley*
1972–1973	Frederick H. Lovejoy, Jr.**
1973–1974	Frederick H. Lovejoy, Jr.** Elias Milgram*
1974–1975	John A. Philips Juanita Lamar*

*(MOPD) Medical Outpatient Chief Resident
**Assistant to Physician-in-Chief

12 Charles Janeway's Scientific Research and Publishing Legacy

Charles A. Janeway was never a Nobel Prize winner. No diseases or syndromes were named after him, albeit a case could be made for the disorder agammaglobulinemia, which some say could have been named after him. Why then do we, and most who knew him, consider him a significant scientist? During his thirty-eight years of publishing he produced 212 papers and book chapters, an average of 5.6 per year. It is said today (in 2006) that one should produce at least two papers per year to ensure an academic career. Many do this only until they achieve tenure. Not only did Janeway exceed this standard, his rate of production scarcely varied throughout his academic life.

With all of Dr. Janeway's contributions to clinical care, his organization and management of a major modern department of pediatrics, and his far-flung international interests and activities, it is sometimes difficult to remember that he originally achieved fame as an experimental scientist. He not only performed such work well; he seemed to revel in it. In a letter to his mother, written in 1941, Janeway wrote, "Work is going well. It is more fun than it's ever been. I'm more and more doing investigative work, which is what interests me most, although I doubt if I would be happy entirely away from patients."[1] Some of Janeway's penchant for science was imbedded in his family background. He came into medicine with a family history and tradition wherein medicine was a blend of clinical skill and research. Further, he arrived on the academic medical scene just as major advances were beginning as a result of new research methods and, most impor-

tantly, new therapeutic agents were being introduced, first the sulfonamides and then penicillin, that gave reason for precise and detailed bacteriologic diagnoses in order to treat patients effectively.

His co authors in the 1930s and 1940s constituted a virtual Who's
Who of academic medicine; many, indeed, became the giants of internal medicine in the post World War II years. Among Dr. Janeway's collaborators who later became heads of departments of medicine at
prestigious universities were A. McGee Harvey, at Johns Hopkins
School of Medicine; W. Barry Wood, at Washington University and
Hopkins; Paul Beeson, at Yale and Oxford; Eugene Stead, at Emory
and Duke; W.T Longcope, at Hopkins; and R.H. Williams, at the University of Washington. Two other collaborators were giants in fields
outside of internal medicine: Gustave Dammin, chair of pathology at
Harvard's Peter Bent Brigham Hospital; and Janeway's mentor, Edwin
Cohn, director of the physical chemistry laboratory at Harvard (although CAJ never co-authored a paper with Cohn). The trend continued in later years; his co-authors in the 1950s through the 1970s also
became some of the outstanding practitioners and researchers in pediatrics in the United States. Among them were Weller, Gitlin, Rosen,
Metcoff, Barness, Cook, Wedgwood, Gellis, Stokes, Wallace, Schwartz,
Shwachman, Scheinberg, and Berenberg, He also had stellar international leaders as co-authors, including Hallman, of Finland; Gomez,
Gordillo, and Cravioto, of Mexico; Hitzig, of Switzerland; Nakasone,
of Japan; and Monkeberg, of Chile (one of the few pediatricians ever
to run for president of his country, albeit unsuccessfully!).

Alan Gregg, in his address entitled "The Natural History of the Academic Life," told that the first decade was for preparation; the second,
for research and patient care; the third, for teaching; and the fourth, for
mentoring and providing wisdom.[2] Dr. Janeway's career, as evidenced
in his published works, follows this pattern. This is most evident in his
later works, which tended toward greater emphasis on educational
philosophy and international issues, the latter being, in our opinion,
driven by his desire to share wisdom with international colleagues and
also to bring the wisdom of those colleagues to pediatricians in the
United States. Even in his later years, however, one still sees glimpses
of Janeway's interest in basic science and research. Perhaps the most
important lesson for today's academics is that CAJ continued writing

throughout his career. The subject matter changed but he maintained his intellectual curiosity throughout his life and continued to share that curiosity with colleagues through his writings. Dr. Janeway's *bibliography* is a long one . Volume of output, however, is not enough; what one writes must be important and must also be written well. According to both of these criteria, CAJ was a monumental success.

The first description of the use of sulfonamides, by Domagk, was published in 1935. Janeway's first paper followed very soon thereafter, in 1937. That paper described, for the first time, three cases he had seen during his residency at Hopkins of acute hemolytic anemia;[3] he tested the three patients with small doses after they had recovered, and he did skin testing to determine whether the response was an allergic one. The only positive response was a small rise in bilirubin, possibly indicative of some hemolysis. He was cautious in his conclusion, noting that he had not proved a causal relation. He paid tribute to the house officer who recognized the complication. This first publication set the stage for much of Janeway's scientific and clinical work. It combined his expertise in infectious diseases with the emerging field of immunology and with his concerns about drug toxicity. Many times in his later work at the Children's, when children had prolonged fever of unknown origins, he would suggest that the patients first be taken off all drugs to determine whether the fever was a drug reaction. Often this proved to be the case. This led him later into experimental work with rabbits (many experiments were recorded in his laboratory notebooks, but not published, as was true of his records of patients given sulfonamides). His most significant later research describes the production of experimental glomerulonephritis in rabbits.[4] In the margins of his bound laboratory notebooks are the names and chart numbers of the patients.[5]

Dr. Janeway's first paper was followed by two clinical descriptions: one of sickle cell anemia associated with congestive heart failure,[6] and another on acute arthritis.[7] He then returned to a series of papers on sulfonamides. The latter work was done when CAJ was a fellow in Dr. Zinsser's laboratory, studying the mechanism of action of sulfonamides.[8] Using beta hemolytic streptococci, he assessed the growth of the organism with sulfonamide and rabbit serum. He noted that the two together were associated with more inhibition of growth than was either alone. In later clinical discussions he often suggested that anti-serum might be useful in severe infection. He made these suggestions, perhaps based on this early work, at a time when most physicians were using only antibiotics. In this study he also demonstrated that with higher doses of sulfonamides there was less phagocytosis, suggesting a toxic effect of the drug on the white blood cells. He also examined the morphology of the bacteria that had been exposed to the drug and noted that the chains became longer and they stained more deeply. After washing of the organisms the effect disappeared, showing that the drug was bound loosely. The next paper was a technical one, demonstrating that the electrical potential of the organism fell with multiplication and was maintained when sulfonamide was added.[9]

Typical of Dr. Janeway's passion for understanding mechanisms as well as outcome were his papers on the measurement of changes in plasma volume in ten patients recovering from acute congestive heart failure using the new technique of dye dilution.[10] Not content with pure laboratory research, Janeway followed these publications with a number of papers on the clinical use of these new drugs, including infections during pregnancy[11] and reviews of medical progress in bacteriology in the *New England Journal of Medicine* on treatment of infections.[12] A year or two later, he published another such review.[13] It is interesting to note that CAJ was selected to write the first of these review articles when he was only two years from his fellowship and only in his early thirties. All these papers demonstrate an enduring quality: his ability to synthesize a complex field for the practitioner and yet include the experimental basis of his reviews. For instance, in the second review,[14] the first section is labelled, "How Drugs [*i.e.,* sulfonamides] Work." He reviewed the oxidation products of sulfa drug that produced methemoglobinemias and cyanosis rather than merely stating that sulfonamide sometimes produced cyanosis in patients. In the third review[15] he wrote of the importance of making a specific bacteriologic diagnosis, given that a specific therapy was then available. The theme that the specific bacteriologic diagnosis and knowledge of the pharmacology of the drugs were necessary for good treatment continued in the two-part review of the sulfonamides in the *New England Journal of Medicine.*[16] In a discussion at a meeting of the New England Pediatric

Society CAJ said, "I am not open minded about it," (*i.e.*, the need for specific bacteriologic diagnosis) but added in his disarming way, "When one is not open minded he is apt to be wrong!"[17]

In an earlier paper, written with Paul Beeson, who was then a resident, they reported an interesting observation: that sulfapyridine seemed to be an antipyretic as well as antimicrobial.[18] In addition to the clinical presentations, Janeway and Beeson gave the drug to rabbits, found a decrease in their temperature, and then speculated on the mechanism. They noted that the ears of the rabbits felt warmer when they were given the drug and suggested that the mechanism of action was peripheral dilatation and increased heat loss. This paper is also typical of CAJ: he was always interested in mechanisms of drug action and side effects. He continued his interest in the sulfonamides with another paper, again with Beeson, of eighty patients with pneumococcal pneumonia treated with sulfathiozole and also immune rabbit serum.[19] Janeway acknowledged that others were using antiserum less but, we suspect on the basis of his earlier work, felt that antiserum enhanced the effect of the sulfa. The paper also included using the Francis test to determine when there were adequate antibodies, either from the antiserum or as a result of the patients own response.

One practical aspect of how to obtain a specific diagnosis was the basis of a paper demonstrating that if a patient had been treated with a sulfa drug the cultures were often sterile, yet bacteria could still be seen on microscopic examination.[20] If para-amino benzoic acid was added to the culture, however, a needed metabolite of the bacteria, the yield of positive cultures was increased. This observation was especially useful in patients suspected of having bacterial endocarditis. In one of his review articles on bacteriology for *The New England Journal of Medicine*[21] Janeway commented on the proper technique for obtaining throat cultures, *i.e.*, a very vigorous swabbing. Most of us can remember, as residents, observing Dr. Janeway seeing a patient we thought had a streptococcal infection, but who had been on antimicrobial therapy and whose original culture had been negative, only to have CAJ come by and vigorously swab the tonsils and obtain a positive culture. Later we would laugh and comment among ourselves that when CAJ did a throat culture, he almost did a tonsillectomy too.

An interesting aside of Janeway's research was his study with

Cheever[22] of the Brown-Pearce rabbit sarcoma, which was believed to be caused by a filterable virus that could be transmitted to other rabbits by the cell free supernate (probably containing a virus) of ground-up tumor. The first time the rabbits received the filtrate, they developed these tumors. What seemed to interest Janeway most, however, was that rabbits who survived failed to develop tumors with a second challenge, presumably owing to an acquired immunity. The future immunologist could be seen at work. In his laboratory book, labelled "Corneal Inocul.," there are a series of descriptions of inoculations of rabbit cornea with lesions from humans having a variety of diseases, and notes indicating that Janeway was looking for viruses. Each patient's name and hospital chart number are meticulously noted, as are the sources of the human material (*i.e.*, herpetic lesion, diarrheal stool, cerebrospinal fluid, etc.). None of the rabbit corneas showed any reaction. It was frustrating to try to isolate viruses before tissue culture methods were available.

Several studies of a variety of infections followed. These included attempts to show the etiologic relation of Listeria monocytogenes bacteria to infectious mononucleosis,[23] with negative results; a study of an outbreak of Salmonella suipestifer,[24] which was followed by CAJ writing the chapter on this disease in *Cecil's Textbook of Medicine;*[25] and an interesting study of three patients with lymphocytic choriomeningitis, in which the investigators trapped mice in the homes of the patients and demonstrated disease when other mice were injected with the brains of the trapped mice.[26] The latter paper is sixty-three journal pages long and has 120 references, a very complete review of the state of knowledge of that disease. This also was followed by a chapter on this disease in later editions of Cecil's text.[27] From time to time Janeway was asked to write reviews of various infectious diseases, but he was about to move into a new field, the plasma proteins.

As the clouds of a looming war were gathering in 1940–41, Professor Edwin Cohn became certain that his ethanol fractionation of plasma would yield purified albumin in sufficient quantity to serve as a useful plasma expander on the battlefield.[28] He convinced Walter Cannon, fellow faculty member at Harvard and head of the National Research Council's Committee on Shock, Transfusion, and Blood Substitutes, to set up a mechanism for testing the Cohn fractions. Can-

non approached Soma Weiss, the newly appointed Hersey Professor of
the Theory and Practice of Physic at the Peter Bent Brigham Hospital.
Weiss decided that Dr. Janeway should "Conduct the needed clinical
testing."[29] CAJ was already in charge of the microbiology and immunology laboratories at the hospital. In a laboratory notebook, starting
October 30, 1941, are multiple recordings of his work with bovine and
human albumin fractions. His work was primarily to determine sterility with cultures and perform safety tests in guinea pigs and rabbits.
Later, starting in early 1942, the records show batches being sent to
Dr.Owen Wagensteen (a Minnesota surgeon), and Drs. Chambers,
Mahoney, Gibson, Blalock and others as part of the multi-center trial
for patients in shock. These studies of patients in shock were reported
later in the war.[30]

Janeway was in charge of this clinical testing and, consistent with his
dedication to patients, he was on call continually for those in the
Boston area. Many of the recordings in his laboratory books are not in
his handwriting but frequently at the end there are notes, "All OK CAJ"
or "Sterility tests OK CAJ" or "Rabbit thermal tests OK CAJ." Or, on
one occasion, "All returned to Oncley, Unsatisfactory CAJ." What had
started out to be a study of 1,000 patients in shock was terminated after the first 200 patients were studied because there was such good response. Toward the end of this laboratory book, in 1944 and 1945,
there are notes about globulin fractions distribution to various physicians, including Dr. Berenberg, Janeway himself, and Dr. David Rut-
stein. In addition to Janeway, the group of physicians involved included
Robert Ebert, Eugene Stead, Andre Cournand, Dickinsen Richards,
John Merrill, James Warren, George Thorne, and, in pediatrics, Joseph
Stokes, Sydney Gellis, William Berenberg, and the future Nobel prize
winning microbiologist John Enders. Although a number of papers resulted from this work, much of it was supported by the military during
the war and was therefore classified and left unpublished.

In early 1941 Dr. Janeway had given small doses of the purified bovine albumin to five test subjects without ill effect, except for one case
of mild serum sickness.[31] The Armour meat packing company in Chicago had set up the fractionation procedure for bovine plasma and
were gearing up for the production of large amounts of purified bo-

vine serum albumin. This early experience (of one patient who had serum sickness) was a portent of worse things to come with the use of bovine serum albumin. Ultimately, two prisoners in the Norfolk prison colony died of serum sickness following such experimental infusions; thereafter, the trials were stopped. Dr. Janeway was devastated by this. He personally visited the prison to counsel the participants and noted later his satisfaction that after the war the two prisoners who had died in the study received a posthumous amnesty.

Meanwhile, purified human serum albumin was being prepared at the pilot plant at Harvard Medical School. In July 1941, Janeway infused this human albumin into eight patients in shock and into three medical students who had been intentionally bled to the point of shock;[32] this was the definitive experimental study by Janeway and his group, one not likely to be approved today by hospital human investigation committees. Volunteer medical students were recruited and, after careful examination, these subjects were rapidly bled of 10 to 20% of their blood volume (in from ten to fifteen minutes) and then given concentrated human albumin intravenously. Blood volumes were measured before and during administration, and demonstrated rapid recovery. A secondary aspect was to mildly dehydrate some of the subjects. These subjects were less able to rapidly replace their blood volume, showing that part of the replaced blood volume was water entering the vascular system from the extracellular space. The details of the procedures and the care to ensure that no harm came to the subjects is exemplary. They were rescued with the purified human serum albumin. CAJ first reported experience with plasma albumin in articles and an editorial in *The New England Journal of Medicine*[33] and predicted an important future for the Cohn fractionation procedure in the war effort.[34]

The first lots of purified human serum albumin were received from Armour on January 26, 1941. Soma Weiss died suddenly and unexpectedly five days later. Janeway was immediately appointed to succeed him as chairman of the Conference for the Study of Albumin. As the commercial preparation of human albumin expanded to involve many meat packing companies, Janeway took charge of vetting these projects. He set up the clinical testing committee.

The results of the Norfolk Prison Colony investigation were heavy blows to the massive efforts that had been invested in the crystalline bovine albumin project. The clinical testing had consumed a year of Janeway's efforts. Yet it became equally clear that the incidence of serum sickness from bovine albumin approached 33%. CAJ organized and chaired a meeting of the National Research Council that ended any further exploration of crystalline bovine albumin as a therapeutic agent. Janeway felt a keen responsibility for these contributors to scientific knowledge, two of whom paid with his life for volunteering.[35] At a meeting of the Conference on Albumin Testing, which Janeway chaired, bovine albumin was then abandoned in favor of human albumin. Certainly this experience planted in CAJ's mind the later landmark experiments on immune complex disease he was to carry out after the war, with Hawn.[36]

By 1943, the fractionation of plasma to produce human serum albumin had been transferred almost entirely to industry. The attention of the Cohn laboratory then focused on the antibody content of Cohn Fraction II+III, which had been studied extensively *in vitro* by John Enders.[37] Probably because of the catastrophe with bovine albumin at the Norfolk Prison, Janeway injected himself with gamma globulin fractions. On March 19, 1943, at 3:30 p.m., he received IV gamma globulin; at 4:10 was admitted to the Peter Bent Brigham Hospital with nausea, vomiting, diarrhea, headache, chills, and a fever of 102°F. He was treated with IV fluids and discharged on March 21 with the diagnosis, "Reaction to staphylococcus toxin in IV gamma globulin." (It is now known that the staphylococcal exotoxin is a super antigen with the properties exhibited by CAJ.) His physicians were Drs. George Thorne and Lewis Dexter.[38]

Janeway's final conclusions about the use of human serum albumin were reported to the National Research Council on November 17, 1943: "The recommendation [appears] justified that 100ml of 25% albumin in the standard unit, which should result in an increase in the volume of plasma by approximately 500ml in the absence of continuing plasma loss or dehydration."[39] As a consequence of this conclusion, every landing craft at the Normandy beachheads in June 1944 was well supplied with 25% human serum albumin. Countless lives of wounded men were saved. This was accurately depicted in the opening of the motion picture, "Saving Private Ryan," in which the landing at Omaha Beach was re-enacted.

Dr. Janeway's second paper on this subject was a review of war medicine. He surveyed the various attempts to have a replacement for whole blood on the battlefield. He noted that "an entirely new approach to therapy with blood plasma has been proposed by Cohn," the use of one component in the serum, albumin. This work was supported by the U.S. Navy and some of the results were published in naval publications. Even in his first reviews of "War Medicine," Janeway took the broad historical perspective of the effect of wars on civilians and noted that preventive programs should also include mental health, nutrition and epidemiology.[40]

In 1944, Lawrence Oncley, an investigator in the Cohn laboratory, succeeded in separating Cohn Fraction II from Fraction III. It rapidly became apparent that sterilizing the 16.6% solution of gamma globulin offered new problems and that heat sterilization, as was performed for albumin, would not be feasible. Concerns were immediately raised about the transmission of hepatitis, but Dr. Janeway laid this to rest when he found evidence of hepatitis in only one child of 1,200 who had received gamma globulin.[41] Two important trials were conducted to study the attenuation and prevention of measles with the Cohn Fraction II (gamma globulin). One was carried out by Joseph Stokes and Sydney Gellis in Philadelphia; the other by Janeway at Philips Academy in Andover and at Milton Academy, CAJ's alma mater. Measles was modified or prevented in 98% of the students who received gamma globulin. The two studies were published jointly.[42]

Before Cohn died, he persuaded Harvard to allow him to patent a number of processes, royalty free, mainly to ensure standards of safety. Janeway was appointed to the commission to control quality. After the war, the second committee in which he was instrumental was the Committee on Blood and Blood Derivatives of the National Research Council. Janeway chaired that committee and was joined by Louis K. Diamond as medical director of the National Blood Program of the American Red Cross. Thus Janeway was, at a very young age, thrust into the center of national war efforts and continued to play a significant role for many years in the successor of the plasma fractionation program, the Protein Foundation, of which he was president from 1955 to 1960, and scientific director from 1960 to 1968. (The foundation was known as the Blood Research Institute, Inc. from 1967 on and continues today as the Center for Blood Research. Its president until 2005 was Dr. Fred Rosen, one of Janeway's most distinguished colleagues.) The time he was so active in the Protein Foundation were the very years that he was also heavily involved in the Iran Foundation, as noted earlier. During the Korean war the need for blood and protein components became critical once more; Janeway, in his capacity as chair of the NRC Committee on Blood and Blood Derivatives, stressed the need for the use of the technical experts on his committee at national meetings with the American Red Cross. The problem of possible transmission of serum hepatitis in pooled plasma and blood led him to study whether this occurred with human serum albumin, and he reported a study done with Paine (later a neurologist at the Children's) demonstrating that it did not.[43]

In many ways Dr. Janeway's pediatric investigations after he became chief at Children's Hospital were but a continuation of the work he did before. Rosen, in a short biographical profile of CAJ, noted that

> Dr. Janeway introduced to pediatrics an important clinical discipline while inaugurating a new era in clinical immunology. With his background in bacteriology, protein fractionation, and experimental hyper-sensitization, which brought early leadership in the investigation of immunological disease, Dr. Janeway's studies of the nephrotic syndrome of childhood established: 1. the usefulness of adrenal cortical steroids in its treatment; 2. the catabolic perturbations in serum proteins (particularly the increased metabolism of albumin and immunoglobulins); and 3. the role of polyanions in the clearance of hyperlipidemia.[44]

After the war, and ensconced as chief at the Children's, Dr. Janeway and his colleagues returned to the laboratory and their work on experimental hypersensitivity. In this experiment they injected bovine serum albumin and bovine serum gamma globulin into rabbits. Those receiving albumin became sensitized and showed inflammation of the arteries (periarteritis), while those receiving gamma globulin developed glomerulonephritis. This was the first experimental production of glomerulonephritis. Additional studies followed, and demonstrated that X-radiation or nitrogen mustard prevented the antibody formation and the subsequent pathologic disease.[45] In the latter study they also demonstrated that, with production of the nephritis, serum complement fell, but did not fall in animals protected by nitrogen mustard or irradiation.

Rosen believes that Janeway's most original scientific contribution was this work on the production of glomerulonephritis in rabbits. He also noted that CAJ's ability to have scientific insight into areas wherein research should be directed was demonstrated by a patient with angioneurotic edema (whom RJH had as a patient but never had an insight as to etiology), in whom Rosen would find the complement disorder after Janeway told him to "go measure complement."[46]

The laboratory at the Children's that Dr. Janeway developed became very productive when David Gitlin arrived in 1950. A comment must be made about the relationship between Janeway and Gitlin, although we are not privy to the inner workings of their relations. Gitlin was a brilliant laboratory research worker. There is no doubt but that CAJ was as productive as he was in the 1950s because of Gitlin. It is one more example of his wisdom and ability that he was able to forge such a productive relation with Gitlin (who had a very different personality than Janeway had). Why Gitlin left for the University of Pittsburgh while at the peak of his career and still being so productive is not clear, although need for higher salary probably was part of the reason.

Their remarkable relationship resulted in voluminous technical and clinical papers. In one of them,[47] the group demonstrated that fibrin is the component of the fibrinoid material seen in the pathology of collagen diseases. They used rabbit antiserum against human fibrin to show this. Other studies of experimental rabbit hypersensitivity that Janeway conducted with Gitlin and others determined the localization of antigen antibody reaction using radioisotopes, and, with Wedgwood, he elucidated the mechanism of action of ACTH in experimental nephritis.[48] These experimental hypersensitivity studies were interspersed with clinical studies of nephrotic syndrome. Among the latter papers were one written with Barness on the natural history of the disease.[49] In Janeway's Howland award address he noted that Barness's review demonstrated how, in many children with nephrotic syndrome, the disease improved after an attack of measles.[50] He had been working on the prevention of measles with gamma globulin and became interested in this relation to a very different disease. He then began a series of studies on nephrotic syndrome and hypoprotenemia; later he worked with Metcoff and Kelsey on clinical, biochemical, and renal hemodynamic features;[51] and with Metcoff, Rance, Kelsey, and Nakasone on the use of ACTH in the treatment of nephrotic syndrome.[52] The studies led to investigations of the plasma proteins in severe malnutrition.[53] These works were the result of Metcoff developing a close working relation with an exceptional group of researchers in Mexico, and undoubtedly were stimulated by Janeway's interest in the health problems of developing countries. This series of studies demonstrates how Janeway let work with colleagues and scientific advances take him into new fields that today are quite different subspecialities of pediatrics. He was never one to be pigeon-holed into one clinical subspeciality, and opposed the barriers often set up by these artificial groupings.

Rosen notes that in 1952 came the discovery of x-linked agammaglobulinemia and its attendant complications of arthritis and other connective tissue diseases.[54] The cellular basis of the disease was defined. This was followed by the discovery of transient hypogammaglobulinemia of infancy, and selective immunogobulin deficiency and the role of the thymus in severe combined immunodeficiency. One of the few papers in which Janeway was the first author was the report of three cases of agammaglobulinemia.[55] In his characteristically generous fashion, Dr. Janeway gave credit to Bruton for publishing the first paper on this new disease, but noted that they had each presented descriptions of the first patients at a meeting of the Society for Pediatric Research in 1952. The disease could as easily have been called Janeway disease (or Janeway, Apt, and Gitlin disease, in recognition of his co-authors) but primacy of publication and publicity was never CAJ's goal. He much preferred to have a disease referred to by the patho-physiological nature rather than by an eponym. A more comprehensive review of the gamma globulins appeared in several contributions Janeway wrote with Gitlin.[56] Interestingly, in one of these articles he describes the condition of Waldenstroms macroglobulinemia, the disorder from which he would die twenty-four years later. Later, when Janeway and his colleagues published a series of papers on the association of collagen diseases and agammaglobulinemia,[57] the multiple serum protein deficiencies in acquired and congenital agammaglobulinemia,[58] the hyper IgM syndrome,[59] and the selective immunoglobulin deficiencies,[60] it became apparent that this group of investigators was plumbing the depths of the whole field of the pathophysiology of the gamma globulins; they were not merely looking at only one such disorder. Papers continued to pour out from this group on the gamma globulins and their relation to lymphoid tissues, including a report of a patient with thymic alymphocytosis who showed delayed hypersensitivity and homograft survival,[61] and another regarding implantation of fetal thymus in a patient with thymic aplasia.[62] These extensive studies led Janeway to several summary papers and chapters on the broader topic of susceptibility to infection as well as serving as the topic for many lectures in foreign countries.[63]

Dr. Rosen recalls another side of Dr. Janeway, a somewhat more competitive one. In 1970 Rosen had retrieved the reagents Dr. Enders had used in a 1933 paper and repeated the experiments on opsonization. He and his colleagues found the mechanism for the phenomenon and sent the manuscript to the *Journal of Experimental Medicine*. Just before the report was published, Janeway had a visit from his close friend and colleague of many years, Dr. Barry Wood, who told him that Hopkins investigators had already discovered the proteins that mediate opsonization. CAJ told him, "Too bad, we already have a paper in press on this and it will be out next month."[64] It is interesting that Janeway still had a friendly competitive relation with Barry Wood. They had played football together in prep school and, in some ways, Wood had exceeded CAJ—he was the last All-American football star from Harvard; he had been a chair of a department of medicine, dean and vice-president of health affairs at a leading university, and was then back as chair of microbiology at their alma mater, Hopkins. We suspect that CAJ still had some longing for the scientific role as a basic science professor that Dr. Park had urged him to seek. It must have given him some satisfaction to have beaten this friendly rival into print on his own basic science turf.

Some papers on Janeway's list of publications appear, at this remove, to be anomalous. A paper on muscular dystrophy was written at a time when Janeway chaired the National Advisory Board of the National Foundation for Neuromuscular Diseases (1954–1968); the text is essentially a call for clinicians to be involved in the care of these patients.[65] It is not clear now why he was appointed to this group, inasmuch as there are no other papers on the topic by him or his group. Another apparent sideline is reflected in two papers on copper metabolism, both published in the prestigious scientific journal *Nature*,[66] about which Dr. Rosen notes,

> In another direction, the role of ceruloplasmin in Wilson's disease was discovered, and in a classic work, the first double-turnover study with radioactive copper bound to labelled apoceruloplasmin proved that ceruloplasmin did not transport copper.[67] Later, the role of beta 1c globulin or the third component of complement (C3) was found to be diminished in membranoproliferative glomerulonephritis, thereby defining that disease. During the 1940s, 1950s, and 1960s, Dr. Janeway maintained an interest in the therapeutic uses of gamma globulin, first in prevention of measles and hepatitis, then in the therapy of immunodeficiency disease. This series of studies, spanning three decades, was a fitting fulfillment of his initial courageous act as the first human being to be injected with human gamma globulin.[68]

From the late 1940s and through the 1950s, most of Janeway's experimental papers were published with his younger colleagues. He usually was the last author. As had been true of his grandfather, CAJ never would allow his name to be the first author on work done primarily by colleagues. In review papers, philosophical treatises, and educational and book chapters, however, he was frequently the only author. In the only paper that the primary author (RJH) published with him, a study of the subsequent careers of graduates of the Children's residency program[69] it was difficult to persuade him to even allow his name on the paper. I wanted his name on it because the paper reflected the period when Dr. Janeway was chief and because he edited each draft extensively; more pragmatically, I knew that if his name was on the paper it had a much better chance of being accepted for publication! The other author (FHL) had a similar experience. Janeway actively encouraged me to submit my first paper to *Pediatrics*, advocated for it actively, helped by editing but refused to add his name to it. Both of us learned that this was entirely characteristic of the man. He was unfailingly generous; sharing came as naturally to him as breathing. It also set an example which we both tried to adhere to throughout our careers and demonstrates how good example is a better teacher than rhetoric.

Janeway continued throughout most of his career to publish review chapters in standard texts and journals. The topics were wide-ranging: plasma proteins; lymphocytic choriomenigitis; salmonella infections; deficiency syndromes of gamma globulin and uses of gamma globulin; nephrotic syndrome; and more general descriptions of infection, immunity, and allergy in children. The clarity of his writing and his high reputation continued to ensure that editors of standard textbooks would call upon him to update chapters he had written previously. As many scientists do, he shifted from early in his career, when his papers were largely experimental science and clinical issues, to reviews and philosophical/educational papers in his later career. But he demonstrated remarkable consistency of production of papers over his entire career, varying from eleven in the five years between 1935 and 1940, when he was twenty-eight to thirty-two years old, and a maximum of thirty-three in the five-year period 1956 to 1960, when he was forty-seven to fifty-two. Even in the period from 1971 through 1979, when CAJ was between sixty-two and seventy years of age, he published twenty papers. Rosen has pointed out that until 1963 CAJ would come once a week to the immunology laboratory and was familiar with what was going on, but after that was not as active in the laboratory. For instance, he never learned the technology of column chromatography. In 1968 he turned the laboratory over to Rosen.

Dr. Janeway published several papers on educational issues as early as 1947. At that time he began to expound his ideas about the nature of pediatrics. In a review paper, probably recruited by the editor of *The New England Journal of Medicine* for the new professor to outline his philosophy, Janeway stated that the justification for pediatrics (as a separate discipline) was not due to any particular disease or region of the body, "but rather from the nature of its patients who are distinguished by an outstanding characteristic, they are constantly growing." The aim of a pediatrician was to assist, to the limit of his abilities, this process of growth so that his patient may increase "in wisdom and stature." CAJ defined the ages of the pediatrician's patients as from conception through adolescence (this at a time when most pediatric services ceased to see children when they were approximately thirteen years old). He outlined two areas in which pediatrics had been deficient: accident prevention and mental health. He proffered a utopian vision of what pediatrics should be saying: "The ultimate standard by which the success or failure of pediatrics must be judged [is] by the extent to which its charges become well integrated, responsible citizens when they graduate to adult life."[70]

Janeway also gave early evidence as to why he supported family health when he wrote, "In society the unit is not the child, but the family, all of whose members are involved whenever illness strikes in the group." In this era, before prevention of any viral infections except measles, he advocated allowing or even encouraging exposure during childhood to rubella, mumps, and chicken pox (through parties to ensure spread of the diseases) and decried the then popular use of quarantine for these diseases. He recognized that generally these disorders were much milder in childhood. His only reference to infant feeding (the one field in which he never did become expert, if that were necessary) was to decry the then popular pediatricians' enthusiasm for inspecting the stools of babies. "The frequency and character of stools, especially in breast fed babies, are far too often carefully supervised." He was an optimist at a time when many were writing dire warnings of the decline of the quality of childhood. It was part of his philosophy of first doing no harm. He urged that we not push the child, that "given time to mature appropriately before being asked to assume various responsibilities, each child will grow up able to utilize his innate abilities . . . The resilience of the human infant and child must be recognized, for many able adults appear to have been most unwisely handled in childhood."[71] In 1947 this was an unusual philosophy, especially when stated by the new Thomas Morgan Rotch Professor of Pediatrics at Harvard, who had been trained as an internist and had a very short exposure to children's disorders.

Janeway was mindful of the need to educate the public as well as the profession. In 1946 he gave a public broadcast sponsored by the Massachusetts Medical Society in Boston on radio station WAAB; the topic was the sulfonamides. CAJ pointed out the great success of these new agents but also warned of potential complications. Another, more comprehensive publication for the enlightened citizenry was the summary paper by Janeway and Gitlin published in *Scientific American* on agammaglobulinemia.[72] In 1962 he appeared on Boston's Channel 2 as part of a televised panel of four interviewees discussing the effects of radiation, especially nuclear fallout from atomic bomb testing. He noted the increase in incidence of leukemia in children but was careful to point out that many factors other than radiation might be responsible.[73]

Dr. Janeway's thoughtful, philosophical papers, while not strictly "scientific" contributions, touched on ways to promote science and educate the next generation of scientists. In 1955 he published a paper that he had presented at the dedication of the Mayo Memorial Building in Rochester, Minnesota October 22, 1954. Therein he paid tribute to the support of research by individuals who created foundations, but he was worried that it (research) "may be driven by demands of where lay people think it ought to go rather than to flow from scientific advances and the imagination of free and creative people." This sounds elitist and, for a man of such democratic beliefs, rings oddly. We think it was stated, however, in response to several new initiatives in research that at the time were not based on sound scientific development of the field. Janeway and others were concerned with the Cystic Fibrosis Foundation's push for therapeutic research at a time when the basic pathological defect was not known. His view of research was that it must be based upon an orderly development of knowledge and could not leapfrog over vacant areas of knowledge, and that such an orderly process was central to a medical school's function. Research, he noted, "is not an entity to be nurtured so much in its own right as much as it is to be related to the advancing frontiers of science in the whole university community. We must recognize the problem of communication between scientists working in different fields."[74]

He noted further that, after preparation of two to three years, the clinical investigator must "maintain contact with the basic science field." While it was even then becoming necessary for teams of basic and clinical scientists to join in research, he warned that such collaboration is not necessarily a productive way to do research. One of his recommendations sounds a bit quixotic, for he thought "Faculty should maintain communication in the faculty dining room," and that "free beer might be the most fruitful gift anyone could make to a medical school." At the 1960 White House Conference on Children and Youth, he wrote that a nation must support creative investigators, and he warned that if scientists are placed in a straitjacket of political and intellectual uniformity, we may lose our capacity for adaption to an ever changing environment and, like the dinosaurs, become extinct. He was concerned that, with affluence, something was missing in life. He felt that

> Man needs to be challenged, to lose himself in a struggle for something bigger than himself in which he believes deeply . . . We cannot afford to allow the difference between our high standard of living and the low levels in many other parts of the world to increase. How to narrow this gap, how to provide equality of opportunity and how, not just for America, but for all the world's youth . . . is the greatest challenge which faces us now.[75]

We doubt that Dr. Janeway would be happy with what has transpired in the ensuing forty-six years. The income inequality between countries has increased and, with it, much of the violence of the twenty-first century. In his Copeland lecture at the Washington Children's Hospital,[76] Janeway surprisingly decried the recent successful "Moon shot, when money could be better used on earth." This does not sound like one who always supported research, but, in context, he went on to decry the technology alone that makes such a feat possible, to the detriment of what he thought of as basic science.

Janeway continued to publish scientific articles late into his career. The last fifteen years of his life, however, saw his writings (often based on lectures given around the world) turn to broad issues of medical education and the environment. As we have noted elsewhere, his personal library contained collections of publications on family planning, renewable agriculture, and ecology. His passion for a peaceful world and his observations of the huge population increases in his travels to the developing world led him to become concerned with overpopulation, limited food supply, and use of dangerous pesticides. He recognized these issues as harmful to health, and foresaw that they would lead to violence and war.

His unpublished Marshall Woods lecture, given on the occasion of the launching of Brown University's re-entry into medical education in 1964, was one of his first efforts to examine where medicine was going. The title was self-explanatory: "Looking Ahead: the Future of Medicine." Janeway began with the broadest view of man. "Mankind must now be accepted as a brief manifestation of biochemical activity on an incredibly thin film of soil on the surface of a small planet dependent on energy from radiation from a star of low magnitude in a huge galaxy." Against this sobering view of mankind he added, "The modern condition, the optimistic view of the inevitability of progress has disappeared. Medicine itself used to look forward to eliminating disease and creating a totally healthy world . . . [but] we now realize that we can only solve one set of health problems at a time and must reconcile ourselves to a likelihood that in solving them we shall probably be creating new ones to challenge our successors."[77]

Janeway offered this view even before AIDS came to worldwide attention. Given this sober view of mankind he then asked, "What is the mission of medicine?" He reviewed some of the major advances in medicine but noted that, at that time, "we appreciate that diseases rarely have a single cause . . . but are the expression of the complex interplay of a number of factors both within the patient himself and in his environment." His own work had illuminated a number of diseases that had single causes, but he realized that the ones left to conquer were different. He may have been remembering H.L. Mencken's waggish comment, "For every complex problem, there is a solution that is simple, neat, and wrong." Janeway outlined the complex genetic, environmental interplay in most diseases, including the "Complex, dynamic socio-economic systems . . . that deeply effect his [man's] life." He was recommending that medical education must include the new sciences of behavior and socio-economics. "While research goes deeper . . . the physician must become more comprehensive and synthetic in his approach." He saw the great potential of new research leading to advances in transplantation, aging, and therapeutics, but he was not an uncritical apologist for research. He foresaw some of the dangers:

> These applications of scientific knowledge to birth, death and disease will have profound consequences upon the morals and mores of society and one can only hope that man will have the wisdom and the capacity to deal with them successfully, as he has so far with the terrible threat of atomic energy . . . More and more man will probably have to control his environment and mold [sic] it to his purposes, but he must remain keenly aware of the interdependence of soil, water, and air with micro-organisms, plants and animals in sustaining the great aspects of life on this planet.

In the same presentation Janeway then addressed the more immediate issue for a new way medical care would be delivered. "I believe that medical practice will be divided into two general types . . . specialists in group clinics or University medical centers and the practice of the speciality of family medicine." He had become a convert of family medicine, partially as result of the Family Health Care Program at Harvard. He concluded with his prescription: "Prune all but the minimum of clinical medicine from the medical school curriculum in order to broaden its scientific content; put more scientific discipline into the post doctoral hospital training; and improve the post doctoral hospital training and improve the post graduates' opportunities for all physicians to enable them to keep up with the increasingly rapid march of medical sciences." Janeway submitted a shortened version of this talk to his friend, Ted Weeks, the editor of *Atlantic Monthly,* in order to achieve more general readership, only to be rejected. Weeks wrote, "Dear Charlie, Though there is considerable improvement in the revision of your paper on the Future of Medicine, the objections against the original, I am sorry to say, hold."[78] Even Dr. Janeway at his best had his defeats.

Dr. Janeway's lectures on family medicine were published in three papers in 1974. In one of them[79] he dealt with the "unforeseen consequence of the Flexner report," first recounting the experience of his own father, Theodore, who, as noted in chapter 1, was the first full-time professor of medicine in the country. Theodore's position was a direct result of the Flexner Report, which had recommended the full-time system. As noted in Theodore's paper to the Association of American Universities, partly quoted in our initial chapter, he had found that not only was the remuneration too small for a full-time professor, but also that the care of patients was an essential part of being a successful clinical professor, and he felt that this was reduced and jeopardized by the full-time system (where at Hopkins all fees received from clinical care were turned over to the medical school).

A second "unforseen consequence" was the concentration of educational experiences in the teaching hospital, which offered very specialized and uncommon clinical conditions. Janeway paid tribute to the magnificent contributions that research, funded largely by the National Institutes of Health, had made to medical progress, but was concerned that the other functions of the medical center, teaching and patient care, had not been equally supported, thus leading to a "devaluation of the importance of teaching or clinical activities." He also, perhaps wistfully, owing to his own large investment in the administrative aspects of research activities, noted that, "Time spent by faculty members in travelling, attending committee meetings, going on site visits and writing grant applications and reports . . . has taken its toll in fatigue, absence from the university and lack of time for personal attention to students." He pointed out that, in response, several schools had developed special teaching programs such as those at Case Western Reserve (Family Clinic) and Cornell (Comprehensive Care Program). He described the Children's Hospital response, with the Family Health Care Program, as a model to supplement its hospital-based teaching, care, and research.

Dr. Janeway had come to the conclusion that the solution to the shortage of primary physicians and overemphasis on hospital-based experience for students was to develop primary care physicians who would work in groups of multidisciplinary professionals with "a fundamental scientific base" that emphasized health promotion, identification of those patients at higher risk, early detection of serious disease, management of emergencies, and rendering continuing care to chronically ill patients. He declared "the family physician must be a specialist . . . in people rather than in a specific disease or therapeutic modality." He recognized that the "future . . . may sound utopian, but I believe it a reality." This is still a vision that the authors believe in, but many other forces have rendered it difficult to achieve. Some family medicine training programs have come close to the ideal offered by Janeway, and primary care pediatrics and internal medicine residencies have become more successful examples, but support for the comprehensive care program envisioned, once these residents are in practice, has not been forthcoming.

In another of his papers on family medicine, Janeway wrote that the field was "for real."[80] In the third of his publications on this topic, he reviewed the experience of the Family Health Care program at Harvard.[81] He noted an important aspect of the Harvard program, the education of fellows, many of whom would become faculty elsewhere, a traditional Harvard role. From 1960 until 1974 there had been forty-three fellows; ten were in primary care practice in pediatrics, internal medicine, and family medicine but twenty-three were in full-time academic careers; eight in pediatrics, seven in family medicine, two each in public health and community hospital teaching, and three in administration (it is not clear what happened to the final one!). It is apparent today that all too few academic family physicians have been trained in the research methods that were part of the Harvard experience. The closing of the program at Harvard had this unfortunate result, since few other places were prepared to educate such fellows in the research base for primary care. The Harvard emphasis on research training for fellows, had the fellowship program been continued, might have resulted in more leaders of family medicine prepared for a research as well as an educational career, and the trajectory of academic family medicine might have been different. This was certainly the vision of Dr. Janeway.

In the late 1950s Janeway became involved in the Association of American Medical College's Teaching Institutes. Dean George P. Berry of Harvard was a guiding organizer of these, along with Dr. Julius Richmond. They probably were the ones who got CAJ involved. He had also become interested in the new field of medical education started by George Miller at the University of Buffalo. Janeway stimulated RJH to attend a two-week seminar on research in teaching in medical schools. Whatever the origins of his interest, CAJ chaired the 1958 seminar, "The Student, the Patient, the Teacher." His own paper was titled, "The Scholar and the Devil's Advocate."[82] He made a chart to summarize his views. According to him, the academician should be:

A Student—Always
A Participant—Active
A Teacher—A Privilege
A Process—Lifelong

In the discussion section of this paper Janeway made an interesting comment:

> as head of a department, having people who can get along with their fellow faculty is extremely important to the peace of mind of the department head, but my own personal experience is that intellectual brilliance and equanimity in interpersonal relationships do not always go along together . . . if we are to rate diplomatic talents as highly as scholarly attainments in clinical departments. I submit that mediocrity may be the result.

This note is fascinating in light of Janeway's own supreme diplomatic skills and intellectual ability. Perhaps he was reflecting on some of the most productive people in his department, who were prickly at best.

At the sixth annual conference on medical education for foreign students, Janeway discussed his concern that pharmaceutical companies supported much of continuing medical education.[83] We noted earlier that Janeway never accepted drug company money for house officer parties or other activities. For the 1960 White House Conference on Children and Youth, he wrote of the need for children to adapt to change and innovation and expressed concern for the emphasis on efficiency in childhood; he thought that children needed leisure. He also decried publically the devastating effect of McCarthyism on children. He ended with a question, "Am I my brother's keeper?" and answered it, "There can be only one answer, yes, for if you are not, there is no future for mankind." He expanded this to the commitment to assist the developing world to "help themselves with dignity and without loss of freedom. This is the greatest challenge which faces us now and in the foreseeable future."[84]

On December 4, 1969, Janeway received the degree, "Doctor Honoris Causa," from the faculty of medicine of Rheims University.

The invitation, his response, and his acceptance speech are all in French. He praised the spirit of freedom and "amitie" between the two countries and talked about the problems of youth in both lands, which he characterized as "grandes problemes" owing to social injustice, war, poverty, overpopulation, and the failure of medicine as it had become "isole et specialise" to deal with these grand problems. His international reputation was at its height.[85]

In 1973 Janeway presented two of the most prestigious awards in pediatrics to long-time colleagues: the Aldrich Award to Ross Gallagher for his initiation of the field of adolescent medicine in a teaching hospital,[86] and the Howland award, the highest award of academic pediatrics, to Louis K. Diamond.[87] Both of these men were among his closest colleagues. Janeway remarked that his own greatest contribution to pediatrics was his support for initiation of adolescent medicine by Gallagher. He noted that both men had been active in general pediatrics before they originated their specialities. This was in line with his belief that good academic physicians should have a general clinical background before launching their careers in subspecialization. In his introduction of Gallagher, CAJ went to some length to describe Gallagher's role in research done in private schools, testing gamma globulin for the prevention of measles, and some of his early publications on biological issues in pediatrics. Dr. Janeway liked people who had shown ability in traditional pediatrics before they branched out into new fields.

Janeway was called upon to write obituary remembrances of colleagues he had worked with, notably Edwin Cohn[88] and S. Burt Wolbach,[89] the long-time chief of pathology at the Children's. He also was the keynote speaker at the opening of the ninth Congress of the International Pediatric Association.[90] In that address he observed that "Pediatrics is a speciality in only one sense of the word, in its subject, i.e., children." He thought that pediatrics might even be called "Pediology," since it incorporated all sciences relating to children, not only the medical sciences. As chairman of the Executive Committee of IPA, he also opened the twelfth Congress and closed it with a summary of the proceedings.[91] He was often called upon for these summations; he could assimilate enormous amounts of material and see the connections between seemingly disparate parts of a congress and draw relevant conclusions. This knack of seeing the interrelations between areas was similar to his clinical ability to perceive the key elements of a patient's problem and avoid being overwhelmed by less relevant details. In recognition of his overall knowledge of research, Janeway was appointed to several research agencies. His *curriculum vitae* lists some of these: Member, Scientific Advisory Committee, Research Institute of the Hospital for Sick Children, Toronto, Canada; Consultant to National Research Council, Assembly of Life Sciences; and member of WHO Expert Advisory Panel on Maternal and Child Health. These are but a small sampling.

Toward the end of his active career, Dr. Janeway served for four years, 1970–1973, on the Advisory Council of the National Institute of Allergy and Infectious Diseases. Advisory councils are composed of senior, well-respected experts. His appointment was evidence that he was still, at that late date in his career, regarded as a national expert in the field of infectious diseases. Dr. Leighton Cluff, chair of Medicine at the University of Florida and later president of the Robert Wood Johnson Foundation, served with him, as did several very well known infectious diseases experts, including Albert Sabin, developer of the oral polio vaccine, Frederick Robbins, and Thomas Weller, Nobel Prize co-winners for their work with John Enders in developing the method for culturing the polio virus and other viruses. Cluff remembered two of Janeway's outstanding characteristics: "he was a moderating force among some very strong personalities, a kind, gentle person, with wisdom and a broad perspective, and he had creative ideas about changes that should take place in the Institute of Allergy and Infectious Diseases." For example, Janeway and Cluff advocated more emphasis on sexually transmitted diseases at a time when such emphasis was not popular. Cluff remembered CAJ's skill as a mediator between strongly held positions, even as he always made his own positions clear.[92]

On March 23, 1973, Janeway testified before the Subcommittee on Public Health and Environment of the House of Representatives on behalf of the "National Research Fellowship and Traineeship Act of 1973." His testimony was in heartfelt response to the Nixon Administration's effort to phase out the research training authority of the National Institutes of Health and the National Institute of Mental Health. He reviewed the major contributions made by trainees, remarked on the small amount proposed ("0.8% of the national budget") and pointedly stated that "The present administration . . . is business minded; no successful major business would think of operating without provision for depreciation of plant and building . . . Yet this is what, in essence, has been proposed for biomedical research." He then focused specifically on the need for pediatrician-scientists to further contributions such as neonatal determination of disorders such as PKU, hereditary hypercholesterolemia, and deafness. As the elder statesman of pediatrics, he took seriously his role as spokesperson for future pediatric researchers.[93]

The prestigious John Howland Award was awarded to Dr. Janeway in 1978. In his acceptance address, Janeway reviewed his family's history in medicine and his associations with colleagues as the basis for his successful career. He then presented the highlights of his work at the Children's. He paid tribute to the contributions of the many scientists who had worked with him at that hospital to improve the health of children. He then noted that new problems among children demanded new educational experiences; experiences with the social-emotional problems of childhood. He spoke with the forward-looking vision that always characterized him, advising his audience,

> But there is promise in the air. Pediatrics and obstetrics, made safer by technology, based on the hard science of the past, now are beginning to be "humanized" in their practice . . . It is essential that we continue to see that the advancement of knowledge which it brings is effectively applied in pediatric education, in pediatric practice, in ways that are most relevant to the needs of children and families, now and in the future.[94]

Two final, thoughtful, summing-up lectures remained. One was the Merriman Lecture, given in 1976 at the University of North Carolina.[95] He spoke of the need for a vision and linked the lecture around the United States' Constitution and its vision and promises, especially those not yet fulfilled: equality, liberty, and freedom. He then catalogued the failures to achieve equality of the races in infant mortality, income, unemployment, and poverty, and noted medicine's failure to deliver equality of services to all. He had clearly assimilated a population view as well as the view of the consummate clinician with concern for each patient. He reiterated his faith in research, especially the need to break down barriers between research disciplines. He elucidated what was becoming his obsession, a world view:

> If we are to have a stable world, it is in our own best interests to be generous to the developing countries, to work as much as possible through international agencies, such as the U.N. Development Fund and do everything possible to encourage building from the bottom up rather than imposing the American model, such as a medical school or tertiary care hospital on an economy not able to support them.

He had learned the lessons from Iran very well.

The Thayer lecture, at his alma mater, Johns Hopkins Medical School, was his final public lecture.[96] It was a fitting summary of his family history and his life and beliefs and, also fittingly, it was stated in his own words. There is no better summary of his life. At the end he discussed the threats to children in the future and iterated the global view he had espoused for four decades:

> The greatest quantitative threat to life and health for the majority of children, three quarters of whom live in the third world, is malnutrition. It is compounded of food shortages, climatic changes, ignorance and poverty, each a potentially solvable problem, but accentuated by the uneven distribution of wealth, the lack of adequate health services and the incredible inexcusable squandering of funds on armaments by all nations, but particularly our own country and the U.S.S.R.

He went on to condemn the proliferation of nuclear arms and their concomitant threat of contamination. His final suggestion was

> To overcome this [i.e., social and technological changes] we must have the courage to include the social sciences, genetics, ecology as sciences of fundamental importance to medicine and health, to think boldly about the organization of government and of our whole commercialized, acquisitive and consumptive society which provides so well for some of our people, but not for all, with little

thought for preservation rather than exploitation of the natural resources which cannot be renewed.

The dedicated laboratory scientist, superb clinician, and exciting educator had come to see the world as an integrated whole. The seeds of this world view were planted in early childhood, nourished by his family and international colleagues, and strongly supported by his wife. Dr. Janeway's life was not a series of separate interests. At various times certain parts were emphasized, but as this book has tried to make clear, one of the most remarkable things about Charles A. Janeway was his ability to carry out all these roles simultaneously.

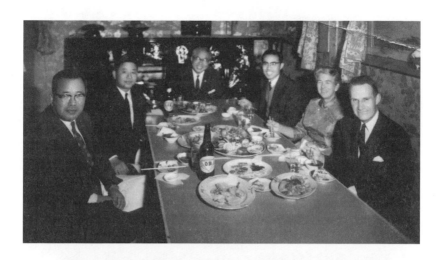

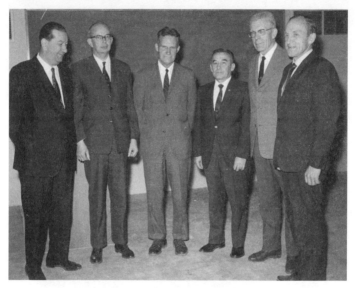

Illustration 13. *Above:* Dr. Janeway's visit to Korea, 1965. Left to right, Unknown pediatrician, Dr. Kwang Wok Ko, unidentified pediatrician, Dr. Se Mo Suh, Betty Janeway, and CAJ. Both Drs. Ko and Suh had trained in Boston and were the hosts of the Janeway's trip. *Below:* Executive Committee, International Pediatric Association, Tokyo, 1965. Left to right, Prof. I. Dogramaci, Turkey, Prof. T. Stapleton, Australia, CAJ, D. L. Benavides, Mexico (President, 12th International Congress of Pediatrics, held in Mexico City, 1968), Prof. Vesterdam, Denmark, Prof. N. Hallman, Finland.

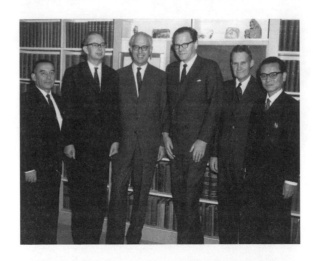

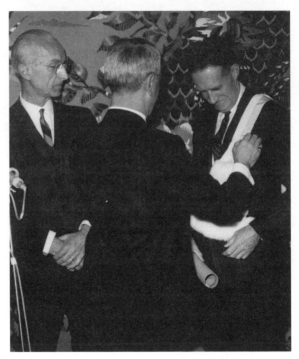

Illustration 14. *Above:* Executive Committee, International Pediatric Association, Boston, Massachusetts, 1966. Left to right, Prof. L. Benavides, Prof. T. Stapleton, Prof. G. Franconi, Switzerland, Prof. B. Vahlquist, Sweden, CAJ, Prof. I. Takatsu, Japan. *Below:* CAJ receiving honorary doctoral degree, Rheims, France, 1969. Others in the photograph are not identified.

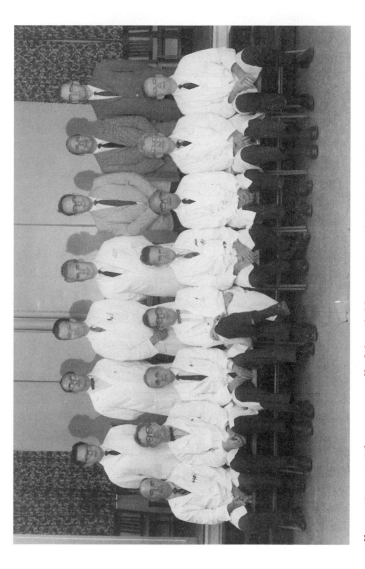

Illustration 15. The senior staff of the Children's Hospital, 1968–1969. Front row, left to right: Drs. Masland, Crigler, Mueller, Rosen, Janeway, Berenberg, Cone, Gerald. Back row, Khaw, Kevy, Fisher, Nelson, Crocker, Perlman, Winter.

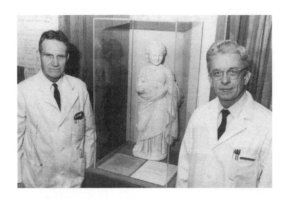

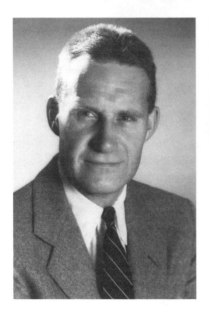
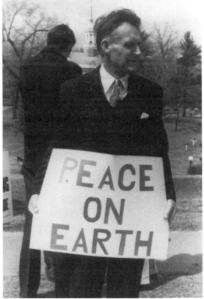

Illustration 16. *Above:* CAJ and Dr. Thomas Cone in 1970, with statue donated to the Department of Pediatrics by the University of Athens, Greece. *Below:* Left, CAJ in 1970; right, Dr. Janeway demonstrating on the Boston Common against the war in Vietnam, 1972.

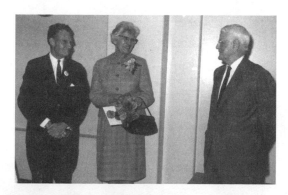

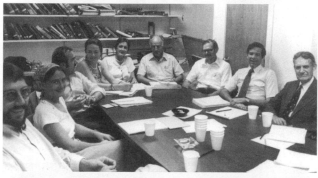

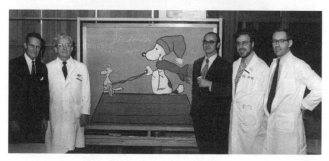

Illustration 17. *Above:* CAJ with Marian Green, for many years the pediatric department administrator at the Children's, and Dr. Richard Smith, head of the department during World War II. The picture was taken ca. 1970. Center: Harvard/Cameroon project staff, 1973. Left to right, Dr. J. Naponick, Ms. S. Colgate, Dr. P. Drouin, Ms. N. Garrett, Ms. L. Cousineau, Dr. R. Arnhold, Dr. R. Chamberlin, Dr. N. Guillozet, CAJ. *Below:* Holiday greetings, 1974. The "Merry Christmas" message has been replaced by a non-religious theme but the traditional blackboard presentation remains. Left to right, CAJ. Drs. Thomas Cone, Sherwin Kevy, John Graef, Frederick Lovejoy, Jr.

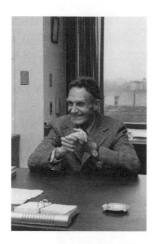
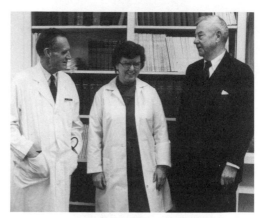

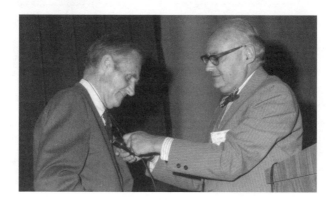

Illustration 18. *Above:* left, CAJ in the new Enders research building, obviously happy about the completion of its construction. He had just been described as a "Premier Physician" in a story in *Children's World* in June 1974; right, CAJ passing the torch to his successor, Dr. Mary Ellen Avery, 1974. Dr. Clement Smith appears on the right. *Below:* CAJ receiving the John Howland Award of the American Pediatric Society from Henry Kempe on April 26, 1978.

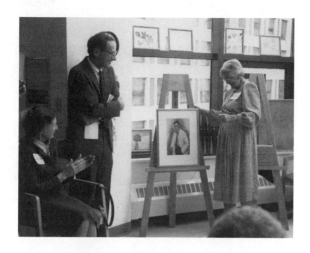

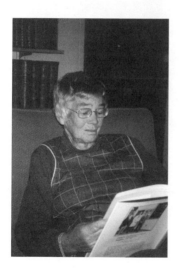

Illustration 19. *Above:* Unveiling Dr. Janeway's portrait, 1988. Left to right, Mrs. Cummings, former neighbor and family friend, Dr Frederick Lovejoy, Jr., Bette Janeway. *Below:* left, Betty Janeway at home in Weston, March 1991; right, An example of CAJ's lecture notes, such as he used on several trips to interntional sites. They were always organized clearly and neatly as shown here.

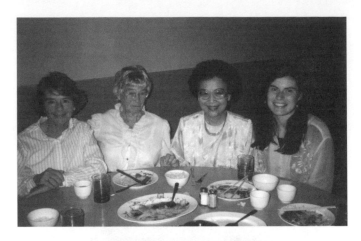

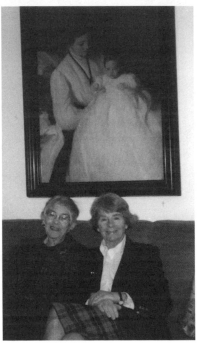

Illustration 20. *Above:* Betty Janeway, second from left, with Muriel Haggerty on the far left and Dr. Sylvia Chang and Betty's granddaughter Katherine (Katie) to the right, 1988. Katie later became a pediatrician at the Children's Hospital Boston. *Below:* Betty Janeway (left) with Muriel Haggerty in Betty's retirement home at Kendall-at-Hanover, Vermont in 1996. They are seated beneath a portrait of Betty's mother holding Betty (about age one).

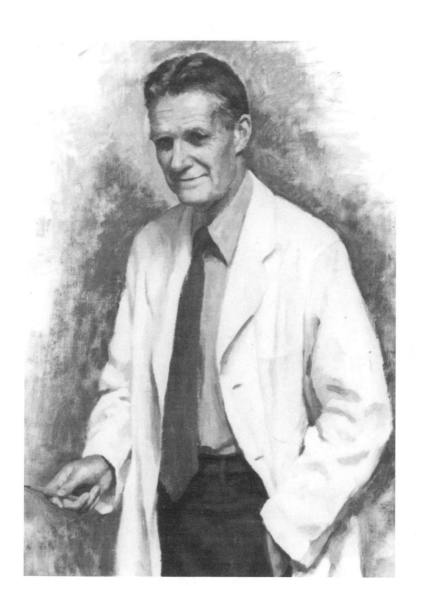

Illustration 21. Dr. Janeway's official portrait by George Augusta at Children's Hospital Boston, showing him in his familiar blackboard pose.

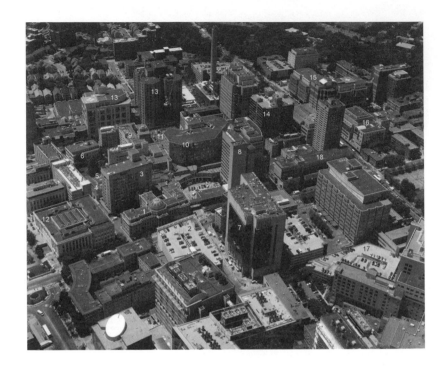

Illustration 22. The view of the Children's Hospital complex and surrounding structures, as it appeared in this 2004 photograph, shows the
enormous growth the Children's Hospital underwent since Dr. Janeway's
initial association with it in the early 1940s, much of it occurring during
Janeway's tenure as chair of medicine.

13 WHAT MANNER OF MAN WAS THIS?
Charles Janeway's Personal Characteristics

WE HAVE MADE many references to Charles Janeway's personal characteristics throughout our biography of him. Nonetheless, it is useful to enlarge here on some of his distinguishing qualities and traits, especially those that do not readily fit within the respective chronological presentation of the book. They are the most important aspects of his life, since they characterize the kind of person he was and show the context in which he was reared and lived. Through a further recital and analysis of his personal attributes and habits, we can gain a better comprehension of why he achieved the great things that he did. The characteristics we describe are based largely upon anecdotes culled from the interviews with many of his associates, students, and friends, as well as from the authors' long-time relations with him. Typical of the reserved, modest man that he was, Dr. Janeway never disclosed his own perception or assessment of the personal qualities that made him tick.

Dr. Janeway's personality, beliefs, intelligence and human warmth, with a touch of Victorian reserve, were enduring qualities that led most of us who knew him to trust him and to love him in a way that we did no other person. Professor John Davis, an early exchange resident from St. Mary's Hospital in London, summed him up as "the epitome of the 'All-American boy,' a WASP, good-looking in a meso-morphic way, intelligent, decent, hard-working, technically competent, unaffectedly friendly, modest, well-meaning and a family man and successful in his work, but not in the European sense an intellectual and absolutely lacking in our cynicism and world weariness." Davis noted also that Dr. Janeway characteristically chose a field that was ripe for development. Davis observed that "when he called you by your Christian name he meant it as the beginning of a life-long friendship in which he was the giver rather than the taker."[1]

Janeway was, as Davis remarked, a good-looking man, but not remarkably so. He was middling in height, about 5'9", weighing 150 pounds. Perhaps the most notable components of his appearance were his eyebrows, which were bushy and very expressive. All who knew him, it seems, commented on the movement of those eyebrows. Whether furrowed in worry or bouncing up and down in pleasure, they dominated his square jaw and highlighted his slightly curly brown hair. Otherwise, he could easily get lost in a crowd. It is, in fact, surprising that he played football in prep school and club football at college; he was rather slight, but he nonetheless played the game. This resolve may say more about his determination than his physical aptitude for the sport.

Several commentators assumed that Janeway was born to wealth. That was not the case. As we noted in chapter 1, his father, Theodore Janeway, died when the son was eight, at a time when Theodore was in the process of leaving Johns Hopkins School of Medicine as chair of the Department of Medicine because he could not afford to live on the full-time salary it mandated. Janeway's mother probably had some inherited wealth, but would have needed a considerable capital inheritance to survive the nearly forty years after the death of her husband. Janeway's frugal nature may have come in part from growing up knowing that, while he came from a prestigious family, it was not a wealthy one.

Dr. Janeway was an incredibly hard worker. He had a habit of writing on the blackboard in his office the dates and times he completed tasks; we and several others can remember some of those times: 2 a.m., 3 a.m. He habitually arose at 5 a.m. to work at home. He worked while riding on trains on the way to New York and Washington in the days before air shuttles. In his library at home was a copy of May-June 1964 issue of *World Health*, which contains short biographies of several leading French pediatricians, including Janeway's close friend, Professor Robert Debre. In that biography Debré described his workaholic life, in which he said he had given up theatre and concerts so as not to lose time from work. Janeway was somewhat like that. Fortunately CAJ, although most would call him a workaholic, did not give up theatre or concerts, and he enjoyed skiing, outdoor work, and getting back to rural or wild places.

In spite of what seems to most of us as working beyond the call of duty, Dr. Janeway sometimes thought of himself as "lazy." In a letter to a former house officer he said, "I am ashamed that your letter has sat on my desk as long as it has, practically two months. The whole trouble is, you ended the letter with the question, 'How do you keep from being lazy?' That frankly is a question I have never been able to solve and, being lazy, I have been putting off thinking about it."[2] CAJ did procrastinate over matters he did not want to decide. I (RJH) remember seeing a pile of unanswered mail on his desk that was easily a foot high. I had discovered that he had not answered a memo of mine for several weeks, so I asked him about the pile. He replied that he worked from the top and every so often threw what was unanswered in the wastebasket. He said, "If it is really important the writer will write again. And anyway, most of the things people ask me to do get solved by themselves if you wait long enough!" Janeway, then, was a bit of an enigma. He was respected and loved even though he was a bit standoffish, in some ways like a classic closed-mouthed New Englander.

Integrity is the word most often used to describe Dr. Janeway by those who knew him. Alexander Nadas recalled,

> With CAJ all the cards were on the table . . . you never questioned whether he was truthful. He was always truthful although at times parsimonious in what he said . . . The adjectives that best fitted him were decency, integrity, broad vision of the job, serious, stick-to-it-iveness, frugality, enormously private person. He had an immense ability to bear his own burdens and to treat you like an adult. He was not an intellectual snob and had great ability to see the other side of things.[3]

David Nathan, at the dedication of the Janeway Professorship, to which Dr. Fred Alt was named its first occupant, told of his own transition from internal medicine to pediatrics because

> I sensed that I was going to have an opportunity to work with a man of unimpeachable integrity, deep intelligence, and a complete commitment to the kind of clinical investigation that I wanted to prac-

tice. He was devoted to patients, to teaching, and to uncovering of new biological principles from the study of patients . . . I felt that I should cast my lot with him, that if just a bit of his tremendous intelligence, honesty, and self-criticism would rub off on me, I would make some sort of contribution too.[4]

Another aspect of Janeway's integrity was his unwillingness to accept money from pharmaceutical firms or companies that made infant milk formulae. According to Dr. Charles Cook, "Charlie was absolutely adamant that no house officer, the Department of Pediatrics, and no staff or faculty member should, under any circumstances, accept anything from drug or formula companies."[5] Today this sort of view might seem extreme to some, but it was utterly typical of the chief. In our opinion, such a position is one of those attributes of a chief's moral compass that stick in most residents' and staff's minds longer than any specific medical information.

Dr. Janeway was a liberal in politics but, consistent with much of his personality, was not adamant about it and was in no sense a revolutionary. His political views seemed to arise from his concern for the less fortunate and unfortunate. Janeway's prep school and college chum, John Whitcomb, shared his recollections with us several times.[6] In college, Whitcomb states, CAJ was considered "to the left politically." Whitcomb attributes this in part to Janeway's participation while at Milton Academy as a counselor at Camp Gannett, where he was influenced by Freda Regolsky, who was interested in liberal causes. At Yale, Whitcomb says, CAJ was a friend of George Brooks, another liberal who later was active in the Pulp and Paper Makers Union. As noted in the chapter on Janeway's college education, he participated in a tie-makers unionization march in New Haven and was arrested and briefly detained. He was also active in Dwight Hall, a liberal Christian group committed to the underserved. Whitcomb also recalled that during the freshman year at Yale, CAJ would disappear from the room many evenings to coach a group of boys at the New Haven Boys Club, a settlement house related to Ms. Rogolsky's activities. Further, Whitcomb recalled, in 1940 Janeway voted for Wendell Wilkie, probably because of Wilkie's "one world" platform. In 1932 he, Betty and the Barry Woods had gone to the inauguration of Franklin Roosevelt, but he was never active in any political party.

In 1952, Janeway voted for Eisenhower because he promised to end the War in Korea.[7] In 1960, when CAJ was in Korea, he became opposed to the North Korean government and to Communism generally because of the stories he heard of North Korea's pressure against South Korea.[8] In Janeway's appointment book for 1976, under November 2, appears a note, "Election Day—Vote for Carter." This voting record demonstrates that he was not a confirmed follower of either political party, but he was not afraid to express his views either, though he usually did so quietly.

Dr. Berenberg recalls that when Dr. Janeway was being considered for the Roche Professorship in 1944, he had a large Roosevelt for President poster on his office door. One of the senior members of the hospital, who was anxious to see Janeway receive the appointment, urged him to remove it, since it might influence some of the right-wing members of the committee.[9] Berenberg believes that CAJ did take down the poster.[10] (Janeway's wife, Betty, believed that he did not remove the poster. For most of their married life Betty was more liberal than CAJ was, but she also was apprehensive that his political views would prevent him from receiving the coveted Harvard chair.[11]) Berenberg went on to say, however, "He continued to wear his Roosevelt for President lapel button." Dr. Nadas remarked that Dr. Janeway subscribed to a bi-weekly newsletter published by I.F. Stone. Stone was a well-known liberal who tended to polarize opinion.[12]

An interesting series of letters exists between Dr. Janeway and his father figure, Dr. Edwards Park. They were exchanged in the late 1940s and early 1950s, and concern the policies of the American Medical Association. Park had drawn up a letter of resignation over the AMA's hiring of a public relations firm to oppose the amalgamation of the national Blue Cross with Blue Shield. The latter then was primarily the insurance program that paid surgeons' fees. This amalgamation was perceived by the national organization as a first step toward a national health program, which it opposed. The AMA assessed members an extra $25 to fight this through a public relations program. Park asked CAJ to sign a petition in opposition to that action. Janeway gave his reasons for not signing and for not resigning from the AMA:

Unfortunately my relations with the Red Cross are such that as Chairman of the Advisory Committee on Blood and Blood Deriva-

tives, I am looked on by the AMA group as one of the leaders of the
development of the National Blood Program. The relations with the
AMA have not always been smooth as one would have desired, and
on occasions we have had to struggle quite hard to overcome opposition on the part of organized medicine. We have been able to do that
to a considerable extent because . . . [we] act as members of the
AMA in good standing . . . I feel that I have no right to jeopardize the
Red Cross Program by taking a public stand on this controversial
issue.[13]

CAJ went on to say that he was writing the AMA to tell them that he
was opposed to their position and submitting a copy for publication in
the *New England Journal of Medicine*.[14] His letter carefully laid out the
reasons he paid the assessment and the reasons he disapproved of the
policy behind it. It was followed by a long rebuttal from the Massachusetts delegate to the AMA and an editorial highlighting both views. It
certainly got the attention of the readers of *The New England Journal*.
Park wrote back, saying that, "whatever you do in the world is done
with gentleness, not devoid of strength," which CAJ took as a "gentle
rebuke," but Park continued, saying that with his own Calvinistic background, "harshness of judgement and the tendencies to develop preju-
dices and take extreme positions have been great faults of mine . . . To
my way of thinking, you are exactly right and are behaving in exactly
the right way and let me urge you never to change but always to be
friendly with everyone but to continue to try in your tactful and
charming way to exert your influence toward improvement."[15]

This characteristic was central to CAJ's character, but it must have
been reassuring to hear it from his father figure, Ned Park. In a following letter, Park told his young protegee, "I envy you your tolerance and
good nature. I think you are right in remaining in the AMA and in en-
deavoring to produce changes in the organization from within. But it is
certainly uphill work." He ended his letter, saying, "I am filled with
pride over you and rejoice over everything you do and in all your successes. I rejoice for yourself and, also in the thought of the pride which
your father would have had in you . . . He was a bit Calvinistic, too, in
his sense of right and wrong. I think you have a sounder makeup than
he."[16]

In 1946 CAJ wrote to his Congressman, to his U.S. Senator, and to

President Truman: "As an ordinary citizen who has no axe to grind, let me urge you to do everything in your power to see to it that we send sufficient food to Europe and to Asia where people are starving and can only look on us as selfish, greedy and potentially enemies unless we ration ourselves."[17] He advocated the imposition once more of food rationing in this country in order to make distribution fair and equitable, and to have enough to share with the rest of the world. His position was an unpopular one, so soon after World War II, but demonstrates Janeway's belief in equality and sharing the nation's beneficence.

Dr. Janeway's concern about international aid and the Vietnam War was high on his agenda in the late 1960s and early 1970s. He had a file labeled "Letters of protest." Several are addressed to President Lyndon Johnson (with copies to Dean Rusk, the Secretary of State). The letters began in January 1964, wherein he said that he, "as a citizen and as someone who has both had experience in the Foreign Aid program and has a deep concern for it" advocated that Rusk support the Foreign Aid bill. The problems of economic development and technical assistance have to be, by their very nature, long-range programs and must be divorced from the short-range diplomatic maneuvering of the Department of State."[18] He was protesting another reorganization of the US AID program that would delay the important work of the agency. He wrote again to the President several months later, supporting the nuclear test ban treaty.[19] By the autumn of 1966 he was becoming less supportive of Johnson, and (with copies of his letter directed to the Secretary of State, the U.S. Ambassador to the U.N. and the Secretary General of the U.N.) wrote, "Although I appreciate the terrible responsibilities which you carry and your own deep desire for peace and a better life for the world's people . . . I am deeply troubled by the apparent inflexibility of this country's foreign policy."[20]

He went on to urge that the forthcoming U.N. General Assembly be used to: 1) admit China (with guarantees of the political independence of Taiwan), 2) support creation of a permanent U.N. peace-keeping force, and 3) internationalize the space program. In 1967, Janeway wrote a four-page letter to Johnson in which he related that he had, as a citizen, "worked hard for your election . . . [He praised Johnson for] "a magnificent record of a series of bold solutions to the domestic problems that have denied equality to many of our citizens—bills on civil rights, education, medical care, conservation, pollution and revival of our cities have given this country a great forward thrust . . . But this . . . has been betrayed by the consequences of our outdated foreign policy based on the concept of a monolithic communist conspiracy for world domination."[21]

He expressed horror that so much of the nation's budget was being used for defense, "the amount being spent on the destruction of Vietnam in one day exceeds the total annual budget of UNICEF and WHO, two of the most constructive agencies in the world today." He went on to rebut all the reasons given for the nation's involvement in Vietnam and said, "I consider the Vietnam policy to be politically indefensible." He added the biting comment that "Charles De Gaulle . . . had the guts to call off the long and hopeless war in Algeria . . . You have the same opportunity." As history shows, these and many other protests did little in the short run to stop the Vietnam War. His letters demonstrate, nonetheless, that Janeway felt personally responsible for stating his views.

Janeway wrote an even stronger letter to Senator Henry Jackson, who had made some motions to run for President. He chastised Jackson for advocating continuance of the same foreign policies, "which have brought this country close to economic bankruptcy and to internal chaos . . . What America needs is a Presidential candidate . . . who will lead the free world into new institutions and policies . . . [including recognizing the world has been made one by modern technology and that the] . . . concept of national sovereignty is totally outmoded . . . The search for national military security . . . is futile."[22] He went on to observe that countries that have followed this course have been doomed to fail, and asked, "When will we get a president who takes the lead in proposing revision of the U.N. Charter to create a limited world government?"

Janeway would not have been happy with the U.S. government's stance since 2000, especially its willingness to essentially act alone in opposition to the role of the U.N. on the matter of Iraq, and abrogating the Kyoto agreement. Although he never visited mainland China, he was an early supporter of getting that nation to join the U.N.; an article in a 1966 issue of the *Saturday Review*, on China, was in his personal library. It is clear that his personal sympathies lay with those countries such as China, whose health successes, despite their political oppression, stood in stark contrast to those of many of the so-called Western-style democracies that he visited in southeast Asia, where there were many fewer health successes.

His personal library also contained a copy of a report from the American Universities Field Staff Reports Service, which advocated that, "Among the laborers in the vineyard of diplomacy are some who insist that if men managing power just keep talking with one another, their differences—which otherwise might precipitate warfare—will be resolved or at least reduced."[23] The essence of this argument was the negotiated peace engineered by the president of the Philippines and the prime minister of Malaysia. CAJ believed in negotiated settlement of disputes, whether within the local hospital or on the international scene. Family planning was central to his belief in a better future for mankind. Several publications on population growth in his library and the Janeways' personal financial support in yearly contributions to family planning organizations document this point.

A letter in Dr. Janeway's personal file in 1967 noted that he had been having $25 per month deducted from his pay and put into U.S. Savings Bonds but, "Since U.S. Savings Bonds are being used to support our military effort in Viet Nam, of which I heartily disapprove, I would like to stop the payroll deduction."[24] Janeway was not a doctrinaire pacifist, however. During World War II he wrote several letters to his mother in which he said that he was glad when the U.S. finally entered the conflict. In an interesting letter to his sister, Nora, which he wrote eight months before Pearl Harbor, Charles asked,

> Have you seen a movie called "Pastor Hall"? It's done by Jimmy Roosevelt . . . it is one of the finest things I have ever seen, being based on Pastor Niemoeller's life. It gives you a little faith in something which I feel very strongly—that even if the Nazis conquered the whole world they still couldn't conquer the human spirit, and I certainly believe implicitly that it is that very weakness which is going to be their ultimate downfall, although that downfall is awfully slow in coming.[25]

Charles and Betty were interested in, went to meetings of, and gave modest amounts of money to the World Association of World Federalists. They also made annual contributions to UNICEF, ecology groups, the NAACP Legal Defense Fund, the Population Reference Bureau, the Northern Student Movement (a program to increase educational opportunities for minority students in Roxbury, Massachusetts), and peace committees. He gave to many medical causes as well as to his various alma maters, and paid his dues regularly to such organizations as Phi Beta Kappa. For someone who lived on a modest income, CAJ gave to many organizations, but especially to "liberal causes" with a world view or program. A review of his reported earnings in the 1940s and 1950s reveals that the Janeways gave about 10% of their gross income every year to non-profit organizations such as these. A modern type of tithing, perhaps? When travelling, Betty took pictures of children and the programs for UNICEF. That organization arranged her visits on the trips abroad, and when she returned she gave talks about UNICEF and solicited funds from those attending. The Janeways' trips encouraged others to give to what they (Charles and Betty) believed were worthy organizations. It seems fair to say that the Janeways were citizens of the world.

Janeway sent a wry letter to the class agent of the 1930 Yale class, who had written to the class and congratulated them for their successful fund raising, but had added in his final paragraph, "In spite of Spock [the radical pediatrician who spoke against the Vietnam War], Coffin [a chaplain at Yale, also an advocate for ending the Vietnam War], admissions policy at Yale [considered by some to be evidence that radicals had taken over Yale] . . . the alumni feel that Yale is worthy of their dollars."[26] In his reply, which he copied and sent to his close friend, John Musser, Janeway told that the reason "that I stretched my contribution was because of Spock, who was a Yale graduate, because Brewster [president of Yale] re-appointed Coffin as Chaplain, and because I know that they have given scholarships to two outstanding students who had to have full support. I am sure we could have a fine debate about this or the Vietnam War . . . I am afraid to see our involvement in Vietnam as bearing many, many resemblances to the action of the Russians in Czechoslovakia, namely an imposition of a government the people don't want."[27] CAJ ended the letter with "Best personal regards from your unreconstructed classmate."

Although Dr. Janeway tended to stay out of the limelight, he was not hesitant to lead a parade of medical students in the common cause for peace during their march from the Harvard Medical School quadrangle to Boston Common to protest the Vietnam War. The act was reported in his local newspaper, the *Weston Town Crier,* which told that,

> One of the leaders of the antiwar movement in the metropolitan area is Dr. Charles A. Janeway of 445 Concord Road, Weston, who spoke to several hundred medical professionals last Friday in Copley Square. Dr. Janeway said "Since this nation is also committed to the proposition that all men are created equal, we must also deplore the terrible loss of somewhere between 500,000 and one million Vietnamese lives, many of them innocent victims of our ill-conceived effort to defend our conception of their freedom. As citizens of the United States we must each of us accept considerable responsibility for these deaths, for the maiming of many thousands more, for the ruthless destruction of land and crops by toxic chemicals whose ultimate effects on the delicate web of life are unknown and for the total destruction of an ancient culture. Our intervention . . . [has been bought] at the price of support for a corrupt government in the South."[28]

Charles and Betty went to Washington at that time to march in a Vietnam War protest, one of the few times Betty appeared to be involved in public protests. If ever she had been concerned that her husband's liberalism was a possible constraint to his career, her worries were gone by the time of the Vietnam War. Janeway's antiwar views were expressed in response to a series of letters to[29] and from an investment firm that was offering a prospectus for investment in oil drilling.[30] CAJ wrote his financial advisor, David Kirkbride, to say that he did not feel competent to judge but, "emotionally I kind of hate to be associated with Texas oil people. I disagree with them so fundamentally on everything from the Vietnam War to many other aspects of American life, that I am not sure that I want to get involved . . . I still believe that one's investments at least should relate somewhat to one's principles."[31] CAJ's liberalism was also evident in the effort to bring under-represented minorities into the Harvard hospitals. Dr. Berenberg told of a time when they were selecting house staff and Dr. Janeway pushed for a Shapiro over a Saltonstall. When Berenberg protested "that it might not be fair," Janeway replied, not to worry, that, in fact, "the Saltonstalls would always get a good job somewhere."[32] Berenberg reported that Janeway, at another time, resigned from the medical school admissions committee because he perceived them to be biased against Jews.[33]

Janeway was not active in party political activities and never ran for public office, as his brother did. However, he was very active on one local issue, fluoridation of the public water supply in Weston. In 1956 he resigned from the town Board of Health because he was going on sabbatical that year but noted that he would continue to chair the Committee on Fluoridation of the Public Water Supply.[34] Fluoridation concerned Dr. Janeway for years. Starting in 1954 he and four others (Dr. David J. Farrell, Dr. Charles Christopher, Mr. James T. Mount and Dr. Paul L. Munson, with CAJ as chair) petitioned the town moderator to appoint a committee to "investigate the matter of fluoridation of the Town's public water supply."[35] Such a committee was appointed March 22, 1954, with Janeway as chairman. The committee made a reasoned study that encompassed more than a decade: there are minutes of many meetings at the Janeways' home on the issue in 1964–65, and reports of several attempts to bring the matter to a vote at the town meeting, but for many reasons it was deferred.

There was vigorous opposition in the Town of Weston. A conservative group declared that fluoridation was a Communist plot to poison Western democracies; such opposition was one reason the committee deferred submission of the matter to a vote. Finally, a letter to a town official[36] and the minutes of a special meeting the committee[37] indicated that the group had decided to petition the Town in the spring of 1967. Shortly thereafter, Janeway was asked by James Dunning, chairman of a committee of the Massachusetts Dental Society, and a leading advocate for fluoridation, not to submit the petition because a similar bill was in the General Court (Massachusetts legislature) and if one was rejected by a town such as Weston, it might jeopardize the passage of the state bill. CAJ replied that the Weston committee would accede to the Dental Society's committee; that even though they believed that they had the votes to pass the petition in Weston they would defer their action that year in hopes that the state bill would pass in order that Commonwealth citizens might soon benefit of this public health measure.[38] The bill passed in the Massachusetts legislature; consequently no more minutes of the local committee exist thereafter.

Dr. Janeway also corresponded actively with the Weston representative in the General Court on other issues. In one letter he said, "I am glad to hear that your acute sense of smell enabled you to smoke out a rider in a bill, which might have undone all the efforts to keep the broken stone activities under control by the town."[39] There was a quarry in Weston that wanted to expand, and CAJ obviously was opposed. On another issue, he told that "I am writing . . . to urge you to . . . oppose the chiropractic bill H2180 . . . It would be a tragic thing if Massachusetts succumbed to their pressure and allowed them to set up an independent body . . . if they wish to practice medicine they should be licensed by the same set of examinations and by the same board which registers doctors and osteopaths."[40] Dr. Janeway was a consistent liberal during his life, but only on rare occasions in later life did he become an activist. His method, as in the solving of problems in the hospital, was to be a voice of reason; he always tried to bring parties together. We doubt that he ever used the words, "conflict resolution," but that was his style; he did not favor confrontation. That did not mean that he did not have very strong feeling on public policy issues, however. He was a respectable rebel.

Almost everyone we interviewed commented on Dr. Janeway's personal concern for other people. Many told poignant stories of the kindnesses he extended, acts that perhaps seemed small when recounted but loomed large to the recipients. Dr. Steven Joseph, who has had a brilliant career in international health and was Commissioner of Health of New York City and Deputy Undersecretary for Defense in Health in the Clinton administration, told Betty that when he started his internship he told CAJ that he wished to go into the Peace Corps for two years after the internship. Dr. Janeway indicated immediately that there would be a place for him in the residency program when he came back. This seemingly small act is larger than it appears: at the time, the residency program was pyramidal; i.e., there would normally be no place for someone who left. Nevertheless, CAJ promised Joseph a place, and a place there later was.[41] Nor was his concern for others restricted to only the professional staff. Dr. Berenberg noted that CAJ always had a quick smile and a greeting for the cleaning woman, the mail delivery man, and other hospital workers. "He did this regularly," Berenberg said, "even when he might pass some other distinguished member of the faculty with simply a nod."[42]

Although Janeway was always considerate of the feelings of others, he did not praise faculty openly and directly. In person he was quite reserved. Toward the end of his life he probably began to regret what had not been said. The letter to Dr. Berenberg, written a little over a year before Janeway died, but when his illness was progressing, which was quoted in Chapter 5, is but one of several attempts he made at that time to amend past oversights. He ended it by saying, "Most of all it is personal aspects of this association of long standing which has meant so much to the department and in my own life. With best wishes to you and Blanche and more gratitude than I can express to you as a friend and wonderful colleague."[43]

Dr. Janeway's personal concern for others was especially noticed when the recipient was a foreign physician. In several of his diaries he noted that, after the hospitality shown him abroad, he must do more for those who come to the United States. Dr. Diamond described one such person, who wanted to obtain from the Jackson Laboratory (at Bar Harbor, Maine) a strain of mice that had inherited immunodeficiency syndrome. Diamond, who had worked at the laboratory, was asked to obtain them and the animals were obtained and shipped at some expense, which CAJ paid.[44] In Diamond's words, this was "Just another example of CAJ's kindness to everyone, especially foreigners."[45]

Dr. Niilo Hallman, CAJ's first post-residency Fellow, was brought to the United States for the International Pediatric Congress in 1947 and stayed on with Janeway in Boston. He was alone for the first six months of his stay; only then did his wife join him while his parents took care of their three children in Finland. After Mrs. Hallman arrived, the two of them worked in a hotel-like apartment house for their room and board. Janeway often took them to his home for dinners and gave them packages of food and cigarettes. (CAJ was then, like many physicians, a smoker.) He arranged for packages to be sent back to Hallman's family in war-ravaged Finland. Hallman's recollection of Janeway was, "first, as a scientific leader of American pediatrics, to whom Europe looked for training, and secondly, as a very kind, generous person."[46] Hallman, after he became chair of pediatrics in Helsinki, sent all of his division chiefs to receive additional training in the U.S.; many came to the Children's. Hallman and Janeway remained very close friends and, on one of his trips to Finland, CAJ was made an honorary member of the Finnish Pediatric Society.

Dr. Richard Goldbloom tells of an episode when he was a resident at the Children's. Goldbloom's father, the distinguished chair of pediatrics at McGill University and Montreal Children's Hospital, was visiting. Janeway, with his typical courtesy, invited the elder Goldbloom to lunch, and the younger Goldbloom related,

> disregarding my lowly status, invited me to join them . . . At 11:30 I received a telephone call from my wife, who was concerned about our two-year-old son, Alan, who had developed a fever and who seemed to have a slightly stiff neck. [This occurred during an epidemic of polio in Boston.] I ran upstairs to Charlie's office and told him I could not join them for lunch. When I mentioned the possibility of a stiff neck, he announced that he was coming out himself to have a look. I protested as vigorously as I could, but he would have none of it. He cancelled the luncheon, hustled me into his Jeep, and we took off at high speed for my apartment, where he examined Alan carefully and reassured me that he did not have polio . . . There are still those who feel that an outstanding level of scientific knowledge, brilliance in research, clinical skill and intense personalized concern are somehow mutually exclusive . . . No one proved the wrongheadedness of that idea better than Charlie Janeway.[47]

A few other examples of Dr. Janeway's personal consideration for others can be mentioned. Dr. Jack Metcoff recalled that when he was just starting as a junior faculty member, he received a typical kindness from CAJ. "We were living in a small apartment on Longwood Avenue, truly in a situation of poverty, and one Friday afternoon Janeway stopped by and invited the two of us out for a lobster dinner at their place in Weston, which was warmly received."[48] One of the authors was also on the receiving end of another of Dr. Janeway's typical kindnesses. The day that our (RJH's) son Rick went into the hospital for his tonsil and adenoid removal, CAJ asked Muriel if he could have a ride in to the hospital. She was glad to oblige but had to leave the baby, John, in my office while she went to see Rick. On arriving at the hospital, Dr. Janeway insisted on carrying John into my office, which was across Blackfan Street, while Muriel parked the car. This small, simple act made Muriel's life less complicated that morning; it was yet another example of CAJ's consideration for others.

Dr. Sophia Chang, a Chinese physician who had a long and successful career practicing in New York City, was an outpatient Fellow at the Children's in 1948. The Chinese Communist revolution occurred then, and she could not return home. She was engaged to be married to another Chinese physician in Boston, but had no family in the U.S. to give her away. How Charles and Betty learned of this situation she does not know, but they offered to give her away and have the reception afterwards. Dr. Chang was forever grateful, in spite of an "embarrassment at the reception. One socially well-connected woman received a fortune cookie that read, "All your good efforts are in vain." Added to that, a small flower girl from the church disliked the food and told Betty that she was a bad cook. Nevertheless, the kindness of the Janeways' offer to a lonely Chinese physician was never forgotten. In the late 1980s, Dr. Chang hosted a lavish party for Betty at a Chinese restaurant while Betty was visiting New York.[49] An earlier letter from both Drs. Chang thanked the Janeways for the "wonderful days of our studies in pediatrics at the Children's Hospital Center under you."[50] Dr. Chang always remembered the Janeways with fondness because they went out of their way to arrange a wedding for a foreign resident who had no other family in America. When I (RJH) met Dr. Chang in New York in the late 1980s, she still remembered this kindness and treated my wife, Betty, her granddaughter Katherine, and me to a wonderful Chinese dinner in remembrance of the Janeways.

Despite Dr. Janeway's aura of aloofness, he conveyed warmth and concern. Dr. McKay was surprised one day when he found a senior pediatric staff physician (a practicing pediatrician in the community) in CAJ's office, crying and discussing with CAJ the reasons why his wife had committed suicide. That this pediatrician felt close enough to confide in Janeway represented to McKay a sensitive side of the man, especially to practicing pediatricians who were not perceived by most to be very close to him.[51]

With regard to Dr. Janeway's clinical skills, Clement Smith once said: "It could be said in all honesty of Charles Janeway, as someone

said of a skilled 18ᵗʰ century English physician, that 'He practiced medicine with such grace that you would have thought he was born to the
art and never had to learn it'."[52] We heard stories of CAJ's excellence as
a clinician from many of his students and colleagues. Closely related to
his personal relations with his staff was his relation with patients.
Dr. Diamond tells the story of an eight-year-old girl referred to Dr.
Janeway from Baltimore with multiple problems:

> Charlie called in several of the specialists for each of her problems.
> He told the parents who each of the specialists were and that they
> would be taking care of each of their areas. The girl began to cry,
> and Charlie asked her what she was crying about. She said, "I under-
> stand Dr. Davies is taking care of my infection, and Dr. Diamond is
> taking care of my blood, but who will take care of me?" Charlie said,
> "Why my dear, I guess you didn't understand. I am your doctor. I am
> taking care of you and all these other doctors are going to help me. I
> will not let anyone do anything that you do not like . . . and even if it
> hurts I know you will not mind because we are going to get you
> better and send you home.[53]

That was typical of him. CAJ took the extra fifteen or twenty minutes
to reassure the child that he was the child's doctor. Diamond recalled,
forty years later, "I can see the expression on the child's face when he
said 'I am your doctor'." Diamond added, "Actually, I think of Charlie
as the pediatric equivalent of William Osler. He was a great teacher, he
was an excellent clinician, he had a cordial feeling for people working
under him . . . Charlie was a master of that."

Charles Janeway was devoted utterly to patients. I (RJH) recall one
incident that may illustrate this. In 1962, at one of the staff meetings,
the new hospital administrator announced that in the future, if any patients in the emergency room did not have health insurance, they were
to be sent to the Boston City Hospital. From a legal and fiduciary view
this was probably sensible, but Dr. Janeway rose to his feet and declared passionately that the day when any patient was sent away from
the Children's was the day the hospital director had his resignation on
his desk. Nothing further was ever heard about this director's new
policy.

CAJ had a sixth sense of what patients needed. When I (RJH) was a
resident, one duty was to select a patient for him to see with students

in the outpatient department. I was embarrassed one day because we had no "exciting" patients, *i.e.*, none with an exotic disorder. I apologized to him that the only patient was an eight-year-old girl from Maine who had an innocent heart murmur but the parents and child seemed very concerned. He went into the examining room and sat on the examining table next to the girl, took her hand and said, "I'll bet that you are worried that you have heart disease like President Eisenhower." (The visit occurred soon after President Eisenhower's heart attack.) The girl's eyes widened and she said, "How did you know?" With that underlying concern dealt with, the family and girl left reassured and pleased. None of the rest of us had thought to ask about her concerns or say such a thing. It was a vivid example of his clinical skill, and reinforced the concept that to be a physician meant going beyond strictly medical matters. Dr. Metcoff recalled that Dr. Janeway often said, "children have ears like elephants; doctors should not discuss another patient in front of kids."[54]

Every resident at the Children's had the experience of being puzzled by a child with prolonged fever with no cause being found. Finally we would ask the chief to see the child. Inevitably he would arrive, pull back the covers, and there was the telltale rash of juvenile rheumatoid arthritis. Probably if we ourselves had waited to pull back the covers we would have seen it too, but we all felt that somehow CAJ had magically made the rash appear. Janeway had a tremendous knack of using a physical examination to reach a prompt diagnosis and of being called at the right time.

Dr. Nelson Montgomery recalled that, when he was an exchange resident from St. Mary's Hospital, London, CAJ was asked to see a four-year-old boy who had a fever but no other signs. The resident staff were concerned. CAJ did a "painstaking examination. Eventually he pressed a point on the right portion of the boy's iliac crest and elicited a sharp pain. An x-ray confirmed osteomyelitis at that site." Montgomery went on to add, "I cannot remember anything that led him to think of, or find, that spot."[55]

Dr. Georges Peter, who had known Dr. Janeway while growing up at Annisquam, came back to the Children's as a resident and Fellow in infectious diseases. Peter remembered CAJ's "uncanny ability to sift the extraneous and synthesize a large amount of material which he could then simplify to a few basic questions and points."[56] One other example of his clinical skill, but even more, of his dedication, was told by Dr. Peter. Peter was sailing at Annisquam, with his wife, when his seven-month-old son, Mark, who was being cared for by Peter's mother, had a febrile convulsion. She knew that Dr. Janeway was playing tennis nearby, and she asked him to look at the baby. CAJ did so, and provided sage advice.[57]

Dr. John Houpis, a pediatrician in Brattleboro, Vermont, told us of a time when he was an intern in Worcester, Massachusetts, and came to the Children's grand rounds to hear Janeway talk about nephrotic syndrome. At that time Houpis had a fifteen-year-old patient who had the disorder; he asked him about the patient. CAJ said that, since he lived in Weston and it was not a very long trip to Worcester, he would come and see the patient. Houpis recalled, "He was extremely nice to me, admonished me slightly in terms of the way I had treated the child . . . but in such a way that I did not take offense."[58] On another occasion Houpis referred to Dr. Janeway a patient who had peculiar bumps on the head. The child died, and the family had another child who also died. As Houpis remembered, "Dr. Janeway was simply marvelous with the family. They had no funds and Dr. Janeway was extremely generous. [He] would be sure they had a place to stay when they came to Boston. He was perceived by the family as a 'Messiah'."

Dr. John Kennell recounted another example of Janeway's clinical acumen. The incident occurred soon after Dr. Neuhouser (Chief of Radiology) had sent a memo saying that he had reviewed 1,000 radiological examinations of skulls and found all to be normal and therefore such examinations were no longer to be done. One holiday weekend when the chief was working in the hospital, a family arrived in the out-patient department. Kennell related that

> Through some process they arrived at Dr. Janeway's office. He immediately dropped everything, obtained one of his characteristically thorough histories and physical examinations, and ordered skull x-rays for the child, who was retarded. I remember being in the x-ray department when the patient and request for x-rays arrived—on this holiday. The radiologist reacted with anger but then proceeded to take the x-ray because the request had come from Dr. Janeway. Well, as you might guess, the skull x-rays were highly revealing. The child had agenesis of the corpus callosum, and a lipoma was clearly visible on the routine skull x-ray.[59]

David Smith, later chair of pediatrics at Rochester, said of Dr. Janeway: "He was one of the best diagnosticians . . . I ever had the chance to make rounds with. Regardless of how well prepared you were . . . or how well you had reviewed the patient's chart or performed the physical exam, Janeway would come and see the patient . . . and always find some additional parameter that had either been overlooked or had not been taken into full account. He did that very graciously."[60] Smith also said that CAJ believed in starting one's research from clinical experiences. Whenever he would see a patient with *Hemophilus influenza* meningitis, Janeway would say that someone should develop a vaccine against this organism. David Smith took this advice and spent his career successfully developing the current vaccine that has almost eliminated this serious illness of children. Most of Janeway's own research grew out of his clinical experiences.

As legendary as were Dr. Janeway's clinical skills, his compassion for patients was no less remarkable. Dr. Kevy noted his obsession for the humane care of children in hospital. He said that children admitted to the metabolic unit were often strapped to the bed for prolonged periods to collect accurate urine and stool outputs, as well as to have multiple blood samples drawn. The house staff rebelled but, rather than complaining, they knew that if they reminded the chief that when they unstrapped the child and held him or her, the child no longer cuddled or hugged them, Dr. Janeway would be so upset that it was an effective way to get a child off the metabolic bed.[61]

CAJ remembered his patients, even unto the second and third generation. His dedication to second-generation patients is exemplified by a letter to the chief resident of the outpatient department at the Children's regarding a four-year-old to be seen because of a heart murmur and a skin rash on her fingers. In his note of referral Janeway states that "the [child's] mother is the first patient at the Peter Bent Brigham Hospital ever to have been cured of subacute bacterial endocarditis. I took care of her there approximately ten years ago and she was treated with sulfonamides and fever therapy and responded very satisfactorily. Her disease arose as a result of an abscessed tooth . . . she is an old friend and I should like to see her . . . give me a call when she is in the outpatient department."[62] On the same day he wrote to the child's mother, telling her that he had arranged the appointment and adding, "When you come in, will you please bring the enclosed note with you, as it will help you, and tell the doctor that you are a friend of mine and that I was anxious to see you, if possible, that day."[63]

As we have repeated many times throughout this volume, Janeway was a fanatic about keeping his hands clean. He had been brought up in medicine in the pre-antibiotic era and was aware of the dangers of spread of infection from staff to patients. As was his customary teaching technique, he did not preach hand-washing but taught it by example. Before he saw a patient, and between every patient, he would wash his hands, frequently longer than necessary, keeping the residents waiting, to impress on them the need for hand cleanliness. This lesson is apropos again today, with antibiotic-resistant bacteriae becoming ever more common.

While Dr. Janeway's diplomatic skills were remarkable and were recognized by all, some believed he went too far to be accommodating. Dr. Diamond noted that Dr. Edwin Cohn was a very strong personality. One exmple of Cohn's rigid manner was provided by Diamond, who told of Cohn ordering him to Washington to start the National Blood Program. Diamond was unhappy about it and after three days was set to return to Boston when he got a call from Cohn, who said, "You're staying in Washington." Diamond said that "Charlie was the only one who never had any real argument with Cohn."[64] Diamond also, on occasion, clashed with Dr. Sidney Farber, another strong personality. Diamond said that he could have had the backing of the head of surgery, Dr. Ladd, to confront Farber, but Janeway said, "Lay low. Things will straighten out." Diamond credited CAJ with keeping the Children's together as one hospital. He believed that "The Children's could have fallen apart at that point and it would have taken years to build it up again," if Janeway had not been willing to mediate between the strong personalities of Farber and Dr. Robert Gross, Ladd's successor as chief of surgery.

Diamond recalled another example of Janeway's diplomacy. An Indian of high caste was a Fellow in the department, and CAJ arranged a dinner for him and several other Indians, who were of lower caste. When the high-caste Fellow found out, he said that he could not come to dinner. Janeway was upset because Betty had gone to considerable trouble to arrange the dinner. Nevertheless, he let the invitation to the other Indians stand and arranged another dinner at another time for the first man. Diamond recalled that his wife was not so accommodating. She said that she would have "just gone along with only the first dinner" and not invited the high-caste man back. He noted that Betty had people, especially the foreigners at the Children's, to dinner once or twice a week. Their guest book is filled with the names of the great and not-so-great pediatricians from all over the world.[65] Part of Janeway's success as a diplomat was his strong sense of privacy. He did not talk about the conflicts at the hospital, even with Betty. As she said, "He tended to compartmentalize his work and his play. He was very discreet and didn't say things that were not nice."[66]

Janeway treated his staff with unfailing courtesy. Muriel Graham Small was one of his three secretaries from 1946 to 1948, and again, part-time, until March 1950. Her sister, Caroline, succeeded her and worked for Dr. Janeway for several years. Mrs. Small wrote of Dr. Janeway:

> This was a very exciting time to be at Children's Hospital. Doctors from all over the world came here, and they all wanted an individual interview and tour of the hospital . . . I helped a lot with the testing of blood products, getting interns to test them on babies. He was a fascinating man, utterly upright and moral. I remember when he was late for an airplane, he wouldn't take a taxi at the door because he had called another company![67]

Mrs. Mildred McTear, a later secretary, noted his kindness, not only in the office but to children. Her daughter, who had married a Norwegian and was living fifty miles south of Oslo, had a child that Mrs. McTear had never seen. When Charles and Betty were in Norway, they went out of their way to visit her and reported back "all about their home and about my first grandchild." On another occasion, Mrs. McTear's son was waiting several days to get into the Dana Farber Hospital. When Janeway found out, he called Dr. Farber and, within a day, "Ken was in Dr. Farber's hospital."[68] Dr. Janeway shared gifts with the staff. Mrs. McTear continued, "Doctors and patients came from many countries to confer with Dr. Janeway. I still have a note he wrote to me after King Saud of Aramco [Saudi Arabia] had brought his child to see Dr. Janeway. I quote, 'I cannot bear to pocket the largess of King Saud without sharing a portion of the windfall with the persons who bear the brunt. With many thanks for everything. [Signed] 'CAJ'."

Dr. Janeway was not known for whimsey, but on January 4, 1961, he penned a poem to his staff who had given him a stereo player for Christmas. It reads:

> To Four Lovely Ladies
> With apologies to
> The muse of Poesie who has
> Really inspired one of your number
> From their problem child.
>
> To you, who throughout thick and thin,
> Face the day with uplifted chin,
> Despite your absent minded boss,
> Who blames you for the papers lost,
> When, searching through his tangled mess,
> You unearth it on his desk,
> To you, who work from dawn to dusk,
> Who comfort frozen Indians forlorn,
> Who answer phone calls while you type,
> And never seem to gripe,
> How can I thank you, ladies fair,
> For making life so easy to bear,
> And then you add to my confusion,
> Adding music to beauty in profusion,
> Food for the stereo's delicate
> Bach fills the air before our dinner,
> So, thank you one and all again.[69]

Ms. Brooks Barnes, the head nurse on the infants' ward, recalled that CAJ was "Very reserved, all business, cool and very serious." However, he would do some very nice things to recognize individuals. For example, he sent Ms. Barnes a letter on her twentieth anniversary at the hospital, thanking her for her service to the institution and the medical service. She also noted that frequently he would send a corsage to her at Christmas time.[70] Ms. Barnes remembered teaching rounds. She emphasized Dr. Janeway's absolute insistence on having patients always there for those rounds. He told Ms. Barnes that students and residents always remember things better if they see the patient for themselves. She recollected further that when he came back from trips abroad he would tell her about parents staying with their children, even sleeping in the hospital. Ms. Barnes felt at the time that parents were not helpful to their hospitalized children, but today admits that "He was ahead of his time and he was right." She also commented on his absolute adherence to "precautions" and hand washing, and that he was strict with any violations.

However much expansion occurred at the Children's during Charles Janeway's time as chief, he was no empire builder. His professional conduct and habits were much like his personal ones. His life was, in Clement Smith's terms, "not elaborate. On trips to Atlantic City for the spring meetings [the research meeting of the American Pediatric Society and the Society for Pediatric Research] . . . Charlie always descended from an upper birth as the train neared North Philadelphia, and we learned that he usually lunched at the YWCA, some distance inland from the boardwalk."[71]

Smith added that the Dean had once remarked, "If Charlie has a fault, it's that he's too darn nice." Smith added that this "was a complaint I never heard him lodge against anyone else on his faculty." Smith summed up his forty years of knowing CAJ:

> In this way, and in so many other matters, the most important things he taught us were the intangible ones, and he taught them not by precept but by example; the rare mixture of intelligence and integrity, of insight and humanity, of generosity and reserve. Generosity endowed him with a unique genius for appreciation, whereas reserve almost completely prevented its spoken expression. It, therefore, appeared in beautifully worded little notes, often received months after some event the recipient thought had gone unnoticed.

Although Dr. Janeway was more formal in demeanor with his faculty and staff than with patients or hospital employees, he supported us almost unfailingly, sometimes against other powerful people at the hospital. We could count on him when we needed him.

Dr. William Cochran, a resident in pediatrics and for nearly the rest of his career a clinical neonatologist on the staff, recounted several instances of Janeway's support. Cochran saw a child in the emergency room for third remission of leukemia but, after discussion with the parents, sent the child home, believing that the child did not need to be admitted to the hospital. Dr. Farber opposed the decision and told

Cochran that he would see that he was fired, and would talk to Dr. Janeway about it. CAJ never told Cochran about the incident. Some time later, the father wrote a beautiful letter of thanks to Cochran. He took it to the chief, who agreed that it was a beautiful letter and said to show it to Dr. Farber. Farber took it and never returned it, Cochran recalled.[72] This seemed typical. Janeway did not confront disagreements, at least not by arguing them or defending them, but tended to let them diminish with time. Many of us came to understand that inaction sometimes was the best way of supporting staff, rather than creating an open conflict.

Farber was brilliant but acerbic. Dr. Janeway's relations with him were never revealed to outsiders. He seems to have admired Farber's accomplishments, and in fact once enthusiastically proposed Farber for an honorary degree from Yale.[73] If Farber appreciated the gesture, there is no evidence of it. Rather, Janeway's files contain documents such as a memo from Farber in which the latter complains that CAJ had not talked to him about space for Dr. Samuel Katz and about appointments that CAJ had made without Farber's knowledge. At the top of the memo Janeway wrote, "Administrative woes."[74] There is no evidence of a response by Janeway. This may be another example of his postponing any action that might only inflame the problem; eventually, it went away.

Dr. Janeway took a very personal interest in helping residents settle when they finished their time at the Children's. Dr. Louis Barness told us that when he was completing his residency and had hoped to stay on the faculty, the chief told him he should go to Doylestown (Pennsylvania) in order to enter private practice. "I was crushed, but went," Barness wrote. After he had been in practice about a year, Barness recalled, Dr. Joseph Stokes, chairman of pediatrics at the University of Pennsylvania, called him to say that Dr. John Mitchell, then dean at Pennsylvania's School of Medicine (and also Secretary of the American Board of Pediatrics and CAJ's brother-in-law), had decided that the university needed a course in pediatric physical diagnosis. "Charlie had called and insisted that I be hired to run the course," Barness wrote. "Stokes did not know me from Adam. Charlie came periodically to Philadelphia [to see his sister and brother-in-law, Dr. Mitchell] and frequently checked on my progress."[75] Barness later wrote the only English textbook on pediatric physical diagnosis and had a distinguished career at Penn, the University of Wisconsin, and the University of South Florida, where he was the first chair of the Department of Pediatrics and received the three highest awards in American pediatrics— the John Howland, the Joseph St. Geme, and the Abraham Jacobi Awards. It all began with a recommendation from Janeway.

CAJ's reputation for integrity gained him great support from other faculty members at Harvard Medical School. Dr. Joel Alpert tells of a time when Janeway supported him for a Mosely Traveling Fellowship. Alpert was to go to England on the exchange program with St. Mary's Hospital, but wanted to go for a year rather than the usual six months and felt that he needed more money. CAJ sent him to Dr. Francis Moore, chair of surgery at the Peter Bent Brigham Hospital. Moore, who chaired the fellowship committee, opined that the fellowship was usually reserved for surgeons, but since it was Dr. Janeway who had called, he agreed to use the slot to support Alpert.[76] There were times when Dr. Janeway did not support the house staff, as an anecdote provided by Alpert when he was an intern demonstrates. After being up all night, Alpert, who was ravenous, grabbed two containers of orange juice from the serving area of the hospital cafeteria, only to be upbraided by the woman behind the counter. Alpert, exasperated, jumped over the counter and took two more. Later he was called to CAJ's office and told to apologize with the admonition, probably in jest, "It is harder to get good cafeteria workers than interns!"

A discordant note about Janeway's support of the staff was mentioned by the brother of David Smith at Dr. Smith's memorial service in Rochester. David's brother told one of us (RJH) that Smith and Janeway had an argument about a patient's diagnosis and that CAJ was reputed to have told Smith to leave pediatrics. This is difficult to believe; perhaps the emotional aura of a memorial service may not be the best time to remember accurately. If the story is true, we suspect that Smith may have misinterpreted Janeway's remarks. It is possible that CAJ felt aggrieved enough to have said this, but, if so, it was out of character.

Charles Janeway's passion for fly fishing seems to have been keen from early adolescence, when he wrote the paper about trout fishing discussed in chapter 1. He went fly fishing whenever he could. Although he was politically liberal and personally had a common touch, he was not always friendly to those who despoiled the environment of his fishing. In a letter to his brother-in-law, Dr. Wise who was also an avid fly fisherman, Janeway complained about his experience during a fishing trip in Colorado.

> Colorado has been discovered, and unless you walk about ten miles off the beaten track, it is hard to get away from fishermen within six feet of you. Being the common man, their manners are somewhat boorish and they heave beer cans and fish entrails into the water . . . and they walk right down through the pool you are fishing from the bottom with a dry fly, letting the worm drift before them and catch out the fish that were put there from the hatchery three days before.[77]

Everyone has a breaking point. Janeway's came when anyone interfered with his fly fishing, or did not treat it with the proper reverence.

The root of the word "humility" is the same as "humus," of the earth. It seems at first blush a strange association to make with Dr. Janeway, who, if anything, looked more the patrician than one of the *hoi polloi*. Nevertheless, his egalitarianism was genuine. In the hospital dining room he would often sit with cleaning or nursing staff rather than the physicians. He liked to be called Charlie, even though his stern and sometimes forbidding presence could make this difficult. Dr. Nadas reported that he never called him Charlie in spite of their very close personal relation over many years.[78] Similarly, Dr. Masland tells of visiting him at home in CAJ's last days, accompanied by his wife. "After several 'Dr. Janeways' from my wife, he looked at her with that quizzical, wonderful look of his and said 'my name is Charlie.' After that my wife apologized and did call him Charlie, although I could tell it wasn't easy for her to do so."[79] People did not forget Janeway's humility. They remembered it as much as his notable achievements, perhaps more so. Charles Cook recalled, "Charlie was a great leader because he had absolute integrity, was terribly gentle with patients and their families, and modest and unassuming and at the same time very bright."[80]

Most house staff did not see much humor in Dr. Janeway. He was always kind but stern. As a resident, Will Cochran was a natural clown. So was Hugh MacNamee. Cochran told of a Saturday rounds when

MacNamee walked toward CAJ with a syphilitic tabetic walk, then went to the incinerator, pulled it open, took out a tongue blade and said, "Ah." The rest of the house staff, apparently mesmerized, also looked in the incinerator, then laughed. At which point Janeway also laughed and then said, "Let's go, Hugh." Expressions of humor on CAJ's part were short, few, and far between.[81]

Within an academic medical center there are many good-natured attempts to "one-up" other staff by showing patients with unusual diagnoses, to try to see how astute or clever the other person is, and, by inference, to show how smart you are. We did not usually play these games with Dr. Janeway, but Dr. Ziai tells of a time when he asked him what he thought a two-year-old's diagnosis was. The child was waddling down the hall with bowed legs. The chief expected some rare disease, and, after pondering, said, "Maybe rickets, probably Vitamin D-resistant rickets." Ziai laughed and said, "No, just a full diaper!" CAJ laughed, too. He could take a joke on himself, although it rarely happened.[82]

Almost every resident at the Children's was invited to the Janeways' home on a Saturday or Sunday, but it was for work as well as hospitality. Richard Grand tells of being invited for lunch by Marian Green, the chief's secretary, and told to bring old clothes. He brought the oldest he had, but they were not particularly old. When he arrived at the Janeways' CAJ said, "You can't paint in those clothes. Why don't you go in and read the *New York Times* and talk to Mrs. Janeway, and when I'm done painting we will have lunch."[83]

Although CAJ was associated with Harvard for more than forty years, he was a true-blue Yale graduate, a Yalie through and through. Masland recalled that when Harvard played Yale at the Cambridge Stadium, "Charlie always sat on the Yale side."[84] (The family was later better balanced: Charles and Betty's late son, Carlie, although a Harvard graduate, became a distinguished Yale Professor of Immunology. Robert Masland commented before Carlie's death, "Charlie would like that.") One of he last trips that CAJ took, at a time when he was quite ill, was to his fiftieth Yale reunion. Dr. Cone tells that he was at that time getting forgetful and, sure enough, Janeway forgot to tell Betty that he was going to this reunion. Betty called Cone to ask if he knew where he was. He did arrive safely in New Haven, where he was met by his classmate David Clements, a pediatrician, who took care of him and notified Betty.[85] Janeway had a large folder in his home files, labeled "Yale," with correspondence about his class, fund-raising, and news of his classmates. He was proud of Yale, in spite of what he perceived as its conservative political views.

Dr. Janeway's frugality was probably what everyone noticed most, after his eyebrows. He drove his battered World War II Jeep for years. It had holes in the canvas top, making winter driving in the Boston area seem like living outdoors in Antarctica. Janeway had a bad back, and in the early 1950s was diagnosed with a ruptured intervertebral disc. The bouncing of the jeep could not have helped. One day, when one of us (RJH) was riding in to the hospital with him from Weston, I asked him why he didn't get a more comfortable car. He said, perhaps in jest, that it was to give the staff something unimportant to talk about so they wouldn't ask him for things difficult to deliver.

Dr. Metcoff told, as did others, of CAJ's trips to the annual spring research meetings of the American Pediatric Society and the Society for Pediatric Research. He always stayed several blocks back from the boardwalk at Atlantic City, in a rooming house or at the YMCA rather than in a hotel. One year the junior staff got together enough money to pay for the sleeper on the train to Atlantic City. CAJ sat up all night in the train.[86] Another anecdote from Dr. Diamond concerned travel to yet another spring research meeting, this one in French Lick, Indiana. CAJ was to give a paper, of which the third author was a foreign Fellow. The research grant paid for one person, the presenter, to go to the meeting. Most of the faculty went by sleeper but CAJ went by coach, once again sitting up all night with the junior fellows in order to pay for the trip for the third author.[87]

The stories of Janeway's frugality at the spring research meetings grow, but most seem valid. His stay at third-floor rooming houses at the Atlantic City meetings were recalled by many. But on one occasion Drs. Rosen, Kevy, and Gitlin had a sumptuous dinner and Gitlin thought it a good idea to bring him back a "doggie bag." They went to CAJ's rooming house and presented him with the bag saying, "Charlie, you don't have to spend money for dinner; we're bringing you a meal."

Dr. Janeway, who was not impressed, "looked Gitlin straight in the eye and said, 'Don't worry, someone already treated me to dinner.' There was little humor in his voice."[88] Another tale about going to the spring research meetings involved Henry Giles, an exchange registrar from St. Mary's. Sidney Gellis asked him if he was going to the meetings, and Giles responded that he could see no way of financing it. According to Giles, Gellis was very sympathetic and proposed that we should lay an ambush for Dr. Janeway in the lunchroom. Gellis would start the conversation, "the value for overseas residents of attending such a meeting and the financial barriers that made it difficult for people like myself to attend." Janeway did not respond, so Gellis put some pressure on him, saying, "Henry's even been considering the possibility of camping out somewhere." At this Janeway livened up considerably, "Oh, really. Quite a coincidence . . . the first time I went to Buck Hills Falls I camped out too." The word "too" was clearly final in every respect.[89]

The house the Janeways bought in Tunbridge, Vermont, as their retirement home was strictly a farmhouse and had few added luxuries. CAJ also used a shaving brush until the end of his life, commenting that it could provide excellent medical history. He recalled the story of a man who had syncopal attacks each day as he shaved this way. This led to making the diagnosis of carotid sinus sensitivity (from pressing on the sensitive area of the neck with the shaving brush). We suspect that he told this story to disarm any criticism that he was so old-fashioned that he was still using a shaving brush. The old house and the old brush likely were excuses: CAJ liked to be old-fashioned in his daily personal life but modern in his professional life. We would say today that he was on the cutting edge of science and medical care, but not at home.

CAJ was as frugal with others' money as he was with his own. We have noted in the chapters on his international activities how he kept detailed notes in his diaries of all expenses, down to the penny. At the end of many trips that were under written by foundations he would show a few dollars that had not been spent and were being returned to the foundation. One anecdote about Dr. Janeway's frugality was told by Dr. Mohsen Ziai. Ziai had an old car, in which only the door on the

driver's side opened. Janeway borrowed it one day and came back saying it was too dangerous to drive (a remarkable comment from a man
who drove a battered Jeep). Ziai replied, "But you don't pay me enough
to buy a better car." (This was at a time when the Children's paid no sti-
pend to residents.) CAJ responded that it was good for house officers to
have limited funds.[90] He softened this view later, when he became a
strong supporter of resident salaries. He supported residents in many
ways and was especially attentive to their educational needs, always
putting residents' rounds as a first priority. But he was probably caught
off guard when the proactive residents of the 1960s appeared. In his
personal file from his home is a letter from Dr. Jan Breslow, then president of the House Officers Association, saying that the house staff
"Were disappointed that [they were] not consulted on our views on
possible program changes." They wanted to be consulted but felt that
"the machinery for evaluating our opinions in the past has been
poor."[91] At the top of the letter CAJ wrote, "The rise of HO independence." He was probably somewhat perplexed by this show of independence, but basically agreed with them.

Dr. Mary Ellen Avery tells of the time she was being recruited as Dr.
Janeway's successor. She stayed with him and Betty in their home in
Weston. She was cold and found that they kept the thermostat at about
55°F. When asked, they said it was to save money.[92] Dr. Louis Barness
told of driving CAJ to the Back Bay rail station for a trip that he had to
take to Washington, only to have CAJ ask Barness to lend him $5.00
and to ask his secretary to wire him money in Washington.[93] This captures something essential and somewhat contradictory about Dr. Janeway: he was frugal, yes, but he also had a peculiar disdain for money.
Stories about CAJ's frugality have taken on a life of their own and undoubtedly have become embellished. One that is retold by many, but
not by anyone to whom it actually happened, was of being invited to
the home in Weston, given a lobster dinner and, after being asked to
contribute something to the dinner, be told, "You know, lobsters are
very expensive!"[94] On at least one occasion, however, Dr. Janeway succumbed to luxury. When he was president of the American Pediatric
Society, he and Betty stayed in the Churchill Suite at the Chateau
Frontenac in Montreal. Most of the time, however, according to Betty,

he preferred to stay at modest hotels. This carried over into skiing. The Janeway family did most of their skiing at Randolph, Vermont, a place that, in Betty's words, "Showed our desire to avoid the crowds and fancy outfits of the ski resorts."[95]

Dr. Janeway was as frugal with departmental money and his faculty's salary as with his own. Both of us can testify to this. I (RJH) was started at $4,000 a year, at a time when I was seven years out of medical school and had three children. Each year I was not told whether an increase was to be paid until I received the July check. Dr. Janeway never would discuss salary. Fred Rosen was perhaps more forceful but, after trying to live on $3,600 a year in the early 1960s, he told Dr. Janeway that he could not live on that amount and, after pleading, received a raise, rather significantly, to $8,000. Later, a salary of $25,000 for him was written into an NIH grant. When the grant was approved CAJ told Rosen that he would have to turn back some of the money because at that level his salary would be so much in excess of any other faculty member's.[96]

Indeed, CAJ's own salary in 1973–74, his last year as chair of the department, was $37,000 ($\frac{1}{3}$ from Children's Hospital and $\frac{2}{3}$ from his endowed chair at the medical school). At the time, the average salary of chairs of pediatrics across the country was over $60,000. Both Betty and Charles did have some inheritance income, and Janeway engaged in a small amount of private practice, but they were in no sense wealthy. As CAJ neared retirement he began to worry about expenses with the prospect of reduced income. He wrote to David Kirkbride, who handled the income and expenses of St. Hubert's, saying that in the future he did not want "further invasion of principal . . . so that if there clearly is not enough income . . . we can see if we can meet it from some other means . . . In this way we'll be able to stay within our sources of income and stop having our capital slowly decline."[97] In 1979, Janeway retired fully from the faculty. Thenceforth he received pension and Social Security income.

Dr. Janeway was embarrassed about discussing money. McKay recalled that he had cared for a child of a wealthy family from Florida. They had arrived at the Children's in two limousines. When it was time for the child to go home, the father came to Janeway's office and asked the secretary how much he owed Dr. Janeway. She said that she would need to ask Dr. Janeway. When she did, he mumbled something like "Twenty-five." When she told the father, he wrote out a check for $25,000. The secretary said that she didn't believe that the doctor had meant such an amount, and they settled for a $250 fee. It is likely that CAJ meant $25.[98]

Dr. Janeway was adamant that clinicians should be able to see private patients, but in his ledgers he never recorded more than a few thousand dollars income a year from such practice. One reason is that he, akin to his grandfather, billed much too little for the reputation he had and, as the above story illustrates, for the wealth of some of his patients. We have speculated as to the origins of this parsimony. It apparently started early, for when the family were at Hopkins, when his father was Chief of Medicine, they went to the hospital cafeteria every Sunday for noon dinner. This practice continued for a time after his father's death. Although Charles and his sister, Francesca, went to private preparatory schools and private colleges, the family probably felt that there was a limited amount available after the death of the children's father, who died when the son was only eight years old. For most of CAJ's professional life he earned less than most who were in academic medicine, which was a notoriously poorly paid field of medicine in any case. Frugality was to some degree necessary, but he carried it to an extreme.

Did Janeway have weaknesses? The answer depends on what one considers a weakness. Several have commented on his difficulty saying "no" or discharging people who did not perform. One of the authors (RJH) recollects that Sidney Gellis, in his inimitable way, once said, "It's a good thing Charlie is not a woman; he can't say no!" Mohsen Ziai recalled a house officer who was inadequate:

> He "hid under the bed" when on call [a euphemism for avoiding work], never wrote out his discharge letters to referring doctors and, in a final act of defiance, stayed up all night, supposedly to dictate over 500 discharge summaries not done during the year. In the morning he handed in a dozen or more discs that proved to be empty. Charlie had at one time during the year decided to dismiss him, and had actually written such a letter, but then decided not to send it. Afterwards, Charlie said that perhaps he had been too kind and should have fired him before.[99]

Dr. Berenberg also noted Janeway's problem in dealing with some unpleasant matters. If someone on the house staff or faculty did something that was inappropriate and had to be reprimanded,

> he would call me to his office and tell me about the episode. If he said "What do you think we should do about it?" I realized that he wanted me to speak to the person involved. He usually ended up by acting a bit surprised that I was willing to do it, but quickly agreed. Another area where he had a problem was in firing people from the staff. From time to time, it became clear that he would have to ask for the resignation of certain members of the staff. Frequently, his technique was to send them advertisements from medical journals about unusual positions such [as in the case of one person] Chief of Pediatrics at Hoboken Hospital. In [that] instance he must have sent a dozen such, without any luck. He then went on to reduce that person's salary to zero, which still did not succeed . . . He still could not ask for that person's resignation, but finally did after about three years.[100]

Diamond also felt that "Charlie wasn't definite enough as to what he wanted. He wouldn't give orders to get things done. He should have said no a few times . . . [to Farber] but that's the way he did things." Looking back, however, Diamond said that compromise was necessary. "He [CAJ] was a diplomat of the first order."[101] Dr. Kevy said, "If Dr. Janeway had a single fault, it was that he was too nice." He went on to describe his write-ups of intern applicants. If he really was rejecting them, he wrote long notes about their good qualities but ended saying that it would probably be in the best interests of the individual to seek an internship elsewhere. If he really liked a candidate his notes were short, such as, "Take him, he's great."[102] Dr. Nadas said much the same, but qualified it as a virtue: "I suppose that at times he was not decisive enough, but not making a decision is in fact making a decision."[103]

Dr. David Nathan, who later held Dr. Janeway's leadership position at Children's, said that Janeway "made no effort to aggrandize the Department of Medicine and, in fact, in certain ways gave it away with the statement, 'they will do a better job'."[104] Nathan thought it was a mistake for CAJ to "dismember the department," e.g., spinning off cardiology as a separate department. He also thought that Dr. Janeway did not recognize sufficiently that neonatology was in trouble, owing, in part, to his own lack of experience with newborns. Kevy likewise noted that the one area in which CAJ was less competent clinically was with small infants. He told of several instances when CAJ would not recognize the severity of an illness in an infant.[105] Nathan also thought that Janeway's commitment to train foreign physicians was not wise, that it "took a tremendous expenditure of effort on many people's part." Since Janeway and Nathan did not agree on this matter, they did not talk much about it. Nathan also believed that, because of CAJ's dislike of conflict, he was unwilling to recognize that there are difficult, indeed dangerous, people in the world who consider only themselves.[106]

One former colleague who is bitter about the way he was handled probably reflects Janeway's unwillingness to attend to unpleasant tasks. This faculty member was not promoted when two others, who had been on the faculty for the same length of time, were. He tried unsuccessfully to get an appointment with the chief until Marion Green told him he could ride home to Weston with Dr. Janeway. When CAJ was unwilling to talk about the promotion, the faculty member resigned in the car and has remained bitter ever since. Dr. Janeway had probably already decided that he would not promote the person but did not want to tell him to his face.

A final criticism concerned Dr. Janeway's declining involvement at the Children's. Nathan believed that CAJ, in his last years, "was not engaged enough in the hospital's affairs; he was too busy on the world scene."[107] We think this criticism is valid, but it should be noted that Janeway was deeply engaged with the hospital and clinical issues during most of his chairmanship. As he became more involved in world health, however, and during his last years was ill, the day-to-day running of a large hospital service was less his priority and was at times impractical. It is difficult to maintain a high level of interest in the same area for twenty-nine years. Few chairs stay that long; perhaps CAJ's experience suggests that this is wise.

In conclusion, there is probably no better word to describe Dr. Janeway's overall character than to label him a man of vision. This is exemplified by one of his last "big" lectures, the Merriman Lecture.[108] Janeway commenced that lecture with a quote from Proverbs 29:18: "Where there is no vision, the people perish." He tied the vision to the

Declaration of Independence, the Articles of the U.S. Constitution and especially its Bill of Rights, and the charter of the United Nations. He said that cumulatively these formed a valid political vision, one that should guide medicine. But he decried the "reality" that we in the U.S. do not have equality. He used health statistics to demonstrate inequality in income, health status, unemployment (although paying tribute to the anti-poverty programs as having reduced poverty). In regard to health, he had by this time realized that health status does not depend primarily on access to health care. The sections of his address echo the Declaration of Independence. As he speaks of "preservation of life," "liberty," "the pursuit of happiness," he examines the reality that as a nation there is a long way to go to achieve these visionary goals. In the concluding section he put forward his own vision for the future: that research is important; that the organization of health care, including the education of health professionals and the role of non-physicians, must be a salient priority; that a need exists for a family focus in care.

He spoke of the future of "predictive medicine," and, finally, noted the importance of a world view for American health workers. He ended with the observation,

> unless, as a nation, we are willing to sacrifice some of our super-prosperity, in the form of superfluous luxuries and consumer goods, in favor of a far greater effort to narrow the gap between the people of the rich and poor nations, we will have betrayed our great heritage, which has given the American people a reputation for generosity, decency and faith in freedom and democracy. This is a challenge for many generations to come, but it is a vision well worth the sacrifices required to reach it.

Words such as these encapsulate our story of this great man and the moral compass that guided him through an illustrious career. Even more important than his words, brilliant though they are, is his example as a human being whom we can try to emulate in many ways outside of our careers. His vision can guide us all as we try to make this world a better place than it was when we entered it, as he did.

NOTES

References are given full citations only upon their initial appearance in the notes below; when subsequently cited, they are referenced more briefly and are followed by the chapter and note numbers of their initial appearance, (1, 1) referring to Chapter 1, Note 1, for example.

Foreword

1. H.C. Schonberg, *The Lives of Great Composers: Franz Joseph Hayden.* (New York: W.W. Norton, 1981), p. 93.
2. C.A. Janeway, "Pediatricians for Peace," *Annales Paediatriae Fenniae* 4 (1957): 624–634 (see Chapter 7, Note 42).
3. Letter from Richard Goldbloom to Robert J. Haggerty, January 23, 1989, authors' files, Charles A. Janeway collection, Children's Hospital Boston, Archives (hereinafter cited as CAJ papers, JCHBA).

Chapter 1

1. Letter from Thomas Stapleton to Elizabeth Janeway, November 13, 1981, CAJ papers, JCHBA. The Stapleton letter quotes Betty's remark.
2. The family history and genealogy were provided to the authors through the courtesy of Dr. Richard Janeway, a distant cousin of Charles A. Janeway and vice president for health affairs at Bowman Gray University School of Medicine, and Dr. Timothy Janeway, an orthopedic surgeon in Pittsburgh, Pennsylvania. The latter told us that he had never

met Charles Janeway but he did meet his eldest daughter, Anne. He added, "We both sang in the Amherst-Smith operatic production of *Lucia di Lammermore* and called each other 'cousin'."

3. *Ibid.*

4. *Ibid.*

5. Frances Whitney, Interview with the authors, New York, New York, 1990 (specific date not recorded), authors' files, JCHBA.

6. *Ibid.*

7. Information regarding the Janeway medal of the American Radium Society accessed at: http://www.americanradiumsociety.org/about/janeway/htm.

8. Information on Edward Gamaliel Janeway derives mainly from J. B. Clark, *Some Personal Recollections of Dr. Janeway* (New York: J. P. Putnam's Sons, 1917), and from his biography in H. A. Kelly and W. L. Burrages's *Dictionary of American Medical Biography* (New York: Appleton & Co., 1928).

9. R. J. Carlisle, *An Account of Bellevue Hospital* (New York: Society of the Alumni of Bellevue Hospital, 1893).

10. Frances Whitney, Interview with the authors, 1990 (1, 5).

11. J. B. Clark, *Some Personal Recollections of Dr. Janeway* (1, 8).

12. L. M. Deppish, "President Cleveland's Secret Operation: The Effect of the Office upon the Care of the President," *Pharos of Alpha Omega Alpha* (Summer 1995): 13.

13. J. Greelman, *On the Great Highway* (Boston: Lathrop Publishing Company, 1901), pp. 415–416.

14. Letter of Dr. Graham Lusk, a friend of the Janeway family and later dean of Cornell University Medical College. The undated, handwritten note from Dr. Lusk was sent by Charles A. Janeway's brother, Edward, to Charles, CAJ papers, JCHBA.

15. J. B. Clark, *Some Personal Recollections of Dr. Janeway* (1, 8).

16. *Ibid.*

17. Memorandum from Dr. Thomas Cone to Charles Janeway, November 25, 1975, CAJ papers, JCHBA.

18. Letter from William Henry Welch to Edward G. Janeway, June 25, 1889, Alan Chesney Archives of the Johns Hopkins Medical Institutions (hereinafter ACAJHI).

19. Letter from George Engel to Charles Janeway, December 22, 1977, CAJ papers, JCHBA.

20. Francesca Janeway Keeler, Interview with the authors, Brookfield, Vermont, February 17, 1990, and letter from Francesca Janeway Keeler to the authors, March 2, 1990, authors' files, JCHBA.

21. W. S. Thayer, quoted from the twenty-ninth *Report of the Superintendent, Minutes of the Johns Hopkins Hospital,* January 31, 1918 (Baltimore: 1918).

22. H.A. Kelly and W. L. Burrage, *Dictionary of American Medical Biography* (1, 8).

23. An obituary published in the *Boston Medical and Surgical Journal* 179 (1918):130 reports that Theodore had nearly completed "an elaborate work on diseases of the heart and blood vessels" at the time of his death.

24. Information concerning Theodore Janeway's relationship with the Rockefeller Foundation was provided by Mr. Erwin Levold, Archivist of the Rockefeller Archive Center, Pocantico Hills, New York.

25. *Ibid.,* and see also H. O. Mosenthal, "Theodore Caldwell Janeway, A.M., M.D.", *Johns Hopkins Alumni Magazine* (May 1918), p. 264.

26. W. S. Thayer, in twenty-ninth *Report of the Superintendent, Minutes of the Johns Hopkins Hospital.* January 31, 1918 (1, 21).

27. Elizabeth Janeway, Interview with the authors, Weston, Massachusetts, January 13–14, 1990, authors' files, JCHBA.

28. D. A. Atchley, "The Uses of Elegance: An Address on receipt of the Gold Headed Cane, UCSF, June 10, 1959," *Annals of Internal Medicine* 52 (1960): 881–889.

29. Letter from Abraham Flexner to William H. Welch, undated, ACAJHI.

30. T. C. Janeway, letter of resignation from Columbia University to Nicholas Murray Butler, president, April 28, 1914, CAJ papers, JCHBA.

31. Letter from T. C. Janeway to Lewellys Barker, June 1, 1914, CAJ papers, JCHBA.

32. T. C. Janeway, "Outside Profesional Engagements by Members of Professional Faculties," *Proceedings of the XIX Annual Conference of the Associations of American Universities,* (1917): 72.

33. Letter from T. C. Janeway to Abraham Flexner, April 20, 1915, CAJ papers, JCHBA.

34. Letter from T. C. Janeway to William H. Welch, November 4, 1917, CAJ papers, JCHBA.

35. Letter from T. C. Janeway to Alexander Lambert, December 3, 1917, CAJ papers, JCHBA.

36. Letter from William H. Welch to T. C. Janeway, October 7, 1917, CAJ papers, JCHBA.

37. Letter from T. C. Janeway to William H. Welch, November 19, 1917, CAJ papers, JCHBA.

38. Letter from Frank Goodnow, president of Johns Hopkins University, to Abraham Flexner, General Education Board of the Rockefeller Foundation, December 1917, CAJ papers, JCHBA.

39. Letter from Victor McKusick to Charles A. Janeway, January 31, 1979, CAJ papers, JCHBA.

40. Anne Janeway, Interview with the authors, Annisquam, Massachusetts, August 8, 1993, authors' files, JCHBA.

41. Francesca Janeway Keeler, Interview with the authors, March 2, 1990 (1, 20).

42. Elizabeth Janeway, Interview with the authors, 1990 (1, 27).

43. The obituary of Eleanora Janeway Mitchell appeared in the *Journal of Pediatrics* 58 (1961): 147–148.

44. Information about Edward G. Janeway was compiled from three newspaper clippings, all in CAJ files, JCHBA: "Janeway: One of Vermont's Grand Old Men of Politics Returns to the Senate," *Vermont Reformer,* January 10, 1972, p. 6; "Janeway Decides to Leave Senate," *Vermont Reformer,* 1976, date unknown; "Edward Janeway Honored by Vermont Council on Arts," *Vermont Reformer,* date unknown.

45. Letter from Edwards Park to C. A. Janeway, May 17, 1956, CAJ papers, JCHBA.

46. Fred Rosen, Remarks offered at "A Celebration of the Life of Charles Alderson Janeway, 1909–1981," delivered at Harvard University Memorial Church, June 18, 1981, CAJ papers, JCHBA.

47. C. A. Janeway, "Medicine, Medical Science and Health: The Thayer Lecture in Clinical Medicine," *The Johns Hopkins Medical Journal* 144 (1979): 94–100.

48. Letter from C. A. Janeway to George Schaefer, November 11, 1974, on the history of the Janeway properties at the Ausable Club, CAJ papers, JCHBA.

49. Letter from Eleanor C. Janeway to Charles A. Janeway, July 29, 1946, CAJ papers, JCHBA.

50. Letter from C.A. Janeway to Edward G. Janeway, September 30, 1947, CAJ papers, JCHBA.

51. Letter from C.A. Janeway to George Schaefer, November 11, 1974 (1, 48).

52. Charles A. Janeway, Jr., Interview with the authors, New Haven, Connecticut, March 3, 1992, authors' files, JCHBA.

53. Letter from Eleanor C. Janeway to Charles A. Janeway, December 17, 1956. CAJ papers, JCHBA.

54. Minutes of the Ausable Club in memory of Eleanor Janeway, August 30, 1956, CAJ papers, JCHBA.

55. C. A. Janeway, "Medicine, Medical Science and Health," the Thayer Lecture (1, 47).

56. John Whitcomb, Interview with the authors, Weston, Massachusetts, January 14, 1990 and subsequent letters from Whitcomb to the authors, June 1, 1990 and June 9, 1990, authors' files, JCHBA.

57. C. A. Janeway, "Medicine, Medical Science and Health," the Thayer Lecture (1, 47).

58. John Whitcomb, Interview with the authors, January 14, 1990 (1, 56).

59. Francesca Janeway Keeler, Interview with the authors, February 17, 1990 (1, 20).

60. *Ibid.*

61. C. A. Janeway, "Trout," unpublished manuscript for school essay, written about 1926, CAJ papers, JCHBA.

62. C. A. Janeway, "Medicine, Medical Sciences and Health," the Thayer Lecture (1, 47).

63. *Ibid.*

64. *Ibid.*

65. *Ibid.*

66. Letter from Sol Liptzin to C.A. Janeway, April 4, 1978, CAJ papers, JCHBA.

67. Letter from Elmore McKee to C. A. Janeway, May 25, 1978, CAJ papers, JCHBA.

68. John Whitcomb, Interview with the authors, January 14, 1990 (1, 56).

69. *Ibid.*

70. *Ibid.*

71. *Ibid.*

72. Charles A. Janeway, Jr., Interview with the authors, March 3, 1992 (1, 52).

73. Information recording in CAJ's Yale yearbook, 1930, CAJ papers, JCHBA.

74. C. A. Janeway, "Medicine, Medical Science and Health," the Thayer Lecture (1, 47).

75. *Ibid.*

76. Letter from Eleanor C. Janeway to William H. Welch, October 22, 1930, CAJ papers, JCHBA.

77. "Dr. Charles A. Janeway, Immunology Specialist," *Boston Globe,* May 29, 1981.

Chapter 2

1. Elizabeth Janeway, Interviews with the authors, Weston, Massachusetts, and Hanover, New Hampshire, on several occasions between 1982 and 2000, authors' files, JCHBA. Much of the information in this chapter derives from these interviews and from interviews with all four Janeway children, copies and records of which are also in the authors' files, JCHBA. Such interviews will not be cited elsewhere in this chapter.

2. Elizabeth Janeway, *Recollections: The Bradleys* (N.p.: Privately printed, 1990), CAJ papers, JCHBA,

3. Letter from C. A. Janeway to John R. Graham, April 3, 1967, CAJ papers, JCHBA.

4. Letter from C. A. Janeway to Eleanor C. Janeway, October 31, 1945, CAJ papers, JCHBA.

5. Letter from C. A. Janeway to Dean E. Cowles Andrus (about accepting him to the Johns Hopkins School of Medicine), undated, CAJ papers, JCHBA.

6. Memorandum from Dean E. Cowles Andrus for the record of Mr. Charles A. Janeway, April 4, 1932, in Charles A. Janeway's record at Johns Hopkins University, ACAJHI.

7. Letter from Dean Graham Lusk to Dean E. Cowles Andrus, March 29, 1932, in Charles A. Janeway's record, ACAJHI.

8. Letter of condolence from Charles A. Janeway to Mrs. Graham Lusk, August 2, 1932, CAJ papers, JCHBA. The letter was subsequently given to Dr. Janeway by his brother Edward, who had received it from Louise (Lusk) Platt.

9. Letter from C. R. Stockard to Dean E. Cowles Andrus, March 30, 1932, in Charles A. Janeway's record, ACAJHI.

10. Records of Cornell University Medical College, from Dr. Ladd, Associate Dean, June 13, 1932, to Johns Hopkins School of Medicine, ACAJHI; copy in JCHBA.

11. Records of the Johns Hopkins School of Medicine, dated June 12, 1934, ACAJHI.

12. C. A. Janeway, "Medicine, Medical Science and Health," the Thayer Lecture (1, 47).

13. Letter from John Whitcomb to F. H. Lovejoy, Jr., June 9, 1993, authors' files, JCHBA (1, 56).

14. Letter from C. A. Janeway to Edwards Park, October 6, 1943, CAJ papers, JCHBA.

15. Charles A. Janeway, Jr., Interview with the authors, March 3, 1992 (1, 52).

16. E. A. Stead, "Soma Weiss at the Peter Bent Brigham: Steering a New Course," *Pharos of Alpha Omega Alpha* (Summer 1996): 19.

17. A resume of Charles A. Janeway's career at Harvard appears in Maxwell Finland and William B. Castle's *The Harvard Unit at the Boston City Hospital* (Boston: The Francis A. Countway Library of Medicine, 1983), v. 2, pp. 206–209, with other material on him appearing elsewhere in that volume.

18. C. A. Janeway, "Medicine, Medical Science and Health," the Thayer Lecture (1, 47).

19. A. M. Harvey and C. A. Janeway, "The Development of Acute Hemolytic Anemia during the Administration of Sulfanilamide," *Journal of the American Medical Association* 109 (1937): 12–16.

20. W. B. Wood and C. A. Janeway, "Change in Plasma Volume during Recovery from Congestive Heart Failure," *Archives of Internal Medicine* 62 (1938): 151–159.

21. C. A. Janeway, "Medicine, Medical Science and Health," the Thayer Lecture (1, 47).

22. Charles A. Janeway, Jr., Interview with the authors, March 3, 1992 (1, 52).

23. C. A. Chandler and C. A. Janeway, "Observations on the Mode of Action of Sulfanilamide in Vitro," *Proceedings of the Society of Experimental Biology and Medicine* 40 (1939): 179–184, and C. A. Chandler and C. A. Janeway, "Treatment of Hemolytic Streptococcal Infections during

Pregnancy in the Puerperium with Sulfanilamide and Immuno-transfusion," *American Journal of Obstetrics and Gynecology* 38 (1939): 187–199.

24. P. Beeson and C. A. Janeway, "The Antipyretic Action of Sulfapyradine," *American Journal of Medical Sciences* 200 (1940): 632–639.

25. C. L. Fox, Jr., B. German and C. A. Janeway, "Effect of Sulfanilamide in Electrode Potential of Hemolytic Streptococcal Cultures," *Proceedings of the Society of Experimental Biology and Medicine* 40 (1939): 187–199.

26. R.H. Williams, W. T. Longcope and C. A. Janeway, "The Use of Sulfanil-amide in the Treatment of Acute Glomerulonephritis," *American Journal of Medical Sciences* 203 (1942): 157–172.

27. C. A. Janeway, "Medicine, Medical Science and Health," the Thayer Lecture (1, 47).

28. *Ibid.*

29. Letter from Hans Zinsser to C. A. Janeway, undated, on yellow, lined memo paper, in pencil, CAJ papers, JCHBA.

30. Letter from Morris F. Shaffer to R. J. Haggerty, January 6, 1993, authors' files, JCHBA.

31. C. A. Janeway, "Medicine, Medical Science and Health," the Thayer Lecture (1, 47).

32. R. Rapport, *Physician: The Life of Paul Beeson* (Fort Lee, New Jersey: Barricade Books, 2001), p. 82.

33. C. A. Janeway, "Medicine, Medical Science and Health," The Thayer Lecture (1, 47).

34. Letter from R.V. Perry, Bursar, Harvard University, to C. A. Janeway, September 30, 1941, CAJ papers, JCHBA.

35. Letter from R.V. Perry, Bursar, Harvard University, to C. A. Janeway, July 31, 1942, CAJ papers, JCHBA.

36. Letter from N.A. Wilhelm, Superintendent, Peter Bent Brigham Hospital, to C. A. Janeway, December 18, 1942, CAJ papers, JCHBA.

37. D. M. Surgenor, *Edwin J. Cohn and the Development of Protein Chemistry, with a Detailed Account of his Work on the Fractionation of Blood during and after World War II* (Boston, Massachusetts: Center for Blood Research, 2002), p. 152.

38. C. A. Janeway, "John Howland Award Acceptance Address," *Pediatric Research* 12 (1978): 1139–1144.

39. James L. Tullis, Interview with the authors, 1991 (Deaconess Hospital, Boston, date not recorded), authors' files, JCHBA.

40. Letter from C. A. Janeway to Robert Wise, October 9, 1943, CAJ papers, JCHBA.

41. James L. Tullis, Interview with the authors, 1991 (2, 39).

42. C. A. Janeway, "John Howland Award Acceptance Address" (2, 38).

43. Letter from C. A. Janeway to Edwards Park, October 6, 1943 (2, 14).

44. Letter from John Romano to R. J. Haggerty, May 23, 1989, authors' files, JCHBA.

45. *Ibid.*

46. Letter from C. A. Janeway to W. B. Wood, February 13, 1942. CAJ papers, JCHBA.

47. Letter from C. A. Janeway to Richard Smith, August 28, 1942, CAJ papers, JCHBA.

Chapter 3

1. The term "Department of Medicine" is used for the pediatric medicine department at the Children's Hospital in Boston in a comparable sense with the hospital's departments of surgery and orthopedics. It consists of the various units caring for children by "medical" means—medication, rehabilitation, etc.—as opposed to separate units for children who are cared for by surgical means. Over the years this distinction has become blurred, for the cardiology in-patient unit (now Department) combines medicine and surgery. The pediatrics department of the Children's was always called the Department of Medicine, we suspect, in the same sense that general hospitals do to distinguish medicine from surgery and its subspecialties. Like most children's hospitals, Boston's was started by surgeons.

2. In Clement Smith's history of the Children's Hospital, cited below, the chapter discussing Dr. Blackfan is titled "The Heroic Era." Dr. Blackfan contributed very significantly to the heroic nature of medicine at the time. Few pediatricians were so well prepared clinically then as Dr. Blackfan was when appointed as chief at the Children's Hospital, Boston. Dr. Blackfan was chairman of the department from 1923 until his tragically early death in late 1941. After a two-year period of pediatric residency at Philadelphia and St. Louis, Blackfan was recruited to the Harriet Lane Home pediatric department at Johns Hopkins, where he spent eight years as chief resident in pediatrics, followed by three years

at Cincinnati as Professor before being recruited to Boston. He was an unexcelled clinician and teacher with small groups at the bedside, and developed the department by recruiting able young men to the hospital. In research, before the era of specialization, he worked across what are now distinct subspecialties. He was best known for his superb clinical skills and teaching ability. In the field of hematology, he and his colleague, Dr. Diamond, described a new blood and congenital anomaly syndrome, now known as the Diamond/ Blackfan syndrome; he also worked with Diamond on erythroblastosis. A second area of his interest was to define the several causes of what is now known as "failure to thrive," work that again involved several other subspecialities. Further, in collaboration with a colleague at the Harvard School of Public Health, Blackfan determined the effect of environment and humidity upon temperature control in premature infants. His superb clinical acumen, his sponsorship of research, and his recruitment of outstanding colleagues set the stage for the flowering of the department under Janeway. See C.A. Smith, *The Children's Hospital of Boston—Better Built Than They Knew* (Boston, Mass.: Little, Brown and Company, 1983), chapter 10, pp. 143–148.

3. The Children's Hospital, Staff Executive Committee, "Minutes," July 31, 1942, a copy of which is in the authors' files, JCHBA.

4. Letter from C.A. Janeway to Richard Smith, August 28, 1942, CAJ papers, JCHBA. This letter spelled out the conditions that Dr. Janeway sought, including the authority to develop a teaching and research unit in infectious diseases at the Children's.

5. Letter from C.A. Janeway to Richard Smith, September 10, 1942, CAJ papers, JCHBA. This letter accepted the appointment, "since the plan as outlined in my previous letter . . . is acceptable to both you and the hospital authorities."

6. C.A. Smith, "Address at Grand Rounds at Children's Hospital, Boston, June 24, 1981," authors' files, JCHBA.

7. A. Nadas, "Introduction of Charles A. Janeway as the Howland Awardee," *Pediatric Research* 11 (1978): 1137–1138.

8. Letter from David W. Bailey, secretary of the Harvard Corporation, to C.A. Janeway, July 24, 1946, CAJ papers, JCHBA.

9. Letter from R.V. Perry, Bursar of Harvard University, to C.A. Janeway, July 31, 1946, CAJ papers, JCHBA.

10. Letter from William Berenberg to F.H. Lovejoy, Jr., May 31, 1989, authors' files, JCHBA.

11. Letter from C.A. Janeway to Edwards Park, August 20, 1943, CAJ papers, JCHBA.

12. C.A. Janeway and C.V. Hawn, "Histological and Serological Sequences in Experimental Hypersensitivity," *Journal of Experimental Medicine* 85 (1947): 571–590.

13. William Berenberg, Interview with the authors, Boston, Massachusetts, February 27, 2003, authors' files, JCHBA.

14. C.A. Smith, *The Children's Hospital of Boston—Better Built Than They Knew* (3, 2).

15. Janeway was called "Dr. Janeway" in the hospital, or "Charlie" by his friends . He never was called "CAJ" by anyone, but he signed his papers and memoranda that way, and his staff and associates often referred to him thus when speaking of him. The authors will, therefore, use the convention from time to time in this text.

16. C.A. Smith, *The Children's Hospital of Boston—Built Better Than They Knew* (3, 2).

17. *Ibid.*

18. These units, as listed by Smith, included Neurology (a separate department), Hematology, Clinical Genetics (a spin-off of Hematology), Infectious Diseases, Immunology (originally a part of Infectious Diseases), Renal, Metabolism (originally a single unit with Renal), Adolescent, Allergy, Cardiology (another separate department), Child Development, Clinical Pharmacology, Cystic Fibrosis (including Cell Biology), Dermatology, Endocrinology, Gastroenterology and Nutrition, Newborn Medicine, Respiratory Diseases, and a Service Division for Handicapped Children.

19. Children's Hospital, Boston, "Report from the Fiscal Years 1953–1955," Children's Hospital Archives, copy in authors' files, JCHBA.

20. Letter from C.A. Janeway to Ms. Antoinette Valenza, June 28, 1978, CAJ papers, JCHBA.

21. Sherwin Kevy, Interview with the authors, Boston, Massachusetts, March 15, 1989, authors' files, JCHBA.

22. C.A. Janeway, "Medicine, Medical Science and Health," The Thayer Lecture (1, 47).

23. C.A. Janeway, "The Department of Medicine. The Children's Hospital.

The First 100 Years," in Children's Hospital Medical Center, Boston, *Annual Report, 1969,* (Boston 1969), pp. 38–58 (cited hereafter as C.A. Janeway, 1969 Annual Report, Children's Hospital, 100th Anniversary).

24. F.H. Lovejoy, Jr., "Memorandum to R.J. Haggerty summarizing interviews with Drs. Fred Rosen, John Graef, and others regarding C.A. Janeway's philosophy on forming divisions," August 27, 2002, authors' files, JCHBA.

25. Fred Rosen, Interview with the authors, Boston, Massachusetts, August 8, 2002, authors' files, JCHBA.

26. C.A. Smith, *The Children's Hospital of Boston—Built Better Than They Knew* (3, 2). Dr. Smith quotes from the annual report of James Gamble, who, as acting chair during wartime (1941), wrote concerning the lack of staff: "In view of this . . . your Executive Committee has consented to the acceptance of women interns. This departure from tradition does not imply a disadvantage to the intern service. On the contrary, quality . . . will be better sustained by taking well-qualified women physicians than by accepting men . . . whose qualifications are below our established standards." Most pediatric services today maintain high standards in part because the majority of interns are women.

27. Jack Metcoff, Interview with the authors, Washington, D. C., May 1989 (specific day not recorded), authors' files, JCHBA.

28. *Ibid.*

29. R. James McKay, Interview with the authors, Boston, Massachusetts, February 3, 1989, authors' files, JCHBA.

30. *Ibid.*

31. Letter from William Berenberg to F.H. Lovejoy, Jr., May 31, 1989, (3, 10).

32. Thomas Weller, Interview with the authors, Boston, Massachusetts, March 15, 1991, authors' files, JCHBA.

33. Letter from Alexander Nadas to C.A. Janeway, December 19, 1965, CAJ papers, JCHBA.

34. Letter from William Berenberg to F.H. Lovejoy, Jr., May 31, 1989 (3, 10).

Chapter 4

1. L. K. Diamond, "Replacement Transfusions as a Treatment for Erythroblastosis Fetalis," *Pediatrics* 2 (1948): 520–524; L.K. Diamond, F.H. Allen, and W.O. Thomas, "Erythroblastosis Fetalis; VII Treatment

with Exchange Transfusion." *New England Journal of Medicine* 249 (1951): 39–49.

2. S. Farber, L. K. Diamond, R.D. Mercer, R. F. Sylvester and V. A. Wolff, "Temporary Remission in Acute Leukemia in Children Produced by Folic Acid Antagonist 4–amethopteroylglutamic Acid (Aminopterin)," *New England Journal of Medicine* 238 (1948): 787–793.

3. David Nathan, Interview with the authors, Boston, Massachusetts, October 10, 1990, authors' files, JCHBA.

4. Louis K. Diamond, Interview with the authors, Los Angeles, California, May 7, 1990, authors' files, JCHBA.

5. William Berenberg, Interview with the authors, October 9, 1990, authors' files, JCHBA.

6. D. G. Nathan, "Remarks on Dr. Janeway's Life and Career on the Occasion of the Appointment of Frederick W. Alt, Ph.D. as the First Charles A. Janeway Professor of Pediatrics, November 19, 1993, *"Harvard Medical Alumni Bulletin* (Spring 1994): 5; and Children's Hospital Medical Center, Boston, *Inside Children's* (Spring 1994), not paginated. Alt, a researcher rather than physician, is a leading investigator of the proteins necessary for the maturation of B and T cells in the immune system; he created a mouse model of agammaglobulinemia, the research topic for which Janeway was best known. In a letter from Charles A. Janeway, Jr. to Dr. Fred Rosen, dated November 23, 1993, the younger Janeway wrote, "I am writing to congratulate you on the successful establishment of a Charles A. Janeway Chair in Pediatric Immunology . . . as it is of direct personal importance to me, I appreciate it greatly . . . in addition I want to congratulate you on your selection for the first Charles A. Janeway Professor . . . although I have always thought Dad's research interests extended to all aspects of the immune system and its interaction with infectious agents, certainly his most notable public accomplishment was his study on immunoglobulin deficiencies . . . I can imagine no one better suited to carry on this line of work than Fred Alt."

7. J. Diamond, "Obituary of Louis K. Diamond," *In Memoriam: Harvard Medical School,* 2001, Vol. 3, not paginated.

8. C.A. Smith, *The Children's Hospital of Boston—Built Better Than They Knew,* (3, 2), pp. 236–239.

9. *Harvard Gazette,* Charles A. Janeway Memorial Minute, March 4, 1983.

10. Fred Rosen, Personal communication to the authors, undated.

11. O.C. Bruton, L. Apt, D. Gitlin and C.A. Janeway, "Agammaglobulin-emia," *American Journal of Diseases of Children* 84 (1952): 632 (abstract of the meeting of the Society for Pediatric Research).

12. O.C. Bruton, "Agammaglobulinemia," *Pediatrics* 9 (1952): 722–727.

13. Leonard Apt, Interview with the authors, Washington, D.C., 1999 (specific date not recorded), authors' files, JCHBA.

14. C.A. Janeway, L. Apt and D. Gitlin, "Agammaglobulinemia," *Transactions of the Association of American Physicians* 66 (1953): 200–202.

15. "Three Physicians Tell of New Disease, Lack of Gamma Globulin," *New York Times,* May 6, 1953.

16. C.A. Janeway, "The Department of Medicine. Children's Hospital. The First 100 Years" (3, 23).

17. *Ibid.,* p. 53.

18. William Berenberg, Interview with the authors, October 9, 1990 (4, 5).

19. John F. Crigler, Interviews with the authors, October 8, 1990 and February 27, 2003, authors' files, JCHBA, and Interview with Julia Heskel of the Winthrop Group, Inc., October 17, 2001, on the history of the endocrinology division at Children's Hospital, Boston; text also available in authors' files, JCHBA.

20. *Ibid.*

21. *Ibid,* Interview of October 8, 1990. In regard to one of the points listed by Crigler, he told us that Janeway once said to him, "Why don't you let me write your papers for you?" All of us as faculty marveled at how easily CAJ could turn an awkward phrase into beautiful English. His meticulous notes and rewriting demonstrated that he spent a great deal of time on this.

22. *Ibid,* interview of February 27, 2003.

23. David Nathan, Interview with the authors, October 10, 1990 (4, 3).

24. J. Brennerman, "The Menace of Psychiatry," *American Journal of Diseases of Children* 42 (1931): 376.

25. B. Crothers, *A Pediatrician in Search of Mental Hygiene* (New York and London: Oxford University Press, 1937), a Commonwealth Fund publication.

26. R. Spitz, "Hospitalism," in Anna Freud, H. Martman, and H. Kris, eds., *Psychoanalytic Study of the Child* (New York: International University Press, 1945). vol. 1.

27. D.G. Prugh, E.M. Staub, H.H. Sands, R.M. Kirschbaum and E.A.

Lennihan, "A Study of the Emotional Reactions of Children and Their Families to Hospitalization and Illness, "*American Journal of Orthopsychiatry* 23 (1953): 70–106.

28. Brooks Barnes, RN, Interview with the authors, Boston, Massachusetts, June 12, 1989, authors' files, JCHBA.

29. Dane Prugh, Interview with the authors, Washington, D.C., May 1989 (specific day not recorded), authors' files, JCHBA.

30. G.E. Gardner, "The History of the Establishment of Departmental Status of Child Psychiatry," *American Journal of Orthopsychiatry* 28 (1958): 523–533.

31. The complete manuscript of the speech, handwritten with several references, is in a folder labeled, "Brogden Lecture, Baltimore Nov. 13, 1958," but apparently was never published, CAJ papers, JCHBA.

32. Letter from Helen Woods to C.A. Janeway, June 9, 1958, CAJ papers, JCHBA.

33. Letter from C.A. Janeway to Helen Woods, November 3, 1958, CAJ papers, JCHBA.

34. C.A. Janeway, "Brogden Lecture, Nov. 13, 1958" (4, 31).

35. John Houpis, Interview with the authors, Brattleboro, Vermont, June 7, 1989, authors' files, JCHBA.

36. Alexander Nadas, Interview with the authors, October 10, 1990 (4, 5).

37. C.A. Janeway, "The Department of Medicine, The Children's Hospital. The First 100 Years," (3, 23).

38. C.A. Smith, *The Children's Hospital of Boston—Built Better Than They Knew,* p. 242 (3, 2).

39. Alexander. Nadas, "Sharon Sanatorium and Children's Hospital: a Partnership Founded in the Spirit of Care," May 1989, Sharon Sanitarium publication in authors' files, JCHBA.

40. *Ibid.*

41. B.F. Massell, *Rheumatic Fever and Streptococcal Infection, Unraveling the Mysteries of a Dread Disease* (Boston: The Francis A. Countway Library of Medicine, Distributed by the Harvard University Press, 1997). Massell's book describes the long effort at the House of the Good Samaritan and elsewhere to treat these diseases, which once were true scourges.

42. Alexander Nadas, Interview with the authors, October 10, 1990 (4, 5).

43. Letter from Alexander Nadas to C.A. Janeway, December 19, 1965, (3, 33).

44. *Ibid.*

45. David Nathan, Interview with the authors, October 10, 1990 (4, 5).

46. D. Fyler, "History of Cardiology at Boston Children's Hospital: the First 50 Years," February 2001; manuscript in CAJ papers JCHBA.

47. E.M. Alderson, J. Rieder and M. Cohen, "The History of Adolescent Medicine," *Pediatric Research* 54 (2003): 143.

48. R. Masland and J. Emans, *History of Adolescent Medicine at Children's Hospital,* a four-page publication of Children's Hospital Boston, 2001, CAJ papers, JCHBA.

49. Robert Masland, Interview with the authors, Boston, Massachusetts, May 1990 (specific day not recorded), authors' files, JCHBA.

50. C.A. Smith, *The Children's Hospital of Boston—Built Better Than They Knew (3, 2),* p. 247. A word should be said here about the Prouty Garden, which has been a special place to generations of staff at the Children's. The garden is located between the Hunnewell and Farley buildings and is formally named the Terrace Garden in Memory of Anne and Olivia Prouty. It exists because of a bequest by Olive Higgins Prouty, the mother of Anne and Olivia, who, when told that a parking lot was contemplated for the land, decided that no such thing should be permitted and donated the funds to establish and maintain the garden. It has become one of the "great" gardens of New England and is especially appreciated by children, parents, and staff who use it as a refuge from the routine of the hospital and the busyness of urban Boston only a few yards away.

51. Letter from J. Roswell Gallagher to Dr. Lester Evans, October 13, 1953, CAJ papers, JCHBA.

52. *Ibid.*

53. Letter from C.A. Janeway to Dr. Lester Evans, president of the Commonwealth Fund, October 13, 1953, CAJ papers, JCHBA.

54. *Ibid.*

55. Robert Masland, Interview with the authors, 1990 (4, 49).

56. Robert Masland, Interview with the authors, Boston, Massachusetts, February 24, 2003, authors' files, JCHBA.

57. *Ibid.*

58. R. Masland and J. Emans, *History of Adolescent Medicine at Children's* (4, 48).

59. Robert Masland, Interview with the authors, February 24, 2003 (4, 56).

60. M. Louis and F.H. Lovejoy, Jr., "Adolescent Attitudes in a General Pediatric Hospital—a Survey of Inpatient Admissions," *American Journal of Diseases of Children,* 1219 (1975): 1046–1049.

61. Children's Hospital, Boston, *Children's Hospital News* 1, no. 2 (May 1948), CAJ papers, JCHBA.

62. R.J. Haggerty, "A Teaching Program for Medical Students and Pediatric House Officers," *Journal of Medical Education* 37 (1962): 531.

63. Letter from C.A. Janeway to R.J. Haggerty, September 27, 1961, authors' files, JCHBA.

64. Letter from C.A. Janeway to R.J. Haggerty, October 25, 1961, authors' files, JCHBA.

65. Letter from C.A. Janeway to Mr. Quigg Newton, president of The Commonwealth Fund, 1963 (specific date not recorded), authors' files, JCHBA.

66. Letter from Joel Alpert to R.J. Haggerty, May 16, 1989, authors' files, JCHBA.

67. L.S. Robertson, J. Kosa, M.C. Heagarty, R.J. Haggerty, and J.J. Alpert, *Changing the Medical Care System: a Controlled Experiment in Comprehensive Care* (New York: Preager Publishers, 1974), pp v-vii.

68. C.A. Janeway, "The Department of Medicine. The Children's Hospital. The First 100 Years" (3, 23).

69. F. H. Lovejoy, Jr., *50th Anniversary of the Massachusetts Poison Center, 1955–2005* (N.p.: Harvard University Printing and Publishing, March 22, 2005), pp. 5–8, CAJ papers, JCHBA.

70. William Berenberg, Interview with the authors, February 27, 2003 (3, 13).

71. C.A. Smith, *The Children's Hospital of Boston—Built Better Than They Knew,* p. 191 (3, 2).

72. Letter from Charles D. Cook to F.H. Lovejoy, Jr., September 15, 2002, authors' files, JCHBA.

73. C.A. Janeway," Department of Medicine," in *Annual Report of the Children's Hospital Medical Center, 1964.*

74. Richard Grand, Interview with the authors, Boston, Massachusetts, July 24, 2002, authors' files, JCHBA.

75. Children's Hospital Medical Center, Boston, *Children's World,* Fall 1981, p. 6.

76. C.A. Janeway, "The Department of Medicine. The Children's Hospital. The First 100 Years" (3, 23).

77. Letter from Charles D. Cook to F.H. Lovejoy, Jr., September 15, 2002 (4, 71).

78. CA Janeway, Department of Medicine, in *Annual Report of the Children's Hospital Medical Center, 1964* (4, 72).

79. Letter from Jeffery Maisels to R.J. Haggerty, March 22, 1989, authors' files, JCHBA.

80. Letter from Melvin Levine to R. J. Haggerty, March 22, 2002, authors' files, JCHBA.

81. Letter from Melvin Levine to R.J. Haggerty, July 31,1989, authors' files, JCHBA.

82. John Graef, Interview with the authors, Boston, Massachusetts, July 22, 2002, authors' files, JCHBA.

Chapter 5

1. Letter from Alexander Nadas to C.A. Janeway, December 19, 1965 (3, 33).

2. Children's Hospital, Executive Committee, "Minutes," John D. Crawford, Secretary, courtesy of The Children's Hospital Archives; copy in the authors' files, JCHBA.

3. C.A. Janeway, "The Department of Medicine. The Children's Hospital. The First 100 Years" (3, 23).

4. Alpert at Boston University; Abelson at the University of Washington and, later, at Chicago; Barness at South Florida; Bromley at Emory; Carver at the University of Toronto and, later, at the Robert Wood Johnson School of Medicine; Cohen at Stanford; Cook at Yale; Daeshner at the University of Texas at Galveston; Goldbloom at Halifax; Johnston at the University of Pennsylvania; Haggerty at the University of Rochester; Katz at Duke; McKay at Vermont; Metcoff, and later, Gotoff at Michael Reese in Chicago; Mortimore at New Mexico; Nankervis at Akron; Nelson at Hershey; Pizzo, who returned to the Children's as Nathan's successor as chair and then went to Stanford as dean; Robbins at Case Western Reserve, where he was later dean; Schwartz at Cleveland Metropolitan General Hospital; Simon at Wake

Forest; Tinglestad at Eastern Carolina; Wallace at Case Western Reserve; and Wheeler at Ohio State, as well as many others. In Janeway's 1964 Annual Report he proudly noted that seventeen current chairs of pediatrics in the U.S. were headed by former trainees at the Children's, "which is close to one fifth of all department chairs in the country."

5. Letter from Edwards Park to C.A. Janeway, June 6, 1955, CAJ papers, JCHBA.

6. Letter from C.A. Janeway to Edwards Park, December 9, 1955, CAJ papers, JCHBA.

7. Letter from C.A. Janeway to Barry Wood, November 7, 1955, CAJ papers, JCHBA.

8. Thomas Cone, Interview with the authors, Boston, Massachusetts, March 12, 1991, authors' files, JCHBA.

9. Letter from Frederick D. Robbins to R.J. Haggerty, May 8, 1989, authors' files, JCHBA.

10. References to the Hopkins history come from E. Park, H. Seidel, L. Wisson and J. Littlefield's *The Harriet Lane Home: A Model and a Gem,* which was courteously provided to the authors in manuscript form prior to its publication by the Johns Hopkins University Press in 2006.

11. H.K. Beecher and M.D. Altschule, *Medicine at Harvard: the First Three Hundred Years* (Hanover, New Hampshire: University Press of New England, 1970), pp. 352–353.

12. C. A. Janeway, Memorandum (undated) to house staff of Children's Hospital, Boston, authors' files, JCHBA.

13. Mary Ellen Avery, Interview with the authors, Boston, Massachusetts, March 12, 1991, authors' files, JCHBA.

14. *Ibid.*

15. The Children's Hospital, Executive Committee, "Minutes" for February 2, 1951.

16. The Children's Hospital, Executive Committee, "Minutes" for November 22, 1957.

17. The Children's Hospital, Executive Committee, "Minutes" for January 3, 1958.

18. The Children's Hospital, Executive Committee, "Minutes" for 1958 (otherwise undated).

19. The Children's Hospital, Executive Committee, "Minutes" for December 13, 1960.

20. The Children's Hospital, Executive Committee, "Minutes" for May 2, 1961.

21. The Children's Hospital, Executive Committee, "Minutes" for October 1, 1963.

22. C.A. Janeway to Dean Robert H. Ebert, September 7, 1973, CAJ papers, JCHBA.

23. Letter from Robert Shenton, secretary to the Harvard Corporation, to C.A. Janeway, April 25, 1975, with a second letter of the same date informing him that he was being "recalled to active duty" as Thomas Morgan Rotch Professor of Pediatrics for the period September 1, 1975, to January 15, 1976, CAJ papers, JCHBA.

24. Letter from Derek Bok, President of Harvard University, to C.A. Janeway, January 15, 1976, CAJ papers, JCHBA.

25. C.A. Smith, "Dr. Janeway and American Pediatrics," *Pediatrics* 59 (1977): 149–150.

26. Letter from Ralph Feigin to C.A. Janeway, August 4, 1978, CAJ papers, JCHBA.

27. Letter from Steven Mueller, President, Johns Hopkins University, to C.A. Janeway, March 23, 1978, CAJ papers, JCHBA.

28. C.A. Janeway, "Medicine, Medical Science and Health," the Thayer Lecture (1, 41)

29. Drs. David Rosenthal and William Maloney, Reports on C.A. Janeway's medical condition, March 30, 1976 and April, 27, 1979, CAJ papers, JCHBA.

30. F. S. Rosen Interview with the authors, 2003 (undated), authors' files, JCHBA.

31. Letter to Editor of the *Lancet,* November 3, 1979, v. 2, p 965; copy in CAJ papers, JCHBA.

32. L.K. Altman, "The Doctor's World: The story of a Rare Disease that Appears in Varying Guises," *New York Times,* October 14, 1980, CAJ papers, JCHBA.

33. F.S. Rosen, Interview with the authors, 2003 (undated), (5, 30).

34. Thomas Cone, Interview with the authors, Boston, Massachusetts, March 12, 1991 (5, 8).

35. Letter from Louis K. Diamond to C.A. Janeway, September 21, 1979, CAJ papers, JCHBA.

36. *Ibid.*

37. Letter from Peter Tizard to C.A. Janeway, June 9, 1979, CAJ papers, JCHBA.

38. Letter from C.A. Janeway to William Berenberg, February 7, 1980, CAJ papers, JCHBA.

39. Letter from Anne Janeway to her mother, Elizabeth Janeway, May 23, 1982, with a copy of Anne's recording of C.A. Janeway's last days, written May 28, 1981, CAJ papers, JCHBA.

40. Letter from Professor Noburo Kobayaki to Elizabeth Janeway (undated), CAJ papers, JCHBA.

41. Letter from Professor A. Izzet Berkel to Elizabeth Janeway, June 18, 1981, CAJ papers, JCHBA.

42. Letter from Professor John Davis to Elizabeth Janeway, February 2, 1982, CAJ papers, JCHBA.

43. Letter from William W. Wolbach to Elizabeth Janeway, June 15, 1981, CAJ papers, JCHBA.

44. "Dr. Charles A. Janeway, Immunology Specialist," obituary, *Boston Globe*, May 29, 1981.

45. W. Berenberg, W. Castle, J. Enders, R.J. Haggerty, D. Nathan, F. Rosen, A.S. Nadas, "Charles Janeway Memorial Minute," *Harvard Gazette*, March 4, 1983.

46. Frederick H. Lovejoy, Jr., Remarks made at receipt of Charles A. Janeway award presentation at Medical Grand Rounds, Children's Hospital on July 24, 1981, CAJ papers, JCHBA.

47. Fred Rosen, Remarks offered at "A Celebration of the Life of Charles Alderson Janeway, 1909–1981," Harvard Memorial Church, Cambridge, Massachusetts, June 18, 1981 (1, 46).

48. Letter from Clement Smith, to "Willy" and "Jan," May 31, 1981, notifying them of Janeway's death, CAJ papers, JCHBA.

49. C.A. Smith, "Dr. Janeway and American Pediatrics" (5, 25).

50. Elizabeth B. Janeway, Report of memorial service, scattering of ashes at Stillwater, New York, written September 14, 1981, authors' files, JCHBA.

Chapter 6

1. Letter from Charles Cummings to C.A. Janeway, August 5, 1968, CAJ papers, JCHBA.

2. Charles Kimball Cummings, III, "Sentiments Expressed at Memorial

Service for C.A, Janeway, Harvard University Memorial Church: A Celebration of the Life of Charles Alderson Janeway 1909–1981, Thursday, June 18, 1981, CAJ papers, JCHBA.

3. Letter from C.A. Janeway to Anne A. Janeway, as reported in her interview with the authors, Weston, Massachusetts, August 8, 1991, CAJ papers, JCHBA.

4. C.A. Janeway, "Statement for Yale Twenty Year Book, March 2, 1950," CAJ papers, JCHBA.

5. *Ibid.*

6. Letter from John Kennell to R.J. Haggerty, February 10, 1988, authors' files, JCHBA.

7. *Ibid.*

8. Letter from Georges Peter to R.J. Haggerty, June 28, 1989, authors' files, JCHBA.

9. C.A. Janeway, "Diary of Vacation in Eastern United States and Canada, August 1952," CAJ papers, JCHBA.

10. C.A. Janeway, "Diary of Vacation in Wyoming, July 1958," CAJ papers, JCHBA.

11. Dr. Janeway was a meticulous record keeper. The authors obtained much information—some of it, it must be said, minutiae—on his international visits from his personal diaries. Those same diaries, as will be seen in later chapters, recorded the activities of him, Betty, and his family on such trips; the picture of a vigorous, intellectually curious, socially conscious, and warm and loving family is consistent throughout.

12. Letter from Marie Du Pan to C.A. Janeway, August 21, 1967, CAJ papers, JCHBA.

13. Letter from William Berenberg to R.J. Haggerty, May 31, 1989, authors' files, JCHBA.

14. Fred Rosen, Interview with the authors, Boston, August 8, 2002 (3, 25).

15. William Berenberg, Interview with the authors, Boston, MA, October 8, 1990 (4, 5).

16. Letter from Richard Smith to C.A. Janeway, February 15, 1977, CAJ papers, JCHBA.

17. Letter from T. Berry Brazelton to C.A. Janeway, undated, written in response to Brazelton's reading of Dr. Janeway's Howland Award address, 1978, CAJ papers, JCHBA.

Chapter 7

1. Charles A. Janeway, Jr., Interview with the authors, March 3, 1992 (1, 52).

2. S. Joseph, "Dr. Janeway and the University Center for Health Sciences in Yaounde, Cameroons," *Pediatrics* 59 (1977): 152–153.

3. C.A. Janeway, Self report of his activities in "Yale 30–Year Class Book," privately distributed by the class, CAJ papers, JCHBA.

4. Ihsan Dogramaci, Interview with the authors, Paris, France, July 27, 1989, authors' files, JCHBA.

5. C.A. Janeway, Self report of his activities in "Yale 30–Year Class Book," (3,3).

6. C.A. Janeway, Introduction (inside front cover) to *Children's World*, a publication of the Children's Hospital Boston, Summer 1979, CAJ papers, JCHBA.

7. Letter from Edwards Park to C.A. Janeway, June 1966, CAJ papers, JCHBA.

8. Letter from Edwards Park to C.A. Janeway, April 6, 1955, CAJ papers, JCHBA.

9. Letter from C.A. Janeway to Eleanor C. Janeway, April 18, 1940, CAJ papers, JCHBA.

10. Guido Fanconi, *The History of the International Pediatric Association* (Basil Switzerland: Schwabe & Co., 1968). This volume was published privately. In the front of his copy, CAJ wrote, "Charles A. Janeway, M.D. This specially bound copy of the history of the IPA was presented to me at a meeting of the Advisory Board at the 12th International Pediatric Congress in Mexico as Chairman of the Executive Committee of the IPA." The front endpaper of the volume is inscribed, "To our President, Charles Janeway," and is signed by all the Advisory Board members. Copy available for inspection in CAJ papers, JCHBA.

11. C.A. Janeway, Travel diary, 1956 sabbatical, part II, pp. 23–24, Betty's letter, p. 12, CAJ papers, JCHBA. Janeway kept detailed diaries, itineraries and notes on almost all of his extensive trips and visits to various parts of the world. The diaries were kept in small note books, often requiring more than one for each sabbatical or trip; these are indicated as part I, part II, etc. Often, his wife, Betty, would add follow-up letters, typing from CAJ's handwritten diary notes and adding to them. Throughout his trips CAJ labeled each country separately. In this first trip (1956), part I referred to England, part II to Norway, and so on. In later diaries he la-

beled each country with a number and pages with letters of the alphabet. The authors have reviewed these materials and have hand paginated them lightly in pencil for future reference. All page numbers indicated in citations to these materials, therefore, are the authors.'

12. C.A. Janeway, Travel diary, 1956 sabbatical, part II, pp. 24–25; Betty's letter, p 12.

13. *Ibid.*

14. C.A. Janeway, Travel diary, 1956 sabbatical, part II, pp. 27–28; Betty's letters, pp. 12–13.

15. C.A. Janeway, Travel diary, trip to Europe, 1961, pp. 28a and 29.

16. A letter exists in CAJ's files in which Dr. Fanconi pleads that a younger person be appointed to take over; see letter from Guido Fanconi to "Dear Colleagues" regarding his desire to relinquish his position as IPA Secretary General, May 12, 1965, CAJ papers, JCHBA.

17. Letter from Bo Vahlquist to C.A. Janeway, May 8, 1965, CAJ papers, JCHBA.

18. C.A. Janeway, Diary, Southeast Asia sabbatical, 1965–66 (hereinafter referred to as Diary, SEA65–66), CAJ papers, JCHBA.

19. Letter from C.A. Janeway to Guido Fanconi, April 2, 1965, CAJ papers, JCHBA.

20. Letter from Professor Thomas Stapleton to C.A. Janeway, May 25, 1964, CAJ papers, JCHBA.

21. Letter from Bo Vahlquist to C.A. Janeway, May 8, 1965 (7, 17).

22. Letter from Guido Fanconi to C.A. Janeway, September 21, 1965, CAJ papers, JCHBA.

23. C.A. Janeway, "Address in Mexico City to International Pediatric Association," *Journal of Pediatrics* 74 (1966): 846–847.

24. C.A. Janeway, Concluding speech in Mexico City to congress, International Pediatric Association; quoted by Bo Vahlquist and published in *IPA Bulletin* No. 11, 1969, CAJ papers, JCHBA. Also reprinted in *Pediatrics* 59 (1977): 151.

25. Ihsan Dogramaci, Interview with the authors, July 27, 1989 (7, 4).

26. Rockefeller Foundation Grant GA MEPH 5623–5100 for $2,000, plus an additional grant for $1,000 to enable the Janeways to travel from Colombo, Ceylon, to Indonesia and back to Madras.

27. C.A. Janeway, Report on India sabbatical to Miss Rhind of the Rockefeller Foundation, March 29, 1957, and subsequent letters between Dr. Janeway and the Foundation after the Janeways' return to

Boston. The several letters are contained in a folder labeled "Rockefeller Foundation Travel Grant 1956," CAJ papers, JCHBA.

28. The events of the voyage were recorded in C.A. Janeway, Travel diary, 1956 sabbatical, pt. I, pp. 1–11, and those in London on pp. 12–16 as well as in letters that Betty Janeway transcribed from it, CAJ papers, JCHBA.

29. C.A. Janeway, Travel diary, 1956 sabbatical, part II, p. 1, Betty's letter, p. 8 (July 15).

30. C.A. Janeway, Travel diary, 1956 sabbatical, part II, pp. 4–18 contain entries during the stay in Norway, and are summarized in Betty's letter, pp. 10–11.

31. *Ibid.*, p. 13D, part 2.

32. C.A. Janeway, Travel diary, 1956 sabbatical, part II, pp. 22–23, and Betty's letter. Apparently Dr. Janeway did not follow his later custom of changing to a part 3 when he went to Denmark and later Germany, which was also covered in part II), although he had changed to part II upon his arrival in Norway.

33. *Ibid.*

34. C.A. Janeway, Travel diary, 1956 sabbatical, part II, pp. 47–48, and Betty's letter, pp. 18–25, contains accounts on the family's stay in Switzerland.

35. C.A. Janeway, Travel diary, 1956 sabbatical, part IV, pp. 1–54, and Betty's letter, pp. 28–35, record the Janeways' experiences in France.

36. C.A. Janeway, Travel diary, 1956 sabbatical, part V, pp. 1–10, and Betty's letter, pp. 36–38, are devoted to Charles and Betty's stay in Turkey.

37. C.A. Janeway, Travel diary, 1956 sabbatical, part 2b, Beirut. In the part of his 1956 travel diaries for the Middle East, Dr. Janeway used a different labeling system, such as 1a, 1b, 2a, 2b, etc. Usually the numbers referred to a different country, but not always. 1 was Turkey, 2 Beirut, 3, 4, 5 Iran (different days), 6 India (New Delhi), 7 Lucknow, 8 Calcutta, 9 Madras, 10 Ceylon, 11 Indonesia, 12 back to Madras, 13 Vellore, 14 back to Madras, 15 Bombay, 16 Rome, 17 Florence, 18–20 Vienna, 21 Amsterdam. They are sometimes confusing and difficult to use.

38. The information of Dr. Janeway's visit to Rome and Florence derives from the diary of his sabbatical, Parts 15 and 17, as outlined in the previous note.

39. C.A. Janeway, Travel diary, 1956 sabbatical, p. 20.

40. C.A. Janeway, Travel diary, 1956 sabbatical, unpaginated notebook la-

beled "England," which the authors have lightly paginated in pencil from 1 to 68, CAJ papers, JCHBA. The sentence quoted appears on p. 3.

41. *Ibid.*, p. 51.

42. The Janeways did not visit Finland during the 1956 sabbatical trip and hence there exists no diary for Finland. C.A. Janeway's paper, "Pediatricians for Peace," his first paper on the international role of pediatricians, was published in a commemorative issue of *Annales Pediatricae Fenniai* 4 (1957): 624–634, honoring Professor Arvo Yippo's seventieth birthday and it is likely that the paper was solicited for that purpose. At the conclusion of the paper it was noted that it had been received on February 23, 1957, adding to the evidence that it was not presented as a talk in Finland.

43. On the front page of the diary kept by Dr. Janeway for the 1961 trip he wrote, "journals to Europe March–April 1960." However, at the tops of all subsequent pages the dates are given as 1961. We have been unable to find appointment books or other sources to clarify this discrepancy. We have labeled the diaries "EU61," based mainly on the internal evidence of happenings at that time, among which are included mention of the Bay of Pigs military misadventure that occurred in 1961 and the fact that Janeway indicates that March 25 was Palm Sunday, as it was in 1961. Pagination, when given, refers to the authors' penciled pages, not Janeway's. The diary can be found in CAJ papers, JCHA.

44. C.A. Janeway, Diary, trip to Iran, December 3–17, 1961, p. 5–6, CAJ papers, JCHBA.

45. *Ibid.*

46. C.A. Janeway, Travel diary, European trip 1962, CAJ papers, JCHBA.

47. C.A. Janeway, Travel diary, European trip May–June 1964, p 3, hereafter designated EU64, CAJ papers, JCHBA.

48. *Ibid.*, p. 4.

49. C.A. Janeway, Travel diary, EU64, p. 12.

50. C.A. Janeway, Travel diary, EU64, p. 14.

51. C.A. Janeway, Travel diary, EU64, pp. 23, 28.

52. C.A. Janeway, Travel diary, EU64, pp. 56–57.

53. C.A. Janeway, Travel diary, EU64, p. 63.

54. C.A. Janeway, Travel diary, EU64, p. 64.

55. C.A. Janeway, Travel diary, EU64, p. 67.

56. C.A. Janeway, Travel diary, EU64, p. 66.

57. C.A. Janeway, Travel diary, EU64, pp. 88, 91.

58. C.A. Janeway, Travel diary, EU64, pp. 120–121.

59. The documentation for this visit is a nine-page summary, a typed statement or report that appears to have been prepared as if for a funding agency, but there is no indication as to who or what that supporting organization was. The authors have designated this document the Australia, New Zealand, Philippines (hereafter ANZP) report; pagination cited is as in the original. It is part of the CAJ papers, JCHBA.

60. C.A. Janeway, Report of ANZP trip, p. 1. CAJ papers, JCHBA.

61. *Ibid.*

62. *Ibid.*

63. C.A. Janeway, Report of ANZP trip, pp. 2–3.

64. C.A. Janeway, Report of ANZP trip, p. 3.

65. C.A. Janeway, Report of ANZP trip, p. 4.

66. C.A. Janeway, Report of ANZP trip, p. 8.

67. C.A. Janeway, Report of ANZP trip, p. 9.

68. As was their custom while on other trips, Dr. Janeway kept a detailed diary of this long journey and Betty supplemented it with a detailed letter. Her letter spans several volumes of her husband's diary and the calendar years 1965–66. Pagination in the diaries, which are in two parts, refer to the authors' penciled entries; page citations in the letter refer to Betty's original pagination. The first reference to the Korean part of the trip appears in CAJ's "diary SEA," p. 1.

69. C.A. Janeway, Diary SEA, p. 9.

70. C.A. Janeway, Diary SEA, p. 11.

71. *Ibid.*

72. C.A. Janeway, Diary SEA, p. 20.

73. C.A. Janeway, Diary SEA, p. 21.

74. C.A. Janeway, Diary SEA, p. 26.

75. C.A. Janeway, Diary SEA, p. 31.

76. C.A. Janeway, Diary SEA, p. 35.

77. C.A. Janeway, Diary SEA, p. 49.

78. C.A. Janeway, Diary SEA, p. 53.

79. C.A. Janeway, Diary SEA, p. 17.

80. C.A. Janeway, Diary SEA, p. 57.

81. C.A. Janeway, Diary SEA, p. 61.

82. C.A. Janeway, Diary SEA, p. 63.

83. C.A. Janeway, Diary SEA, p. 64.

84. C.A. Janeway, Diary SEA, pp. 78–80.

85. C.A. Janeway, Diary SEA, pp. 84.

86. C.A. Janeway, Diary SEA, p. 85–88.

87. C.A. Janeway, Diary SEA, p. 116.

88. C.A. Janeway, Diary SEA, p. 144.

89. C.A. Janeway, Diary SEA. This appears on page 1 of a letter that Dr. Janeway wrote on p. 144 of his SEA diary and dated December 30, 1966; it is not paginated, and the authors have penciled in the page number. The Rockefellers in this case were John D. Rockefeller, Jr. and his wife Blanchette, the latter Betty's roommate at Vassar.

90. C.A. Janeway, Diary SEA, p. 149.

91. C.A. Janeway, Diary SEA, pp. 150–151.

92. C.A. Janeway, Diary SEA, p. 157.

93. C.A. Janeway, Diary SEA, p. 101.

94. C.A. Janeway, Diary SEA, pp. 172–173.

95. C.A. Janeway, Dairy SEA, p. 176.

96. C.A. Janeway, Diary SEA, p. 178.

97. C.A. Janeway, Diary SEA, p. 187.

98. C.A. Janeway, Dairy SEA, p. 185.

99. E.B. Janeway, Letter to family from Hong Kong, December 30, 1965, p. 3.

100. C.A. Janeway, Diary SEA, part 2, pp. 20–21.

101. C.A. Janeway, Diary SEA, part 2, p. 12, E.B. Janeway letter, p. 19.

102. *Ibid.*

103. C.A. Janeway, Diary SEA, part 2, p. 24.

104. E.B. Janeway, Letter, p. 23 of the diary (C.A. Janeway's handwritten entry in Betty's letter).

105. C.A. Janeway, Diary SEA, part 2, p. 36.

106. C.A. Janeway, Diary SEA, part 2, p. 37.

107. E.B. Janeway, Letter, p. 26 of the diary.

108. *Ibid.*

109. C.A. Janeway, Diary Egypt, pp. 9–10.

110. C.A. Janeway, Diary Egypt, p. 7.

111. C.A. Janeway, Diary Egypt, p. 38.

112. C.A. Janeway, Diary Egypt, p. 7.

113. C.A. Janeway, Diary Egypt, pp. 9–10.

114. C.A. Janeway, "Asia: Home to Half the World's Children," in A. Dorfman, ed., *Year Book of Pediatrics* (Chicago: Year Book Medical Publi-

cations 1968): p. 26 (abstract). Delivered at the Symposium on Child Health Care, University of Chicago, 1966 (date not recorded); reported in *News of Children's Hospital Medical Center,* Boston, October-November 1966, pp. 3–4.

115. *Ibid.*

Chapter 8

1. Letter from C. A. Janeway to John Weir, September 19,1955, CAJ papers, JCHBA.
2. Letter from M.C. Balfour to C. A. Janeway, April 10, 1956, CAJ papers, JCHBA.
3. As noted before, Dr. Janeway wrote extensive diaries of most of his trips; these often were supplemented with letters from Betty, some of them written jointly with Janeway himself. The letters generally were taken, sometimes verbatim, from the diaries. Since the first India trip formed a part of Janeway's 1956 sabbatical, we have designated it 1956 sabbatical—India, or as a letter. Janeway paginated his diary of the India trip with reference to the city he was visiting at the time; that is, with number-letter combinations. Hence the New Delhi pages began with 5, Delhi with 6, Calcutta with 8, Madras with 9, and so on. The diaries, as noted earlier, are found in the CAJ papers, JCHBA. This quote comes from a letter from CAJ to family and friends, describing the trip to Pakistan and India, p. 1, CAJ papers, JCHBA.
4. C.A. Janeway Diary, 1956 sabbatical—India, p. 5b.
5. C.A. Janeway Diary, 1956 sabbatical—India, p. 5g.
6. *Ibid.*
7. C.A. Janeway Diary, 1956 sabbatical—India, p. 5i.
8. *Ibid.*
9. C.A. Janeway Diary, 1956 sabbatical—India, p. 5j.
10. *Ibid.*
11. *Ibid.*
12. *Ibid.*
13. C.A. Janeway Diary, 1956 sabbatical—India, letter, p. 1.
14. *Ibid.,* Letter, p. 2.
15. *Ibid.,* Letter, p. 3.
16. C.A. Janeway Diary, 1956 sabbatical—India, p. 6n.

17. C.A. Janeway Diary, 1956 sabbatical—India, p. 6q.

18. C.A. Janeway Diary, 1956 sabbatical—India, letter, p. 3.

19. C.A. Janeway Diary, 1956 sabbatical—India, p. 6i.

20. *Ibid.*

21. The authors' files (JCHBA) contain a letter from Dr. Samuel Katz to R.J. Haggerty, dated March 26, 1990, in which Katz wrote of receiving a frantic call from Marion Green, Dr. Janeway's administrative assistant, asking him to do something with Dr. Taneja. Dr. Katz related, "After showing Dr. Taneja our laboratories, I asked him if there was something he might like to do in virology/infectious diseases . . . He spoke of the great problems with measles among the children in India . . . Therefore without any previous planning, funding or additional space, I acquired a laboratory partner for the next six months."

22. C.A. Janeway Diary, 1956 sabbatical—India, p. 6g.

23. *Ibid.*

24. C.A. Janeway Diary, 1956 sabbatical—India, p. 6k.

25. *Ibid.,* p. 6m.

26. C.A. Janeway Diary, 1956 sabbatical—India, p. 6m.

27. Elizabeth Janeway, Letter to family from Lucknow, India, p. 1, CAJ papers, JCHBA.

28. C.A. Janeway, Diary, 1956 sabbatical—India, p. 7l.

29. C.A. Janeway, Diary, 1956 sabbatical—India, p. 8a.

30. Elizabeth Janeway, Letter from Benares, India, p. 3, CAJ papers, JCHBA.

31. Elizabeth Janeway, Letter from Calcutta, India, p. 1, CAJ papers, JCHBA.

32. C.A. Janeway, Diary, 1956 sabbatical—India, p. 8.

33. C.A. Janeway, Diary, 1956 sabbatical—India, p. 8n.

34. Elizabeth Janeway, Letter from Madras, India, p. 3, CAJ papers, JCHBA.

35. Letter from N. Sundaravalli, undated, to R. J. Haggerty, included in a letter of October 12, 1993 from P. Chandra to R. J. Haggerty that is cited in note 64. Dr. Chandra told that Dr. Sundaravalli was an associate of Dr. Achar and that "She is a shy lady . . . trained by both Dr. Achar and Dr. Janeway." She was president of the Indian Academy of Pediatrics in 1986. Her letter is filed with Dr. Chandra's in the authors' files, JCHBA.

36. *Ibid.*

37. *Ibid.*

38. C.A. Janeway, "Medical Research, Medical Education, and the University," Scientific Souvenir, pp. 1–6, December 1957, CAJ papers, JCHBA.

39. C.A. Janeway, Diary, 1956 sabbatical—India, p. 9a.

40. C.A. Janeway, Diary, 1956 sabbatical—India, p. 9f.

41. *Ibid.*

42. C.A. Janeway, Diary, 1956 sabbatical—India, p. 9d.

43. *Ibid.*

44. C.A. Janeway, Diary, 1956 sabbatical—India, p. 9e.

45. *Ibid.*

46. Elizabeth Janeway, Letter from Madras, India, p. 3.

47. *Ibid.*, p. 3–4.

48. C.A. Janeway, Diary, 1956 sabbatical—India, p. 10i.

49. C.A. Janeway, Diary, 1956 sabbatical—India, p. 10e.

50. C.A. Janeway, Diary, 1956 sabbatical—India, p. 11a.

51. C.A. Janeway, Diary, 1956 sabbatical—India, p. 11c.

52. C.A. Janeway, Diary, 1956 sabbatical—India, p. 11d.

53. C.A. Janeway, Diary, 1956 sabbatical—India, p. 11g.

54. C.A. Janeway, Diary, 1956 sabbatical—India, p. 11h.

55. C.A. Janeway, Diary, 1956 sabbatical—India, p. 11h.

56. *Ibid.*

57. C.A. Janeway, Diary, 1956 sabbatical—India, p. 13a.

58. C.A. Janeway, Diary, 1956 sabbatical—India, p. 13c.

59. C.A. Janeway, Diary, 1956 sabbatical—India, p. 13d.

60. C.A. Janeway, Diary, 1956 sabbatical—India, p. 13f.

61. C.A. Janeway, Diary, 1956 sabbatical—India, p. 13g.

62. Letter from John Webb to R. J. Haggerty, December 27, 1989, authors' files, JCHBA.

63. C.A. Janeway, Diary, 1956 sabbatical—India, p. 12d–e.

64. Letter from P. Chandra to R. J. Haggerty, December 10, 1993, authors' files, JCHBA.

65. C.A. Janeway, Diary, 1965 sabbatical—India, p. 12e.

66. C.A. Janeway, "A Tribute to a Pioneering Professor of Pediatrics," *Journal of the American Medical Association* 214 (1970): 1–6. This was also issued as a separate publication by Orient Longmans that same year.

67. Elizabeth Janeway, Letter from Madras, India, p. 5.

68. C.A. Janeway, Diary, 1959 sabbatical—India, p. 12e.

69. Elizabeth Janeway, Letter from Bombay, India, December 13–18, 1956, p. 5.

70. *Ibid.*

71. C.A. Janeway, "Report on Medical Education in the Far East.," Letter

from C. A. Janeway to the Rockefeller Foundation, February 6, 1957, CAJ papers, JCHBA.

72. Elizabeth Janeway, letter, December 19, 1956, p. 1.

73. C.A. Janeway, Diary, SEA, p. 49, CAJ papers, JCHBA. This is the same diary referred to earlier on the 1965–66 trips to the Far East; only those pages that were relevant to the India portion of that trip are cited here.

74. C.A. Janeway, Diary, SEA, pp. 50–51.

75. C.A. Janeway, Diary, SEA, p. 53.

76. C.A. Janeway, Diary, SEA, p. 56.

77. C.A. Janeway, Diary, SEA, p. 59.

78. C.A. Janeway, Diary, SEA, p. 61.

79. C.A. Janeway, Diary, SEA, p. 62.

80. Elizabeth Janeway, Letter, January 15–22, 1956, p. 4.

81. C.A. Janeway, Diary, SEA, p. 63.

82. *Ibid.*

83. C.A. Janeway, Diary, SEA, p. 67.

84. Elizabeth Janeway, Letter, January 15–22, 1956, p. 4.

85. C.A. Janeway, Diary, SEA, 68.

86. C.A. Janeway, Diary, SEA, p. 70.

87. C.A. Janeway, Diary, SEA, p. 71.

88. C.A. Janeway, Diary, SEA, p. 73.

89. C.A. Janeway, Diary, SEA, p. 74.

90. C.A. Janeway, Diary, SEA, p. 75.

91. C.A. Janeway, Diary, SEA, p. 81.

92. C.A. Janeway, Diary, SEA, p. 83.

93. C.A. Janeway, Diary, SEA, p. 84.

94. C.A. Janeway, Diary, SEA, p. 83.

95. Elizabeth Janeway, Letter, January 23–29, 1956, p. l.

96. Elizabeth Janeway, Letter, January 15–22, 1956, p. 4.

97. Elizabeth Janeway, Letter, January 23–29, 1956, p. 1.

98. Letter from C.A. Janeway to Ihsan Dogramaci, September 1, 1977, CAJ papers, JCHBA.

99. Note from C.A. Janeway to Organizing Committee, XV Congress of International Pediatric Association, July 13, 1977, CAJ papers, JCHBA. Manuscript published as C.A. Janeway, "Perspectives in Pediatrics—1977: A View from a Developed Country," *Bulletin of the International Pediatric Association* (1978): 23–31.

100. Letter from C.A. and Elizabeth Janeway to their children, October 21, 1977, p. 4., CAJ papers, JCHBA.
101. Letter from C.A. and Elizabeth Janeway to their children, October 30, 1977, p. 2, CAJ papers, JCHBA.
102. *Ibid.*
103. *Ibid.*
104. *Ibid.*
105. Letter from C.A. and Elizabeth Janeway to their children, November 3O, 1977, p. l, CAJ papers, JCHBA.
106. Letter from Anne Janeway to Jayant Patil, Director, Kosbad Agricultural Institute, September 1977, CAJ papers, JCHBA.
107. C.A. and Elizabeth Janeway to their children, November 30, 1977, p. 6.
108. *Ibid.,* p. 8.
109. *Ibid.,* p. 9.
110. *Ibid.,* p. 10.
111. Letter from C.A. Janeway to O.P. Ghai, September 29, 1977, CAJ papers, JCHBA.
112. Letter from C.A. Janeway to Snehalata Deshmukh, September 29, 1977, CAJ papers, JCHBA.
113. Letter from O.P. Ghai to C.A. Janeway, August 18, 1977, CAJ papers, JCHBA.

Chapter 9

1. Mohsen Ziai, Personal communication to the authors, May 1987.
2. Dr. Forkner, a Harvard medical graduate and a leading New York City internist, became the physician of the Royal Family of Saudi Arabia in 1938 and of the Royal Family of Iran in 1949, as well as physician to many of their people at all economic levels. From 1953 to 1958, he served as President of the Iranian Foundation. In the autobiographical statement that he contributed to Max Finland and William B. Castle's *The Harvard Medical Service at the Boston City Hospital* (Boston: Francis A. Countway Library of Medicine, 1983, v. 2, pp. 117–124), he tells that he presented a memorandum to the medical school's resources committee in 1977 (i.e., 1957) concerning the great need of training able young Iranian students for leadership, out of which developed the participation of Harvard in the building of a great university on the shores of the

Caspian Sea, although the project was halted in 1979 by the anti-American agitation that took place.

3. K.E. Livingstone, Excerpts from a talk, "A Postcard from Iran," presented to the Portland (Maine) City Club, November 17, 1961. Dr. Livingstone was a neurosurgeon who had spent some time in Shiraz. There are three reports in Dr. Janeway's files from Dr. Livingstone to the Executive Committee of the Iranian Foundation, dated July 1, 1961, July 20, 1961, and August 14, 1961, made as consultant to the Foundation, CAJ papers, JCHBA.

4. Mohsen Ziai, Personal communication to the authors, May 1987 (9, 1).

5. J.A. Halstead, "Aspects of Medical Education in Iran," *New England Journal of Medicine* 262 (1960): 707–711. Unfortunately, many of the bills for water were not paid. Water costs were often too expensive for the average family. Financial crises plagued the operation from the beginning. Ultimately, Nemazee's exuberance led him to spend over $12,000,000 to build, equip and to run the hospital, nursing school and water works.

6. C.A. Janeway, "Projected Future of the Iranian Foundation," approved by the then Executive Committee of the Foundation, July 22, 1963, CAJ papers, JCHBA.

7. Translation of the Vaghf Trust by Mr. Nemazee, November 11, 1959, CAJ papers, JCHBA.

8. Letter from R. Taba-Tabai to Mrs. Grimson, July 29, 1959, with an attached letter from Bettina Warburg to C.A. Janeway, November 11, otherwise undated, but undoubtedly 1959, CAJ papers, JCHBA; includes two translations of the original Iran Trust agreement, one by Mr. Nemazee and one by Mr. Taba-Tabai.

9. Several documents reviewing the history of the project were clipped together in Dr. Janeway's file with a hand-written covering note, "Report of the President of the Iranian Foundation, March 21, 1963–[March] 20, 1965." In the packet are many letters beween Janeway and Mr. Nemazee, and others, outlining the history of the entire enterprise. These documents may be found in the CAJ papers, JCHBA.

10. Letter from Campbell McMillan to R. J. Haggerty, February 18, 1986, authors' files, JCHBA.

11. In 1970, only 28% of the people of Iran were literate. A good short summary of Iran's history appears in "University of Shiraz Faculty of Medicine, Present and Future," privately printed in 1957, a copy of which is in CAJ's papers, JCHBA.

12. C.A. Janeway, Diary, 1956 sabbatical, Part V (Iran), p. 15. As usual, CAJ kept detailed diary notes of his visit to Iran, and Betty also added notes to the diary, often following the diary entries with long, typed letters that she sent back to family and friends. Page numbers given are those of CAJ and EBJ; CAJ often did not paginate his diaries, but in this case he did.

13. C.A. Janeway, Diary, 1956 sabbatical, Pt. V, p. 48 (letter of EBJ, based on CAJ's diary entries; page numbers are EBJ's).

14. C.A. Janeway, Diary, 1956 sabbatical, Part V, p. 4c.

15. C.A. Janeway, Diary, 1956 sabbatical, Part V, p. 4f.

16. C.A. Janeway, Diary, 1956 sabbatical, Part V, p. 4j.

17. C.A. Janeway, Diary, 1956 sabbatical, Part V, p. 4f.

18. C.A. Janeway, Diary, 1956 sabbatical, Part V, p. 4g.

19. C.A. Janeway, Diary, 1956 sabbatical, Part V, p. 4h.

20. C.A. Janeway, Diary, 1956 sabbatical, Part V, p. 4s.

21. C.A. Janeway, Diary, 1956 sabbatical, Part V, p. 4m.

22. C.A. Janeway, Diary,1956 sabbatical, Part V, p. 4o.

23. C.A. Janeway, Diary, 1956 sabbatical, Part V, p. 4q.

24. C.A. Janeway, Diary, 1956 sabbatical, Part V, pp. 4r–4s.

25. C.A. Janeway, Diary, 1956 sabbatical, Part V, p. 26.

26. C.A. Janeway, Diary, 1956 sabbatical, Part V, p. 5d.

27. C.A. Janeway, Diary, 1956 sabbatical, Part V, p. 27.

28. *Ibid.*

29. *Ibid.*

30. Iran Foundation, *Annual Report, 1957* (New York: Iran Foundation, 1958), CAJ papers, JCHBA.

31. Iran Foundation, *Annual Report, 1960* (New York: Iran Foundation, 1960), p. l, CAJ papers, JCHBA.

32. *Ibid.*

33. Ziai's rememberance of Janeway's commitment to the Shiraz project was revealed later when Ziai reported that he "had almost reached the end of my rope and wanted to emigrate to the United States. I wrote to [Dr. Janeway] and some of his old friends about possible opportunities. I found out, years later, that he had contacted some of the individuals with whom I might have been likely to communicate, telling them that it would be best to try to keep me where I am. This may sound like harsh treatment by someone who should be on your side, but I must confess that looking back on my career . . . I have derived considerable

satisfaction and find myself more seasoned and perhaps happier professionally than I would have been otherwise." (RJH knows this to be true because Janeway contacted him when he was chair at Rochester to suggest that he not accede to Ziai's requests.) Letter from Moshen Ziai to R. J. Haggerty, February 22, 1989, author's files, JCHBA.

34. Iran Foundation, *Annual Report, 1959–1960* (New York: Iran Foundation, 1960), p. iii, Preface.

35. C.A. Janeway, Diary, August 18, 1963, p. 2b. (It should more properly be moved to his 1963 trip to Iran. It is such a nice summary of his motivation that it needs to be mentioned here.

36. C.A. Janeway, "Report of the Iran Foundation and Its Friends," October 27, 1958 (hereafter referred to as "Iran Report 58," p. 1, CAJ papers, JCHBA.

37. C.A. Janeway, Diary, 1958 trip to Iran, p. 9, CAJ papers, JCHBA.

38. C.A. Janeway, Iran Report 58, p. 4.

39. C.A. Janeway, Iran Report 58, p. 3.

40. C.A. Janeway, Diary, 1958 Trip to Iran, p. 9.

41. C.A. Janeway, Diary, 1958 Trip to Iran, pp. 9–10.

42. C.A. Janeway, Diary, 1958 Trip to Iran, p. 57.

43. C.A. Janeway, Diary, 1958 Trip to Iran, p. 59.

44. *Ibid.*

45. The names and associations were confusing then, and may be confusing to the reader now. The Western-style university referred to here was to be called Pahlavi University, thus carrying the Shah's family name. The University of Pennsylvania was involved with this institution, primarily to assist in its development. The municipal hospital (Saadi Hospital) and its medical school were to be part of Pahlavi University. Nemazee Hospital, its nursing school, the waterworks, and the vocational school would not be part of the university and were to be called collectively, Shiraz Medical Center. Further, another new hospital, an eye hospital called Khalili, was to be named for another Iranian benefactor and was a separate institution that nonetheless came under the aegis of the Nemazee Medical Center. Nemazee Hospital and its affiliates were called Shiraz Medical Center in some publications and the Saadi Hospital and its medical school were called Shiraz University Medical Center after Pahlavi University was started.

46. C.A. Janeway, Diary, 1958 Trip to Iran, p. 66.

47. C.A. Janeway, Diary, 1958 Trip to Iran, p. 73.

48. C.A. Janeway, Iran Report 58, p. 7.

49. Iran Foundation, *Annual Report, 1960–1961* (New York: Iran Foundation, 1961), p. 3, CAJ papers, JCHBA.

50. *Ibid.,* p. 12.

51. Letter from Mohamed Namazee to Mehdi Nemazee, his cousin, June 6, 1960, CAJ papers, JCHBA.

52. Attachment to letter from Mohamed Nemazee to the Iran Foundation, dated as Dr. Janeway received it, July 6, 1960, CAJ papers, JCHBA.

53. Letter from C.A. Janeway to Mohamed Nemazee, November 5, 1958, CAJ papers, JCHBA.

54. An interesting sidelight that illustrates the cultural differences in Iran was the relation of the Khalili eye hospital to a potential source of revenue. The donor, Mr. Khalili, who "owned" a small village nearby, agreed to "pour the earnings back into the village" and make it a model of Village Community Service." He also agreed to "help the Khalili Hospital through a gift of real estate in Teheran." Other villages owned by Mr. Nemazee were to be a source of income as well as places of community improvement. Dr. Mehra's background in public health and his vision of where the enterprise should go placed high priority on such community grass-roots activities in Shiraz and some of these villages. Such feudal concepts made sense in the Iranian context, but were confusing to Americans.

55. Iran Foundation, *Annual Report, 1961–1962* (New York: Iran Foundation, 1962), p. 98, CAJ papers, JCHBA.

56. C.A. Janeway, Report to Board of Trustees of Iran Foundation of trip of December 3–17, 1961, p. 2, CAJ papers, JCHBA. The report extends to twenty pages, with five pages of recommendations.

57. *Ibid.,* p. 4.

58. C.A. Janeway, Diary, Trip to Iran of December 3–17, 1961, CAJ papers, JCHBA. Complaints related mainly to low morale or to much turnover of visiting professors, or from Iranians who often felt that they had been "sold a bill of goods" in regard to housing, research facilities, and low pay, as well as poor administration. The diary is dated 1 / 15 but is without page numbers; the page cited here is the seventh in sequence. Henceforth, the diary will be referred to without page numbers.

59. *Ibid.*

60. *Ibid.*

61. *Ibid.*

62. *Ibid.*
63. *Ibid.*
64. *Ibid.*
65. *Ibid.*
66. These recommendations had little chance of being realized. The entire Iranian administrative structure was monolithic, and it was almost impossible for any institution to be free of political influence in that country.
67. Board members were mainly high government officials; the university was, in fact, still tied closely to the current government.
68. University of Pennsylvania, Report to the Pahlavi Board of Trustees, July 3, 1963, CAJ papers, JCHBA.
69. Iran Foundation, *Annual Report, 1962–1963* (New York: Iran Foundation, 1963), pp. 1–2, CAJ papers, JCHBA.
70. Letter from Mohamed Nemazee to C.A. Janeway, undated, but received June 4, 1963, CAJ papers, JCHBA.
71. Letter from C.A. Janeway to Mohamed Nemazee, June 23, 1963, CAJ papers, JCHBA.
72. Memo from Bettina Warburg to the Executive Committee of the Iran Foundation, and Minutes of Meeting of the Medical Advisory Council of the Iran Foundation, June 24, 1964, CAJ papers, JCHBA.
73. Iran Foundation, Minutes of the Board of Directors, July 22, 1963, CAJ papers, JCHBA.
74. Letter from C.A. Janeway to Mohamed Nemazee, August 3, 1963, p. 2, CAJ papers, JCHBA. The letter was accompanied by a six-page Appendix A, "Projected Future of the Iran Foundation," and a one-page Appendix B, "Duties and Responsibilities of the Director Of the Shiraz Medical Center."
75. Cablegram from Torab Mehra to C.A. Janeway, July 31, 1963, CAJ papers, JCHBA.
76. In an uncharacteristic act of forgetfulness, in July 1964, in a handwritten note Janeway acknowledged a check for $1,000 from John Musser to the Iran Foundation with his note, "Check sent 12/20/63; lost in my drawer, found 7/16/64; sent to Iran Foundation 7/16/64." This episode must have been especially embarrassing, as John Musser had been the best man at Janeway's wedding! They were Yale classmates and life-long friends.

77. C.A. Janeway, Diary, Trip to Iran August 9–26, 1963, not paginated, CAJ papers, JCHBA.

78. *Ibid.*

79. *Ibid.*

80. *Ibid.*

81. C.A. Janeway, Report to the Board of the Iran Foundation, May 4, 1964, CAJ papers, JCHBA.

82. C.A. Janeway, Position Paper to the Board of the Iran Foundation, May 4, 1964, CAJ papers, JCHBA.

83. C.A. Janeway, Diary, Trip to Iran August 19–26, 1963.

84. Iran Foundation, *Annual Report, 1963–1965* (New York: Iran Foundation, 1965), CAJ papers, JCHBA.

85. Letter from Torab Mehra to C.A. Janeway, June 19, 1964, CAJ papers, JCHBA.

86. Letter from Mohamed Nemazee to C.A. Janeway, September 15, 1964,, CAJ papers, JCHBA.

87. Letter from C.A. Janeway to Mohamed Nemazee, November 8, 1964, CAJ papers, JCHBA.

88. Iran Foundation, Minutes of the Executive Committee, November 16, 1964, CAJ papers, JCHBA. The allusion is to a report of Mr. Robert Williams on a recent visit to Shiraz.

89. Dorothy Sutherland, Report to the Iran Foundation on a Visit to Shiraz, December 20–21, 1964, CAJ papers, JCHBA.

90. Letter from Campbell McMillan to R. J. Haggerty, February 14, 1986 (9, 10).

91. C.A. Janeway, Diary of 1966 Trip to Iran, pp. 1–13, CAJ papers, JCHBA.

92. C.A. Janeway, Diary of 1966 Trip to Iran, p. 15.

93. C.A. Janeway, Diary of 1966 Trip to Iran, p. 16.

94. C.A. Janeway, Diary of 1966 Trip to Iran, p. 23.

95. C.A. Janeway, Diary of 1966 Trip to Iran, p. 28.

96. *Ibid.*

97. Letter from Torab Mehra to Dr. Stobbe (otherwise unidentified or unknown), November 18, 1965, CAJ papers, JCHBA.

98. Moshen Ziai, Personal communication to R. J. Haggerty, May 1987 (9, 1).

99. C.A. Janeway, Diary of 1975 Trip to Iran, p. 1, CAJ papers, JCHBA.

100. C.A. Janeway, Diary of 1975 Trip to Iran, p. 6.

101. C.A. Janeway, Diary of 1975 Trip to Iran, p. 7.

102. J.J. Ellis, *Founding Brothers* (New York: Alfred A. Knopf Publishing Group, 2002).

Chapter 10

1. C.A. Janeway, Diary, trip to Africa, February–March 1971 (hereafter Diary, Africa71), p. 1, 2, CAJ papers, JCHBA.
2. C.A. Janeway, Diary, Africa71, p. 4.
3. *Ibid.*
4. C.A. Janeway, Diary, Africa71, p. 26.
5. C.A. Janeway, Diary, Africa71, p. 29.
6. C.A. Janeway, Diary, Africa71, p. 32.
7. C.A. Janeway, Diary, Africa71, p. 36.
8. C.A. Janeway, Diary, Africa71, p. 38.
9. C.A. Janeway, Diary, Africa71, p. 60.
10. C.A. Janeway, Diary, Africa71, pp. 60–61.
11. C.A. Janeway, Diary, 1971 trip to South America (hereafter SA71), p. 1, CAJ papers, JCHBA. As noted earlier, the first few physical pages of this volume are devoted to Janeway's 1967 briefing at the State Department. The authors have paginated the descriptions of the South America trip separately; page 1 of the trip to Colombia follows the description of the State Department briefing.
12. *Ibid.*
13. C.A. Janeway, Diary, SA71, pp. 5, 14.
14. C.A. Janeway, Diary, SA71, p. 7.
15. C.A. Janeway, Diary, SA71, p. 10.
16. C.A. Janeway, Diary, SA71, p. 16.
17. C.A. Janeway, Diary, SA71, p. 19.
18. C.A. Janeway, Diary, SA71, pp. 22–23.
19. C.A. Janeway, Diary, SA71, pp. 28–30.
20. C.A. Janeway, Diary, SA71, p. 29.
21. *Ibid.*
22. C.A. Janeway, Diary, SA71, p. 30.
23. C.A. Janeway, Diary, SA71, p. 31.
24. C.A. Janeway, Diary, SA71, p. 33.
25. C.A. Janeway, Diary, SA71, pp. 34–37.
26. C.A. Janeway, Diary, SA71, pp. 43–44.
27. C.A. Janeway, Diary, SA71, p. 44.

28. *Ibid.*

29. C.A. Janeway, Diary, 1972 trip to Egypt (hereinafter (Egypt72), p. 3, CAJ papers, JCHBA. Page numbers are the authors'.

30. C.A. Janeway, Diary, Egypt72, p. 6.

31. C.A. Janeway, Diary, Egypt72, p. 7.

32. C.A. Janeway, Diary, Egypt72, p. 8.

33. *Ibid.*

34. C.A. Janeway, Diary, Egypt72, p. 13.

35. C.A. Janeway, Diary, Egypt72, p. 22.

36. C.A. Janeway, Diary, Egypt72, p. 14.

37. C.A. Janeway, Diary, Egypt72, p. 20.

38. C.A. Janeway, Diary, Egypt72, p. 21.

39. C.A. Janeway, Diary of trip around the world, hereafter RTW73, CAJ papers, JCHBA. In this diary, Janeway lists the dates of the trip as starting on "9/29" and on the first two pages continues to identify the date as 9/30; only on the fourth page does he give the correct date as September 1. It was the second time his dating on the front page of a diary was incorrect. One wonders whether the error this time owed to his impending Waldenstrom's hypergammaglobulinemia or his upset over the neck pain that Betty was beginning to suffer.

40. C.A. Janeway, Diary, RTW73, p. 4.

41. C.A. Janeway, Diary, RTW73, p. 3.

42. C.A. Janeway, Diary, RTW73, p. 5.

43. C.A. Janeway, Diary, RTW73, p. 6.

44. C.A. Janeway, Diary, RTW73, p. 18.

45. C.A. Janeway, Diary, RTW73, p. 12.

46. C.A. Janeway, Diary, RTW73, p. 19.

47. C.A. Janeway, Diary, RTW73, pp. 30, 30a.

48. C.A. Janeway, Diary, RTW73, pp. 32, 32a.

49. C.A. Janeway, Diary, RTW73, p. 40a.

50. C.A. Janeway, Diary RTW73, p. 44.

51. Material in this section, concerning Janeway's work on the Cameroon project, derives mainly from R.J. Haggerty and R.W. Chamberlin, "Doctor Janeway and the Cameroon Project," *Pharos of Alpha Omega Alpha* (Autumn 2000): 11–16. By this time, Cameroon was a unified nation but was still thought of colloquially as "the Cameroons;" the authors have carried on that convention in this chapter, as that is the term that Dr. Janeway used. Cameroon is in western Africa, on the Gulf of Guinea

and extending north to Lake Chad. It comprises the former French and British Cameroons, which, in 1919, became League of Nations mandates of former German territory that had been occupied by French and British troops during World War I. In 1946 the mandates were made trust territories of the United Nations. British Cameroons consisted of two noncontiguous sections lying on the eastern border of Nigeria, the more southerly extending to the coast. French Cameroons was administered as a separate territory with the capital at Yaounde. In 1960, French Cameroons became the Cameroon Republic. In 1961 the southern section of British Cameroons was joined to the Cameroon Republic to form the Federal Republic of Cameroon. In 1972, that nation became known as the United Republic of Cameroon, at which time the northern section passed to Nigeria. Information obtained from www.encyclopedia.com/html/C/Cameroons.asp, accessed August 4, 2004.

52. G.L. Monekosso, "University Centre for Health Sciences in Cameroon," *Lancet* I (May 6, 1972): 1005–1006.

53. C.A. Janeway, "Caring for Mother and Child in Cameroon. 1. Setting Up a Program," *Harvard Medical Alumni Bulletin* (November/December 1975): 20–21.

54. *Ibid.*

55. S.C. Joseph, "Hospital Diagnosis of Children Aged 0 to 5 Years in Yaounde, Cameroon," *Environment and Child Health* (August 1974): 191–195.

56. Letter from R.W. Chamberlin to C.A. Janeway, undated, CAJ papers, JCHBA. Chamberlin, co-author of the reference in note 51, is a pediatrician who worked on the Cameroons Project in 1977–1978; he is the source of much of the descriptive material in this chapter.

57. C.A. Janeway, Final Summary Report Harvard-CUSS, A.S. Aid Contract #625-11-550-531 for the period November 29, 1973 through December 31, 1979, submitted April 23, 1980, CAJ papers, JCHBA.

58. The lack of a separate diary is quite uncharacteristic of Dr. Janeway. It was probably lost subsequently, since diaries of former trips and the later trips to the Cameroons are so complete that it is unlikely that Janeway did not make a similar one upon his first visit to a new project.

59. C.A. Janeway, Diary, 1975 trip to Cameroon (hereinafter Cameroon 75), p. 1, CAJ papers, JCHBA.

60. C.A. Janeway, Diary, Cameroon 75, p. 6.

61. Letter from Bernard Guyer to R.J. Haggerty, March 28, 1990, authors' files, JCHBA.

62. C.A. Janeway, Diary, Cameroon 75, p. 9.

63. C.A. Janeway, Diary, Cameroon 75, p. 26.

64. C.A. Janeway, Diary, Cameroon 75, p. 31.

65. C.A. Janeway, Diary, Cameroon 75, p. 32.

66. C.A. Janeway, Introduction to *Children's World,* Summer 1979, CAJ papers, JCHBA.

67. D.E.J. Kelland, *The Dr. Charles A. Janeway Child Health Center: A Special Place . . . 1966–1991, The First Twenty-five Years* (St. Johns, Newfoundland, The Children's Hospital Corporation, 1991).

68. *Ibid.* Further information on the history of the founding of the institution is contained in a letter from Campbell McPherson to C.A. Janeway, December 1, 1967, CAJ papers, JCHBA.

69. *Evening Telegram,* St. John's, Newfoundland, Wednesday, August 9, 1966, page 3, and Thursday, August 10, 1966, page 3.

70. C.A. Janeway's handwritten notes in folder labelled, "Hospital St. Johns Newfoundland," CAJ papers, JCHBA.

71. Letter from Richard Goldbloom to R.J. Haggerty, February 28,1989, authors' files, JCHBA.

72. Letters from Drs. Donald and Elizabeth Hillman to R.J. Haggerty, September 28, 1990 and October 18, 1990, authors' files, JCHBA.

73. Matthew 57; King James Version.

74. C.A. Janeway, "Perspectives in Pediatrics—1977: A View from a 'Developed' Country." *Bulletin of the International Pediatric Association* (1978): 23–31.

75. C.A. Janeway, letter to Ihsan Dogramaci April 3, 1978, CAJ papers, JCHBA.

76. Professor Michel Mancieux, Interview with the authors, Paris, France, July 1989, authors' files, JCHBA.

77. *Ibid.*

78. Letter from C.A. Janeway to Robert Debré, October 28, 1956, CAJ papers, JCHBA.

79. *Ibid.*

80. *Ibid.*

81. Pierre Royer, Interview with the authors, Paris, France, July 1989, and letter from Royer to R.J. Haggerty, March 6, 1990; authors' files, JCHBA.

82. Letter from Mildred McTear to the authors, June 10, 1989, authors' files, JCHBA.

83. C.A. Janeway, Speech at Rheims, France, December 4, 1969, unpublished, CAJ papers, JCHBA.

84. Letter from P.M.S. Blackett to C.A. Janeway, undated, CAJ papers, JCHBA.

85. Letter from A. Petros-Barvasian to C.A. Janeway, November 21, 1978, CAJ papers, JCHBA.

86. Letter from Gustavo Gordillo to R.J. Haggerty, June 13, 1986, authors' files, JCHBA.

87. G.D. Harlow and G.C. Maerz, eds. *Measures Short of War: The George F. Kennan Lectures at the NWC 1946–47* (Washington, DC: National Defense University Press, 1991).

Chapter 11

1. C.A. Janeway, "Control of Influenza and Measles," *Acta Paediatrica* 36 (1947), This paper was part of the Transactions of the 5th International Congress of Pediatrics.

2. C.A. Janeway, "Report of Medical Progress: Bacteriology," *New England Journal of Medicine* 221 (1939): 339–345.

3. C.A. Janeway, Radio talk, Station WAAB, Boston, 1946, on sulfanamides.

4. C.A. Janeway, "Medical Research, Medical Education and the University," Scientific Souvenir, p 1–6 to the Eighth Annual Conference of the Indian Association of Pathologists and the Committee of the Indian Association of Pathologists and the committee meetings of the Indian Council of Medical Research, December 1957, CAJ papers, JCHBA.

5. C.A. Janeway, "Some Shortcomings of Medical Education in a Free Society," *Acta Paediatrica Scandinavica*, Supplement 172 (1967): 93.

6. *Ibid.*

7. C.A. Janeway, "Pediatricians for Peace" (1, 2).

8. C.A. Janeway, "The Student, the Patient, and the Teacher," *Journal of the Association of American Medical Schools* (1959), Chapter 9: 107. This was contained in the Report of the First Institute of Clinical Teaching.

9. C.A. Janeway, "The Department of Medicine. The Children's Hospital. The First 100 Years," pp. 53–54 (3, 23).

10. C.A. Janeway, Keynote Address, Conference for Indian Students, State University of New York, Albany, New York, June 18–20, 1959.

11. C.A Janeway, "The Department of Medicine," Annual Report of the Children's Hospital Medical Center, 1966.

12. C.A. Janeway, Address at Meeting of Pediatric Department Chairmen, held at Arden House, New York, N.Y., 1964, unpubished manuscript, JCHBA.

13. C.A. Janeway, "Medical Education after Medical School in the United States of America," *Indian Journal of Medical Education* 4 (1965): 1.

14. C.A. Janeway, "Growth and Development of American Pediatrics in North America," *Pediatric Research* 5 (1971): 560.

15. Francisco Tome, Personal communication with R. J. Haggerty, 1992, authors' files, JCHBA.

16. R.J. Haggerty and C.A. Janeway, "Evaluation of a Pediatric House Officer Program," *Pediatrics* 26 (1960): 858.

17. F.H. Lovejoy, Jr. and D. G. Nathan, "Careers Chosen by Graduates of a Pediatric House Officer Program, 1974–1986," *Academic Medicine* 67 (1992): 272–274.

18. C.A. Janeway, "The Department of Medicine," in Annual Report of the Children's Hospital Medical Center, 1964, pp. 43–64 (4, 72).

19. C.A. Janeway, "The Department of Medicine," in Annual Report of the Children's Hospital Medical Center, 1970, pp. 14–23.

20. C.A. Janeway, "The Department of Medicine,"in Annual Report of the Children's Hospital Medical Center, 1964, pp. 43–64 (4, 72).

21. C.A. Janeway, "The Department of Medicine," in Annual Report of the Children's Hospital Medical Center, 1970, pp. 14–23.

22. Letter from Frederick Robbins to R. J. Haggerty, May 8, 1988, authors' files, JCHBA.

23. Julius H. Richmond, Interview with the authors, Boston, Massachusetts, March 11, 1991, authors' files, JCHBA.

24. David Smith, Interview with the authors, Rochester, N.Y., December 1994 (day not recorded), authors' files, JCHBA.

25. Quotation accessed online January 13, 2006, http://www.medicine. mcgill.ca/oslerwebn/quotes.htm.

26. C.A. Janeway, "Goals and Constraints in the Education of Physicians," *Australian Pediatric Journal,* Supplement no. 3, 1973, based on Dr. Janeway's lecture as Felton Visiting Professor at the Royal Children's Hospital, Melbourne.

27. C.A. Janeway, "The Decline of Primary Medical Care: an Unforseen Consequence of the Flexner Report," *The Pharos of Alpha Omega Alpha* 37, no. 3 (1974): 74.

28. C.A. Janeway, "Pediatrics 1984: An Attempt to Look into the Crystal Ball," 3rd Annual Edgar P. Copeland Lectureship, *Clinical Proceedings of the Children's Hospital,* 9, no. 2, February 1963.

29. C.A. Janeway, "Family Medicine and Primary Care at HMS: Family Medicine at Harvard," *Harvard Alumni Bulletin* (May-June 1974): 8–10.

Chapter 12

1. Letter from C.A. Janeway to Eleanor C. Janeway, March 18, 1941, CAJ papers, JCHBA.

2. This stands in contrast with William Osler's famous and controversial observation in his essay "The Fixed Period" that "The teacher's life should have three periods, study until twenty-five, investigation until forty, at which age I would have him retired on a double allowance. Whether Anthony Trollope's suggestion of a college and chloroform should be carried out or not I have become a little dubious, as my own time is getting so short." The essay is printed in his *Acquinimitas, with Other Addresses.*

3. A.M. Harvey, C.A. Janeway, "The Development of Acute Hemolytic Anemia during the Administration of *Sulfanilamide (Para-aminobenzine-sulfanamide),*" *Journal of the American Medical Association* 109 (1937): 12–16.

4. C.V.Z. Hawn, C.A. Janeway, "Histological and Serological Sequences in Experimental Hypersensitivity," *Journal of Experimental Medicine* 85 (1947): 571–576; L. Schwab, F.C. Moll, T. Hall, H. Brean, M. Kirk, C.V.Z. Hawn, C.A. Janeway, "Experimental Hypersensitivity in the Rabbit. Effect of Inhibition of Antibody Formation by X-radiation and Nitrogen Mustards on the Histologic and Serologic Sequences and on the Behavior of Serum Complement, Following Single Large Injections of Foreign Proteins," *Journal of Experimental Medicine* 91 (1950): 505–526; H. Latta, D. Gitlin, C.A. Janeway, "Experimental Hypersensitivity in the Rabbit. The Cellular Localization of Soluble Azoproteins (Dye-Azo-Human Serum Albumins) Injected Intravenously," *American Medical Association Archives of Pathology* 51 (1951): 260–277; D. Gitlin, H. Latta, W.H. Batchelor, C.A. Janeway, "Experimental Hypersensitivity in the

Rabbit. Disappearance Rate of Native and Labelled Heterologous Proteins from the Serum after Intravenous Injections," *Journal of Immunology* 66 (1951): 451–461.

5. Dr. Janeway's laboratory notebooks of his research experiments, which are not numbered or titled except for the dates of observations, have been deposited in JCHBA.

6. J.T. King, Jr., C.A. Janeway, "Sickle Cell Anemia with Cardiac Complication," *International Clinics* 3 (1937): 41–46.

7. C.E. Wainwright, C.A. Janeway, "Diagnosis of Acute Arthritis," *International Clinics* 3 (1937) 55–63.

8. C.A. Chandler, C.A. Janeway, "Observations on the Mode of Action of Sulfanilamide in Vitro," *Proceedings of the Society for Experimental Biology in Medicine* 40 (1939): 179–184.

9. C.L. Fox, Jr., B. German, C.A. Janeway, "Effect of Sulfanilamide on Electrode-potential Hemolytic Streptococcal Cultures," *Proceedings of the Society for Experimental Biology in Medicine* 40 (1939): 184–189.

10. W.B. Wood, C.A. Janeway, "Change in Plasma Volume during Recovery From Congestive Heart Failure," *Archives of Internal Medicine* 62 (1938): 151–159.

11. C.A. Chandler, C.A. Janeway, "The Treatment of Hemolytic Streptococcal Infections During Pregnancy and the Puerperium with Sulfanilamide and Immunotransfusion," *American Journal of Obstetrics and Gynecology* 38 (1939): 187–199.

12. C.A. Janeway, "Report of Medical Progress: Bacteriology," *New England Journal of Medicine* 221 (1939): 339–345; C.A. Janeway, "Report of Medical Progress: Bacteriology," *New England Journal of Medicine* 223 (1940): 100–104.

13. C.A. Janeway, "Recent Advances in Bacterial Chemotherapy," *Bulletin of the New England Medical Center* 3 (1941): 121.

14. C.A. Janeway, "Report of Medical Progress: Bacteriology." 1940.

15. C.A. Janeway, "Recent Advances in Bacterial Chemotherapy" (12, 13).

16. C.A. Janeway, "The Sulfonamides. I. Their Mode of Action and Pharmacology," *New England Journal of Medicine* 227 (1942): 989–995; C.A. Janeway, "The Sulfonamides. II. Their Clinical Use," *New England Journal of Medicine* 227 (1942): 1029–1044.

17. C.A. Janeway, "The Use of Sulfonamides in the Treatment of Respiratory Infections in Children," *New England Journal of Medicine* 229 (1943): 201–207. (This reported the proceedings of the society's symposium.)

18. P. B. Beeson, C.A. Janeway, "The Antipyretic Action of Sulfapyridine," *American Journal of Medical Science* 200 (1940): 632–639.

19. C.A. Janeway, P. B. Beeson, "The Treatment of Pneumococcal Pneumonia with Special Reference to the Use of Sulfathiazole, Intramuscular Serum, the Francis Test and Histaminase," *New England Journal of Medicine* 224 (1941): 592–598.

20. C.A. Janeway, "Method for Obtaining Rapid Bacterial Growth in Cultures from Patients under Treatment with Sulfanilamides," *Journal of the American Medical Association* 116 (1941): 941–942.

21. C.A. Janeway, "Report of Medical Progress. Bacteriology. The Significance of Bacteriologic and Immunologic Procedures in the Diagnosis and Treatment of Infections," *New England Journal of Medicine* 224 (1941): 813–821.

22. F.S. Cheever, C.A. Janeway, "Immunity Induced Against the Brown-Pierce Carcinoma," *Cancer Research* 1 (1941): 23–27.

23. C.A. Janeway, G.J. Dammin, "Studies on Infectious Mononucleosis. II. The Relationships of the Organisms of the Genus *Listerella* to the Disease, as Studied by the Agglutination Reaction," *Journal of Clinical Investigation* 20 (1941): 233–239.

24. N.E. Goulder, M.F. Kingsland, C.A. Janeway, "*Salmonella suipestifer* Infection in Boston. A Report of Eleven Cases, With Autopsy Findings in a Case of Bacterial Endocarditis Due to this Organism, and a Study of the Agglutination Reactions in the Infection," *New England Journal of Medicine* 226 (1942): 127–138.

25. C.A. Janeway, "*Salmonella suipestifer* Infection," In "The Infectious Diseases," *Cecil's Textbook of Medicine,* 7th edition. (Philadelphia: W.B. Saunders Co.; 1947), pp. 236–238.

26. C.A. Janeway, "Infection with the Virus of Lymphocytic Choriomeningitis," *Bulletin of the New England Medical Center* 4 (1942): 201.

27. C.A. Janeway, Lymphocytic choriomeningitis, In "The Infectious Diseases," *Cecil's Textbook of Medicine,* 7th edition, 1947; C.A. Janeway, Lymphocytic choriomeningitis, section under "Viral Diseases," The Infectious Diseases, *Cecil and Loeb's Textbook of Medicine,* 8th edition (Philadelphia: W.B. Saunders Co., 1950), pp. 51–53; C.A. Janeway, "Lymphocytic choriomeningitis," In section under "Viral Diseases," the Infectious Diseases, *Cecil and Loeb's Textbook of Medicine,* 9th Edition (Philadelphia: W.B. Saunders Co.; 1955), p. 53; C.A. Janeway, "Lymphocytic choriomeningitis," In section under "The Infectious Diseases,"

Cecil and Loeb's Textbook of Medicine, 10ᵗʰ edition (Philadelphia: W.B. Saunders Co.; 1959), pp. 48–49.

28. D.M. Surgenor, *Edwin Cohn and the Development of Protein Chemistry,"* Chapter 6, pp. 89–112 (2, 37).

29. *Ibid.,* p. 105.

30. C.A. Janeway, S.T. Gibson, L.M. Woodruff, J.T. Heyl, O.T. Bailey, L.R. Newhouser, "Chemical, Clinical, and Immunological Studies on the Products of Human Plasma Fractionation. VII. Concentrated Human Serum Albumin," *Journal of Clinical Investigation* 23 (1944): 465–490.

31. C.A. Janeway, P.B. Beeson, "The Use of Purified Bovine Albumin Solutions as Plasma Substitutes," *Journal of Clinical Investigation* 20 (1941): 435 (abstract).

32. J.T. Heyl, C.A. Janeway, "The Use of Human Albumin in Military Medicine. Part I. The Theoretical and Experimental Basis for its Use," *U.S. Naval Medical Bulletin* 40 (1942): 785; J.T. Heyl, J.G. Gibson, 2ⁿᵈ, C.A. Janeway, "Studies on the Plasma Proteins. V. The Effect of Concentrated Solution of Human and Bovine Serum Albumin on Blood Volume after Acute Blood Loss in Man," *Journal of Clinical Investigation* 22 (1943): 763–773.

33. C.A. Janeway, "The Treatment of Traumatic Shock," *New England Journal of Medicine* 225 (1941): 389–390 (editorial); C.A. Janeway, "War Medicine, with Special Emphasis on the Use of Blood Substitute," *New England Journal of Medicine* 225 (1941): 371–375.

34. J.T. Heyl, J.G. Gibson, 2ⁿᵈ, A. Shwachman, L. Wojcik, C.A. Janeway, "Quantitative Studies of the Effect of Concentrated Solutions of Human and Bovine Serum Albumin on Blood Volume after Acute Blood Loss in Man," *Journal of Clinical Investigation* 21 (1942): 639 (abstract).

35. As a demonstration of Janeway's empathy for these volunteers, he and the dean of the medical school, C. Sidney Burwell, visited the sick prisoners to demonstrate their concern. In CAJ's files at home there is a letter from Private Francis O'Connor, dated December 5, 1944, thanking him for seeing his sister's child and extending Christmas greetings. At the top of the letter, in Janeway's handwriting, is written, "One of Norfolk Prisoners."

36. C.V.Z. Hawn, C.A. Janeway, "Histological and Serological Sequences in Experimental Hypersensitivity," *Journal of Experimental Medicine* 85 (1947): 571–590.

37. J.F. Enders, "Concentrations of Certain Antibodies in Globulin Frac-

tions Derived from Human Blood Plasma." *Journal of Clinical Investigation* 23 (1944): 510–530.

38. Patient records, Peter Bent Brigham Hospital, Boston, Mass. Copy in JCHBA

39. F.S. Rosen, Personal communication to the authors. The document referred to is a wartime work, and as such was not publicly available at the time. Dr. Rosen shared the contents with the authors, but in so far as we can determine, this document is not available to the general public; authors' files, JCHBA.

40. C.A. Janeway, "Military Medicine: Its Preventive Aspects," *Medical Clinics of North America* (September 1941): 1459–1476.

41. C.A. Janeway, "Use of Concentrated Human Serum Gamma Globulin in the Prevention and Attenuation of Measles," *Bulletin of the New York Academy of Medicine* 21 (1945): 202–222.

42. S.S. Gellis, J. Neefe, J. Stokes, Jr., L.E. Strong, C.A. Janeway, "Chemical, Clinical, and Immunological Studies on the Products of Human Plasma Fractionation. XXXVI. Inactivation of the Virus of Homologous Serum Hepatitis in Solutions of Normal Human Serum Albumin by Means of Heat," *Journal of Clinical Investigation* 27 (1948): 239–244; C.W. Ordman, C.G. Jennings, C.A. Janeway, "Chemical, Clinical, and Immunological Studies on the Products of Human Plasma Fractionation. XII. The Use of Concentrated Normal Human Serum Gamma Globulin (Human Immune Serum Globulin) in the Prevention and Attenuation of Measles," *Journal of Clinical Investigation* 23 (1944): 541–550.

43. R.S. Paine, C.A. Janeway, "Human Albumin Infusions and Homologous Serum Jaundice," *Journal of the American Medical Association* 150 (1952): 199–202.

44. F.S. Rosen, "Charles A. Janeway; Profiles in Pediatrics II," *Journal of Pediatrics* 125 (1994): 167–168.

45. D. Gitlin, H. Latta, W.H. Batchelor, C.A. Janeway, "Experimental Hypersensitivity in the Rabbit. Disappearance Rate of Native and Labelled Heterologous Proteins from the Serum after Intravenous Injections," *Journal of Immunology* 66 (1951): 451–461.

46. F.S. Rosen, "Charles A. Janeway; Profiles in Pediatrics II" (12, 44).

47. D. Gitlin, J.M. Craig, C.A. Janeway, "Studies on the Nature of Fibrinoid in the Collagen Diseases," *American Journal of Pathology* 33 (1957): 55–78.

48. R.J. Wedgwood, C.V.Z. Hawn, C.A. Janeway, "The Mechanism of Action of ACTH in Experimental Nephritis Due to Foreign Protein," in

Proceedings of the Second Clinical ACTH Conference (Philadelphia: The Blakiston Company, 1951)., v. 1, p. 108.

49. L.A. Barness, G.H. Moll, C.A. Janeway, "Nephrotic Syndrome. I. Natural History of the Disease," *Pediatrics* 3 (1950): 486–503.

50. C.A. Janeway, "John Howland Award Acceptance Address" (2, 38).

51. J. Metcoff, W.M. Kelsey, C.A. Janeway, "Nephrotic Syndrome in Children. An Interpretation of its Clinical, Biochemical, and Renal Hemodynamic Features as Variations of a Single Type of Nephron Disease," *Journal of Clinical Investigation* 30 (1951): 471–491; J. Metcoff, W.M. Kelsey, C.P. Rance, C.A. Janeway, "Effects of ACTH on the Pathologic Physiology and Clinical Course of the Nephrotic Syndrome in Children," *Proceedings of the Second Clinical ACTH Conference* (Philadelphia" The Blakiston Company, 1951), v. 1, p. 148.

52. J. Metcoff, C.P. Rance, W.M. Kelsey, N. Nakasone, C.A. Janeway, "Adrenocorticotrophic Hormone (ACTH) Therapy of the Nephrotic Syndrome in Children," *Pediatrics* 10 (1952): 543–566.

53. F. Gomez, R. Ramos-Galvan, J. Cravioto, S. Frenk, C.A. Janeway, J.L. Gamble, J. Metcoff, "Intracellular Composition and Homeostatic Mechanisms in Severe Chronic Infantile Malnutrition. I. General Considerations," *Pediatrics* 20 (1957): 101–120; J. Metcoff, S. Frenk, G. Gordillo, F. Gomez, R. Ramos-Galvan, J. Cravioto, C.A. Janeway, J.L. Gamble, "Malnutrition. IV. Development and Repair of the Biochemical Lesion." *Pediatrics* 20 (1957): 317–336.

54. F.S. Rosen, "Charles A. Janeway; Profiles in Pediatrics II" (12, 44).

55. C.A. Janeway, L. Apt, D. Gitlin, "Agammaglobulinemia" (4, 14).

56. D. Gitlin, C.A. Janeway, "Agammaglobulinemia. Congenital, Acquired, and Transient Forms," Chapter in *Progress in Hematology* (New York: Grune and Stratton; 1956); D. Gitlin, W.H. Hitzig, C.A. Janeway, "Multiple Serum Protein Deficiencies in Congenital and Acquired Agammaglobulinemia," *Journal of Clinical Investigation* 35 (1956): 1199–1204; D. Gitlin, C.A. Janeway, "Agammaglobulinemia." *Scientific American* 197 (1957): 93–104.

57. C.A. Janeway, D. Gitlin, "The Gamma Globulins," in S.Z Levine, ed., *Advances in Pediatrics* (New York: Year Book Medical Publishers, Inc.; 1957), v. 9, pp. 65–125.

58. C.A. Janeway, D. Gitlin, J.M. Craig, D.S. Grice, "Collagen Disease in Patients with Congenital Agammaglobulinemia," *Transactions of the Association of American Physicians* 69 (1956): 93–97.

59. P.A.M. Gross, D. Gitlin, C.A. Janeway, "The Gamma Globulins and their Clinical Significance. III. Hypergammaglobulinemia," *New England Journal of Medicine* 260 (1959): 121–125.

60. A. Cruchaud, F.S. Rosen, J.M. Craig, C.A. Janeway, D. Gitlin, "The Site of Synthesis of the 19S Gamma Globulins in Dysgammaglobulinemia," *Journal of Experimental Medicine* 115 (1962): 1141–1148.

61. D. Gitlin, F.S. Rosen, C.A. Janeway, "The Thymus and Other Lymphoid Tissues in Congenital Agammaglobulinemia. II. Delayed Hypersensitivity and Homograft Survival in a Child with Thymic Alymphoplasia," *Pediatrics* 33 (1964): 711–720.

62. C.S. August, F.S. Rosen, R.M. Filler, C.A. Janeway, B. Markowski, H.E.M. Kay, "Implantation of a Foetal Thymus Restoring Immunological Competence in a Patient with Thymic Aplasia (DiGeorge's syndrome)," *Lancet* 2 (December 1969): 1210.

63. D. Gitlin, F.S. Rosen, C.A. Janeway, "Undue Susceptibility to Infection," *Pediatric Clinics of North America* 9 (1962): 405–423; F.S. Rosen, C.A. Janeway, "Immunological Competence of the Newborn Infant," *Pediatrics* 33 (1964): 159–160; C.A. Janeway, "Infection, Immunity and Allergy in Relation to Pediatrics," In *Nelson's Textbook of Pediatrics,* 7th edition (Philadelphia: WB Saunders Co.; 1964), pp. 431–438.

64. F.S. Rosen, Memorandum to R.J. Haggerty, October 5, 2004, authors' files, JCHBA.

65. J. Cohen, R. Schwartz, C.A. Janeway, "Muscular Dystrophy. A Problem for Clinician and Community," *New York State Department of Health* 33 (1956): 5.

66. D. Gitlin, C.A, Janeway, "Turnover of the Copper and Protein Moieties Ceruloplasmin," *Nature* 185 (1960): 693; D. Gitlin, C.A. Janeway, "Absorption and Excretion of Copper in Mice," *Nature* 188 (1960): 150–151.

67. S.P. Gotoff, F.X. Fellers, G.F. Vawter, C.A. Janeway, F.S. Rosen, "The Beta$_{1C}$ Globulin in Childhood Nephrotic Syndrome," *New England Journal of Medicine* 273 (1965): 524–529.

68. F.S. Rosen, Memorandum to R.J. Haggerty, October 5, 2004 (12, 64).

69. R.J. Haggerty, C.A. Janeway, "Evaluation of a Pediatric House Officer Program" (11, 16).

70. C.A. Janeway, "Pediatrics," *New England Journal of Medicine* 236 (1947): 867–873 and 901–908.

71. *Ibid.*

72. D. Gitlin, C.A. Janeway, "Agammaglobulinemia" (11, 56).

73. Reported in the *Boston Globe,* September 24, 1962.

74. C.A. Janeway, "Pediatric Research in the Age of the Common Man and the Exceptional Child," *Journal of the American Medical Association* 157 (1955): 1289–1291.

75. C.A. Janeway, "A Physician's View of Change," in Eli Ginsberg, ed., *Values and Ideals of American Youth* (New York: Columbia University Press; 1961), pp. 1–25.

76. C.A. Janeway, "Pediatrics 1984: An Attempt to Look Into the Crystal Ball," *Clinical Proceedings of the Children's Hospital of the District of Columbia* 29 (1963): 33.

77. This lecture was never published, but is in the CAJ papers, JCHB, both as given at Brown University as the Gordon Woods Lecture on October 28, 1964 under the title, "C.A. Janeway, Looking Ahead: The Future of Medicine," and as subsequently submitted to the *Atlantic Monthly.*

78. Letter from "Ted" [Weeks], Editor, *Atlantic Monthly* to C.A. Janeway, May 20, 1965, CAJ papers, JCHBA.

79. C.A. Janeway, "The Decline of Primary Medical Care: An Unforseen Consequence of the Flexner Report," *The Pharos of Alpha Omega Alpha* 37 (1974): 74–80.

80. C.A. Janeway, "Family Medicine—Fad or For Real?" *New England Journal of Medicine* 291 (1974): 337–343.

81. C.A. Janeway, "Family Medicine and Primary Care at Harvard Medical School," *Harvard Medical Alumni Bulletin* 48, no. 5 (May–June 1974): 8–11.

82. C.A. Janeway, "The Scholar and the Devil's Advocate," *Journal of Medical Education* 34 (1959): 79–80. The intitute was held at Swampscott, Massachusetts, on October 7–11, 1958, and its proceedings were published under the title, *Report of the First Institute on Clinical Teaching, Association of American Medical Colleges,* Helen Hofer Gee and Julius B. Richmond, editors.

83. C.A. Janeway, "Medical Education After Medical School," *Proceedings of the 6th Annual Conference on Medical Education for Foreign Scholars in the Medical Sciences.* University of Chicago, June 24–27, 1962; pp. 54–75.

84. C.A. Janeway, "A Physician's View of Change" (11, 75).

85. Dr. Janeway's acceptance speech is preserved in the CAJ papers, JCHBA.

86. C.A. Janeway, "Pediatrics and the Adolescent. Presentation of the C. Anderson Aldrich Award to J. Roswell Gallagher," *Pediatrics* 51 (1973): 454–457.

87. C.A. Janeway, "Presentation of the Howland Award to Louis K. Diamond," *Pediatric Research* 7 (1973): 853–857.

88. C.A. Janeway, "Edwin Joseph Cohn, B.S., Ph.D," *Harvard Medical Alumni Bulletin* 28, no. 2 (January 1954): 16–23; C.A. Janeway, "Edwin Joseph Cohn," *Hebrew Medical Journal* 1 (1955): 162.

89. C.A. Janeway, "S. Burt Wolbach," *Transactions of the Association of American Physicians* 67 (1954): 30–35.

90. C.A. Janeway, "General Summary. Scientific Program of the Ninth International Paediatric Congress," *Journal of Pediatrics* 57 (1960): 125–127.

91. C.A. Janeway, "The International Paediatric Association," *Journal of Pediatrics* 74 (1969): 846–847; C.A. Janeway, "Summary of the Conference," *Journal of Pediatrics* 75 (1969): 1292.

92. Leighton Cluff, Memorandum to the authors, November 29, 1988, authors' files, JCHBA.

93. C.A. Janeway, Testimony to Sub-committee on Public Health and Environment of House of Representatives, March 23, 1973. Copy in authors' files, JCHBA.

94. C.A. Janeway, "John Howland Award Acceptance Address" (2, 38).

95. C.A. Janeway, "Vision and Reality. Medicine Faces Our Third Century." Presented October 13, 1976 and privately published by the University of North Carolina; a copy of manuscript is available in the CAJ papers, JCHBA.

96. C.A. Janeway, "Medicine, Medical Science, and Health," The Thayer Lecture (1, 47).

Chapter 13

1. Letter from John Davis to R.J. Haggerty, September 27, 1989, authors' files, JCHBA.

2. Letter from C.A. Janeway to Lt. A. B. Stimson, November 8, 1945, quoted by Dr. Matthew Eisenberg in presentation of the Janeway Teaching Award, Children's Hospital, Boston, June 21, 1989, JCHBA.

3. Alexander Nadas, Interview with the authors, October 10, 1990 (4, 36).

4. David G. Nathan, Remarks on the occasion of his appointment of Dr. Fred Alt as first Charles A. Janeway Professor, Children's Hospital, Boston, November 19, 1993, JCHBA.

5. Letter from Charles D. Cook to F. H. Lovejoy, Jr., September 15, 2002 (4, 71).

6. John Whitcomb, Interview with the authors, January 14, 1990, and subsequent letters from Whitcomb to R.J. Haggerty, June 1, 1990, and June 9, 1990 (1, 56).

7. Elizabeth Janeway, Interview with the authors, January 13–14, 1990 (1, 27).

8. *Ibid.*

9. Letter from William Berenberg to R.J. Haggerty, May 31, 1989 (3, 10); also, William Berenberg, Interview with the authors, Boston, Massachusetts, October 8, 1990 (4, 5).

10. Letter from William Berenberg to R.J. Haggerty, May 31, 1989.

11. Elizabeth Janeway, Interview with the authors, January 13–14, 1990 (1, 27).

12. Alexander Nadas, Interview with the authors, October 10, 1990 (4, 36).

13. C.A. Janeway to Edwards Park, January 28, 1949, CAJ papers, JCHBA.

14. C.A. Janeway, "Payment under Protest" (letter to the Editor), *New England Journal of Medicine* 244 (April 19, 1951): 612.

15. Letter from Edwards Park to C.A. Janeway, June 5, 1951, CAJ papers, JCHBA.

16. Letter from Edwards Park to C.A. Janeway, June 12, 1951, CAJ papers, JCHBA.

17. Letter from C.A. Janeway to President Harry S. Truman, Senator Leverett Saltonstall, and Congressman Peter Holmes, April 9, 1946, CAJ papers, JCHBA.

18. Letter from C.A. Janeway to President Lyndon B. Johnson, January 17, 1964, CAJ papers, JCHBA.

19. Letter from C.A. Janeway to President Lyndon B. Johnson, October 7, 1964, CAJ papers, JCHBA.

20. Letter from C.A. Janeway to President Lyndon B. Johnson, September 27, 1966, CAJ papers, JCHBA.

21. Letter from C.A. Janeway to President Lyndon B. Johnson, May 23, 1967, CAJ papers, JCHBA.

22. Letter from C.A. Janeway to Senator Henry Jackson, December 18, 1971, CAJ papers, JCHBA.

23. A.M. Ravenholt, "Dream or Achievable Reality?" *American Universities Field Staff Report Services: SouthEast Asia Series* 12 (1964): 105.

24. Letter from C.A. Janeway to the Payroll Office of Harvard University, January 28, 1967, CAJ papers, JCHBA.

25. Letter from C.A. Janeway to Eleanor Janeway Mitchell, April 18, 1941, CAJ papers, JCHBA.

26. Letter from John A. Lindeke to C.A. Janeway, August 20, 1968, CAJ papers, JCHBA.

27. Letter from C.A. Janeway to John Lindeke, August 28, 1968, CAJ papers, JCHBA.

28. *Weston Town Crier,* Weston, Massachusetts, November 20, 1969.

29. Letter from C.A. Janeway to Herman Koester, January 23, 1967, CAJ papers, JCHBA.

30. Letter from Rollin M. Gallagher, Goodale, Bertman and Co., to C.A. Janeway, May 17, 1967, CAJ papers, JCHBA.

31. Letter from C.A. Janeway to David Kirkbride, May 18, 1967, CAJ papers, JCHBA.

32. William Berenberg, Interview with the authors, October 9, 1990 (4, 5).

33. *Ibid.*

34. Letter from C.A. Janeway to Edward Dixon, Town Clerk, Town of Weston, Massachusetts, June 7, 1956, CAJ papers, JCHBA.

35. Weston, Massachusetts, "Annual Report," 1954, pp. 143–146, CAJ Papers, JCHBA.

36. Letter from C.A. Janeway to Herman Koester, Chairman of the Board of Selectmen, Town of Weston, Massachusetts, January 2, 1967, CAJ Papers, JCHBA.

37. Town of Weston, Massachusetts, Committee to Investigate the Matter of Fluoridation of the Town's Water Supply, C.A. Janeway, secretary, "Minutes of a Special Meeting on Fluoridation, "January 30, 1967," CAJ papers, JCHBA.

38. Letter from C.A. Janeway to J. Dunning, DDS, February 7, 1967, CAJ papers, JCHBA.

39. Letter from C.A. Janeway to Edward M. Dickson, March 16, 1965, CAJ papers, JCHBA.

40. *Ibid.*

41. Letter from Stephen Joseph to Elizabeth Janeway, June 9, 1989, CAJ papers, JCHBA.

42. Letter from William Berenberg to F.H. Lovejoy, Jr., May 31, 1989 (3, 10).

43. Letter from C.A. Janeway to William Berenberg, February 7, 1980 (5, 37).

44. Louis K. Diamond, Interview with the authors, May 7, 1990 (4, 4).

45. Letter from Louis K. Diamond to R.J. Haggerty, June 6, 1990, authors' files, JCHBA.

46. Niilo Hallman, Interview with the authors, Paris, France, July 25, 1989, authors' files, JCHBA.

47. Letters from Richard Goldbloom to R.J. Haggerty, January 23 and February 28, 1989, (10, 72)

48. Jack Metcoff, Interview with the authors, May 1989 (3, 27).

49. Sophia Chang, Interview with the authors, New York City, May 17, 1991, CAJ papers, JCHBA.

50. Letter from Sophia and Charles Chang to Charles and Elizabeth Janeway, July 17, 1968, CAJ papers, JCHBA.

51. James McKay, Interview with the authors, February 3, 1989 (3, 29).

52. Clement Smith, Address at Grand Rounds at Children's Hospital, Boston, June 24, 1981 (3, 6).

53. Louis K. Diamond, Interview with the authors, Los Angeles, California, September 27, 1990, authors' files, JCHBA.

54. Jack Metcoff, Interview with the authors, May 1989 (3, 27).

55. Nelson Montgomery, Interview with the authors, New York City, November 9, 1989, authors' files, JCHBA.

56. Letter from Georges Peter to R.J. Haggerty, June 28, 1989, authors' files, JCHBA.

57. *Ibid.*

58. John Houpis, Interview with the authors, June 7, 1989 (4, 35).

59. Letter from John Kennell to R.J. Haggerty, February 10, 1988, authors' files, JCHBA.

60. David Smith, Interview with the authors, December 1994 (11, 14).

61. Sherwin Kevy, Interview with the authors, March 15, 1989 (3, 21).

62. Letter from C.A. Janeway to Chief Resident, Outpatient Department, Children's Hospital, Boston, January 24, 1951, CAJ papers, JCHBA.

63. Letter from C.A. Janeway to Mrs. A. Obuchon, January 24, 1951, CAJ papers, JCHBA.

64. Louis K. Diamond, Interview with the authors, May 7, 1990 (4, 4).

65. *Ibid.*

66. Elizabeth Janeway, Interview with the authors, Weston, Massachusetts, March 10, 1991, authors' files, JCHBA.

67. Letter from Muriel Graham Small to R.J. Haggerty, March 9, 1994, authors' files, JCHBA.

68. Letter from Mildred McTear to R. J. Haggerty, July 19, 1989 (10, 83).
69. *Ibid.*
70. Brooks Barnes, Interview with the authors, July 12, 1989 (4, 28).
71. C.A. Smith, Address at Grand Rounds at Children's Hospital, Boston, June 24, 1981 (3, 6).
72. William Cochran, Interview with the authors, March 1991, CAJ papers, JCHBA.
73. Letter from C.A. Janeway to C. Lohmann, Secretary of the University, Yale University, May 26, 1953, CAJ papers, JCHBA.
74. Memo from Sidney Farber to C.A. Janeway, April 27, 1954, CAJ papers, JCHBA.
75. Letter from Louis Barness to R.J. Haggerty, September 13, 1990, authors' files, JCHBA.
76. Joel Alpert, Interview with the authors, Boston, Massachusetts, March, 1989, and subsequent letter to R.J. Haggerty, May 16, 1989, authors' files, JCHBA.
77. Letter from C.A. Janeway to Robert Wise, August 30, 1963, CAJ papers, JCHBA.
78. Alexander Nadas, Interview with the authors, October 10, 1990 (4, 36).
79. Robert Masland, Interview with the authors, May 1990 (4, 49).
80. Letter from Charles D. Cook to F.H. Lovejoy, Jr., September 15, 2002 (4, 71).
81. William Cochran, Interview with the authors, March, 1991 (13, 72).
82. Mohsen Ziai, Interview with the authors, Boston, Massachusetts, March 1989 (specific day not recorded), authors' files, JCHBA.
83. Richard Grand, Interview with the authors, July 24, 2002 (4, 73).
84. Robert Masland, Interview with the authors, May, 1990 (4, 49).
85. Thomas Cone, Interview with the authors, March 12, 1991 (5, 18).
86. Jack Metcoff, Interview with the authors, 1989 (3, 27).
87. Louis K. Diamond, Interview with the authors, May 7, 1990 (4, 4).
88. Sherwin Kevy, Interview with the authors, March 15, 1989 (3, 21).
89. Letter from Henry Giles to R.J. Haggerty, November 22, 1989, authors' files, JCHBA.
90. Mohsen Ziai, Interview with the authors, March 1989 (13, 82).
91. Letter from Jan Breslow to C.A. Janeway, November 3, 1969, CAJ papers, JCHBA.
92. Mary Ellen Avery, Personal communication to R.J. Haggerty, undated.
93. Letter from Louis Barness to R.J. Haggerty, September 13, 1990 (13, 75).

94. Personal communication to the authors by several former residents.

95. Elizabeth Janeway, Interview with the authors, March 10, 1991 (13, 66).

96. Fred Rosen, Interview with the authors, October 9, 1990, CAJ papers, JCHBA.

97. Letter from C.A. Janeway to David Kirkbride, April 4, 1974, CAJ papers, JCHBA.

98. R. James McKay, Interview with the authors, February 1989 (3, 27).

99. Mohsen Ziai, Interview with the authors, March, 1989 (13, 82).

100. William Berenberg, Interview with the authors, October 9, 1990 (4, 5).

101. Louis K. Diamond, Interview with the authors, May 7, 1990 (4, 4).

102. Sherwin Kevy, Interview with the authors, March 15, 1989 (3, 21).

103. Alexander Nadas, Interview with the authors, October 9, 1990 (4, 36).

104. Letter from David Nathan to R.J. Haggerty, November 19, 1993, authors' files, JCHBA.

105. Sherwin Kevy, Interview with the authors, March 1989 (3, 21).

106. David Nathan, Interview with the authors, October 10, 1990 (4, 3).

107. *Ibid.*

108. C.A. Janeway, "Vision and Reality: Medicine Faces Our Third Century" (12, 95).

About the Authors

Robert J. Haggerty is Professor of Pediatrics and Chair Emeritus at the University of Rochester School of Medicine and Dentistry. He was subsequently President of the William T. Grant Foundation, which supports research on ways to improve the mental health of school-age children and to assist them in utilizing their full potential. A graduate of Cornell University and its Medical College, he completed his residency under Dr. Janeway at the Children Hospital in Boston. He served as Editor of *Pediatrics in Review* for ten years and is now its Editor Emeritus. He is the author of more than 150 original papers and editor or author of three books, one of which, *Ambulatory Pediatrics*, is now in its fifth edition, as well as author of nearly 200 book chapters, editorials and abstracts. He has been Visiting Professor and/or named lecturer at more than fifty institutions.

Frederick H. Lovejoy, Jr., is the William Berenberg Professor of Pediatrics at the Harvard Medical School and Associate Physician-in-Chief and Deputy Chair of the Department of Medicine at Children's Hospital Boston. A graduate of Yale University, he received the M.D. degree from the University of Virginia School of Medicine. He was an intern and resident at Bellevue Hospital in New York prior to serving as a senior resident and ultimately Chief Resident at Children's Hospital Boston and he founded the Massachusetts Poison Control System. As a consequence of his training at the Children's during Dr. Janeway's tenure, he has maintained a leadership role for the residency program at the Children's Hospital, Boston for over thirty years. He has authored over 130 original papers, over fifty chapters, and several books. He has also served on several editorial boards and has been a visiting professor and given many named lectures both nationally and internationally.

Index